Immune & Infectious Disorders

Nursing
TimeSavers

Immune & Infectious Disorders

Springhouse Corporation
Springhouse, Pennsylvania

Staff

Executive Director, Editorial
Stanley Loeb

Senior Publisher
Matthew Cahill

Art Director
John Hubbard

Clinical Manager
Cindy Tryniszewski, RN, MSN

Senior Editor
Michael Shaw

Clinical Project Manager
Mary Chapman Gyetvan, RN, MSN

Clinical Editors
Carole Basile, RN,C, BSN, CCRN; Cynthia C.
Burlew; RN; Arlene Coughlin, RN, MSN; Kathy
Craig, RN, BA; Tina Dietrich, RN, BSN, CCRN;
Mary Jane McDevitt, RN, BS; Elizabeth Wister,
RN, BA

Editors
J. Allen Canale, Marilyn Cummins, Neal Fandek,
H. Nancy Holmes, Judd L. Howard, Richard
Koreto, Ann Lenkiewicz, Judith A. Lewis,
Art Ofner

Copy Editors
Cynthia C. Breuninger (supervisor), Priscilla
DeWitt, Jennifer George Mintzer, Nancy Papsin,
Doris Weinstock

Designers
Stephanie Peters (associate art director), Matie
Patterson (senior designer), Kaaren Mitchel,
Amy Smith

Illustrators
Jackie Facciolo, Robert Jackson, Judy Newhouse

Manufacturing
Deborah Meiris (director), Pat Dorshaw (manager), Anna Brindisi, Kate Davis, T.A. Landis

Production Coordinator
Patricia McCloskey

Editorial Assistants
Maree DeRosa, Beverly Lane, Mary Madden

Indexer
Barbara Hodgson

Library of Congress Cataloging-in-Publication Data
Immune & infectious disorders.
  p. cm. — (Nursing timesavers)
  Includes index.
  1. Immunologic diseases—Nursing—
Handbooks, manuals, etc.
  2. Communicable diseases—Nursing—
Handbooks, manuals, etc.
  3. Infection—Nursing—Handbooks, manuals,
etc. I. Springhouse Corporation. II. Series.
  [DNLM: 1. Immunologic Diseases—
  Nursing. 2. Communicable Diseases—
  Nursing. WY 153 I33 1994]
RC582.I44 1994
610.73'699—dc20
DNLM/DLC   93-50136
ISBN 0-87434-698-3   CIP

Contents

Contributors and consultants vi
Foreword vii

Chapter 1
Applying the nursing process to immune disorders 1

Chapter 2
Exploring chief complaints in immune disorders 39

Chapter 3
Caring for patients with immunodeficiency disorders 51

Chapter 4
Caring for patients with hypersensitivity disorders 81

Chapter 5
Caring for patients with autoimmune disorders 107

Chapter 6
Caring for patients with transplant complications 147

Chapter 7
Applying the nursing process to infectious disorders 161

Chapter 8
Exploring chief complaints in infectious disorders 183

Chapter 9
Caring for patients with viral infections 189

Chapter 10
Caring for patients with bacterial and chlamydial infections 225

Chapter 11
Caring for patients with infections of varying etiology 275

Appendices and Index
Quick reference to treatments for immune and infectious disorders 324
Quick reference to drugs used in immune disorders 326
Quick reference to drugs used in infectious disorders 332
Transmission prevention guidelines 344
Universal precautions 346
Guidelines for minimizing infection 348
Checklist of reportable diseases 352
Index 353

Contributors and consultants

Contributors

Heather A. Flyge, RN, MSN, OCN
Clinical Coordinator, Ambulatory Infusions/Oncology Services, Jersey Shore Medical Center, Neptune, N.J.

Constance J. Galaviz, RN, MS, CIC
Manager, Epidemiology and Infection Control, Lutheran General Hospital, Park Ridge, Ill.

Holly Wainwright, RN, BS, CIC
Nurse Epidemiologist, MacNeal Hospital, Berwyn, Ill.

M. Linda Workman, RN, PhD, FAAN, OCN
Associate Professor, Frances Payne Bolton School of Nursing, Case Western Reserve University, Cleveland

Consultants

Joyce K. Anastasi, RN, PhD
Assistant Professor; Director, AIDS Program, Columbia University School of Nursing, New York

Patricia Bussard, RN, BA, CIC
Manager, Infection Control and Employee Health, St. Francis – St. George Hospital, Cincinnati

Regina S. Cunningham, RN, MA, OCN
Chief Nursing Officer, Cancer Institute of New Jersey, New Brunswick, N.J.

Marsha L. Davidson, RN, MSN, CETN
Enterostomal Nurse/Clinical Educator, Bryn Mawr (Pa.) Hospital

Douglas D. DeCarolis, PharmD
Clinical Pharmacy Specialist, Fairview Southdale Hospital, Edina, Minn.

Angela M. DeMichele, MD
Resident, Internal Medicine, Hospital of the University of Pennsylvania, Philadelphia

Melissa M. Furio, BS, PharmD
Assistant Director, Clinical Pharmacy Services, Bryn Mawr (Pa.) Hospital

Robert Gross, MD
Resident, Internal Medicine, Hospital of the University of Pennsylvania, Philadelphia

Catherine M. Handy, RN, MA, OCN
Clinical Nurse Specialist, Oncology, St. Vincent's Hospital and Medical Center, New York

Lynne Kreutzer-Baraglia, RN, MS
Administrative Dean, West Suburban College of Nursing, Oak Park, Ill.

Ann Lee, RN, MSN, CRNP
Heart and Lung Transplant Coordinator, University of Pittsburgh Medical Center

Susan G. MacArthur, RN, BA, BS, CIC
Department Head, Epidemiology, University of Connecticut Health Center, John Dempsey Hospital, Farmington, Conn.

Carol A. Mason, RN, BS, CIC
Manager, Infection Control and Environmental Safety, Central DuPage Hospital, Winfield, Ill.

Theresa A. Moran, RN, MS
Clinical Nurse Specialist, AIDS/Oncology, San Francisco General Hospital

Geri B. Neuberger, RN, MN, EdD
Associate Professor, Medical-Surgical Nursing, University of Kansas School of Nursing, Kansas City, Kan.

Beverly A. Post, RN, MS
Clinical Services Education Coordinator, Louis A. Weiss Memorial Hospital, Chicago

Paula T. Rieger, RN, MSN, OCN
Oncology Nurse Specialist, Clinical Immunology and Biological Therapy, M.D. Anderson Cancer Center, Houston

Nancy V. Runta, RN, BSN, CCRN
Infection Control/Occupational Health Practitioner, North Penn Hospital, Lansdale, Pa.

Regina Shannon-Bodnar, RN, MS, MSN, OCN
Director, Patient Care Services, Hospice of Baltimore

Ellen Stefanosky, RN, MSN, CCTC
Transplant Coordinator, Thomas Jefferson University Hospital, Philadelphia

Barbara J. Taptich, RN, MA
Director, Heart Institute, St. Francis Medical Center, Trenton, N.J.

Linda Thomson, RPh, BS, PharmD
Clinical Pharmacist, Infectious Diseases, Thomas Jefferson University Hospital, Philadelphia

Foreword

Never has it been more important for nurses to have comprehensive, up-to-date information on immune and infectious disorders. Consider the following health care trends:
• The population of immunocompromised patients is growing because of the AIDS epidemic and the increasing number of patients receiving immunosuppressive therapy.
• Disorders that were presumed to be under control, such as tuberculosis, are reemerging in frightening numbers and with increasingly drug-resistant strains.
• The incidence of nosocomial infections is increasing, partly because of the growing use of hi-tech, invasive procedures.

Caring for today's patients requires many diverse clinical skills. Your responsibilities may range from providing emergency treatment for anaphylaxis to planning long-term care for the patient with a chronic condition, such as rheumatoid arthritis or systemic lupus erythematosus (SLE); from administering immunosuppressant drugs to a transplant patient to providing emotional support to a newly diagnosed AIDS patient. Under all circumstances, you must be prepared to act quickly and efficiently.

Immune & Infectious Disorders, the latest book in the Nursing TimeSavers series, can help you meet the challenge of providing expert care under high-pressure circumstances. It provides up-to-date information, distills the most important facts from a complex body of knowledge, and clearly highlights your nursing responsibilities. Small enough to be easily transported to the workplace, this handbook was developed by nursing professionals — all with years of bedside know-how — who understand the professional demands and time constraints you deal with every day.

The book is divided into two sections: The first covers immune disorders; the second covers infectious disorders. Each section begins with an introductory chapter explaining how to use the nursing process to provide expert care. You'll learn how to identify patient problems, develop a plan of care, set outcomes for the patient, determine the necessary interventions, and evaluate whether outcomes have been achieved. You'll also find concise coverage of key nursing diagnoses used in caring for patients with immune and infectious disorders.

Each section includes guidelines for assessing chief complaints. For instance, if your patient says, "My joints ache" or "I have lost a lot of weight lately," you can look up a list of questions to ask and techniques to perform. For each chief complaint, you'll find a list of potential causes.

Chapters 3 through 6 cover the most frequently encountered immune disorders, including AIDS, asthma, anaphylaxis, blood transfusion reactions, rheumatoid arthritis, SLE, and transplant rejection. Chapters 9 through 11 cover the most frequently encountered infectious disorders, including viral hepatitis, influenza, pelvic inflammatory disease, Lyme disease, tuberculosis, pneumonia, wound infection, and meningitis. To save you time, each disorder is organized according to the nursing process with five easy-to-spot text headings:

• *Assessment.* This section tells you what health history data, physical examination findings, and diagnostic test results to expect.

• *Nursing diagnosis.* In this section, you'll find the most common nursing diagnoses and related etiologies for each disorder.

• *Planning.* This section provides a list of expected patient outcomes for each nursing diagnosis. This feature will ensure that your documentation includes accurate outcome statements.

• *Implementation.* In this section, you'll find complete, step-by-step nursing interventions as well as guidelines for patient teaching.

• *Evaluation.* This section provides criteria by which to judge the effectiveness of your nursing care and gauge your patient's progress toward meeting expected outcomes.

Throughout the book, you'll see special graphic devices called logos that direct you to important and timesaving information. The *FactFinder* logo, for instance, highlights key points about a disorder, covering such topics as risk factors, incidence, and prognosis. The *Timesaving tip* logo alerts you to ways to save time as you proceed with your nursing care. The *Assessment TimeSaver* logo helps you organize and expedite the initial step of the nursing process. The *Treatments* logo summarizes the latest medical therapies for each disorder. The *Teaching TimeSaver* logo provides suggestions and guidelines for teaching patients. And the *Discharge TimeSaver* logo signals a checklist of teaching topics, referrals, and follow-up appointments to promote your patient's well-being after hospitalization.

Additionally, *Immune & Infectious Disorders* includes valuable appendices on common treatments and drugs. The first appendix outlines current procedures for managing immune and infectious disorders, complete with concise descriptions, indications, and complications. The second and third appendices provide information on common drugs used to treat immune and infectious disorders. Each of these appendices includes generic names, classifications, indications, and adverse reactions. Common and life-threatening adverse reactions are clearly marked. Other appendices cover transmission prevention guidelines, universal precautions, guidelines for minimizing infection, and a checklist of reportable diseases.

By giving you current clinical information in a focused, quick-reference format, *Immune & Infectious Disorders* can save you time and help you provide better care for your patients. Become familiar with this tool and use it at home or at work. A better understanding of immune and infectious disease care will enhance your confidence and increase your chances for success in today's fast-changing world of health care. *Immune & Infectious Disorders* is a valuable text for nurses.

Joyce K. Anastasi, RN, PhD
Assistant Professor of Nursing
Director, AIDS Program
Columbia University School of Nursing
New York

Applying the nursing process to immune disorders

Assessment   2

Nursing diagnosis   24

Planning   29

Implementation   33

Evaluation   35

The immune system plays a vital role in preserving health. It provides continuous physiologic surveillance and defends against invasion by foreign substances. The immune system also helps to maintain homeostasis by governing degradation and removal of damaged cells. Lastly, it discovers and disposes of abnormal cells that continually arise within the body. (See *Understanding the inflammatory response*, opposite, and *Understanding the immune response*, pages 4 and 5.)

Caring for the patient with an immune disorder can be complex and challenging. When the immune system fails to function properly, the physiologic effects can be devastating. Because the immune system consists of billions of circulating cells and generalized structures throughout the body, an immune disorder can affect numerous other systems or may signal problems originating elsewhere in the body.

By using the nursing process to structure your care, you can provide the accurate assessment and expert intervention needed in immunologic care. You'll use the nursing process to:

• identify treatable patient problems
• identify preventable patient problems
• develop a plan that addresses the patient's actual and potential problems
• determine what kind of assistance the patient needs and who can best provide it
• select outcomes for the patient and determine whether they have been achieved
• accurately document your contribution to achieving patient outcomes.

The five steps of the nursing process — assessment, nursing diagnosis, planning, implementation, and evaluation — help you address specific patient needs in an orderly and timely way. Keep in mind, however, that these steps are dynamic and flexible and often overlap.

Assessment

Assessment, the first step of the nursing process, is critical. The quality of assessment data will determine the success of subsequent nursing process steps. A complete nursing assessment usually includes taking a health history, performing a physical examination, and reviewing the results of diagnostic tests. You can identify immune system problems while performing a complete assessment or while investigating a patient complaint.

Health history

During the health history, you'll explore the patient's chief complaint and other symptoms, and assess the impact of the illness or complaint on him and his family. You'll also gather information to guide diagnosis and treatment.

Include the patient's family members or close friends when taking the history. They may be able to help you corroborate information you obtain from the patient. (See *Making the most of your interview time*, page 6.)

Obtain biographical data, including age, sex, race, and ethnic background. Keep in mind that some immune disorders occur more frequently in certain populations. For example, systemic lupus erythematosus (SLE) appears more often in women than in men.

Understanding the inflammatory response

The inflammatory response is a complex process through which many parts of the body overcome the stress of wounds and return the body to homeostasis. Its primary function is to bring phagocytic cells (neutrophils and monocytes) to the inflamed area to destroy bacteria and dispose of dead and dying cells. The acute phase of the inflammatory response typically lasts 2 weeks. The subacute phase also usually lasts 2 weeks.

Cardinal signs of inflammation

Inflammation produces four cardinal signs: redness, swelling, heat, and pain. The first three signs result from local vasodilation, fluid leakage into the extravascular space, and blockage of lymphatic drainage. Pain results from swelling and pressure and from chemical irritation of pain receptors.

The illustration below traces the steps of the inflammatory response.

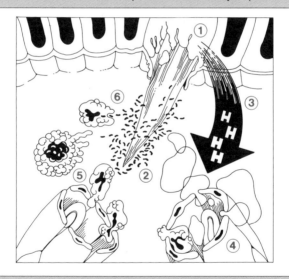

Key
1. Splinter punctures epidermis.
2. Bacteria are introduced and implanted in tissue.
3. Injured cells release histamine and kinins, causing capillary dilation.
4. Dilated capillaries make skin hot and red; escaping fluid from blood vessels causes swelling; kinins and other substances produce pain.
5. Neutrophils and monocytes migrate through vessel walls toward bacteria.
6. Neutrophils and monocytes destroy bacteria by phagocytosis.

Understanding the immune response

When foreign substances invade the body, two types of immune responses reinforce white blood cells' defense: humoral (antibody-mediated) and cell-mediated immunity.

Both types of immunity involve lymphocytes that share a common origin in stem cells of the bone marrow. These lymphocytes undergo differential development to become B cells and T cells.

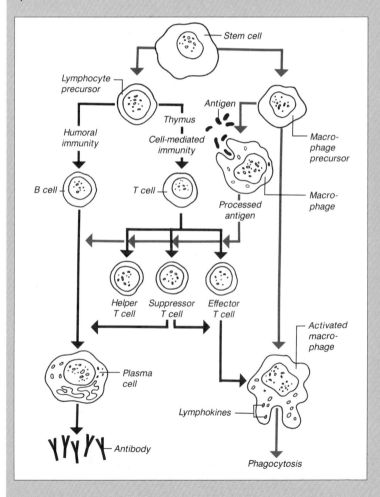

Humoral immunity

In humoral immunity, antigens stimulate B cells to differentiate into plasma cells and produce circulating antibodies that destroy bacteria and viruses before they can enter host cells.

Cell-mediated immunity

In cell-mediated immunity, T cells move directly to attack invaders. Three T-cell subgroups trigger the response to infection. Helper T cells spur B cells to manufacture antibodies. Effector T cells kill antigens directly. Both helper and effector T cells produce lymphokines (proteins that induce an inflammatory response and mediate the delayed hypersensitivity reaction). Suppressor T cells regulate both humoral and cell-mediated immune responses.

Macrophages present antigens to B cells and T cells. This stimulates B cells to mature into antibody-producing plasma cells and sensitizes T cells, making them capable of interacting directly with the foreign material.

Each time foreign substances invade the body, T cells and B cells preserve a "memory" of the encounter, which provides long-term immunity to many significant diseases.

Chief complaint

Document the chief complaint in the patient's own words. Ask about its onset, duration, frequency, location, setting, and aggravating and alleviating factors. Ask the patient if he has experienced adverse effects from any treatment. If the patient has trouble identifying his signs and symptoms, ask if he has any of these common immunologic complaints: fever, fatigue, joint pain, swollen glands, weight loss, and skin rash. You might ask him, "What made you seek medical care today?" (For more information, see Chapter 2, Exploring chief complaints in immune disorders.)

Illnesses and treatments

Find out if the patient has any disorders or has undergone any procedures that could affect his immune system or influence his recovery.

Consider asking such questions as:
• Have you received treatment for cancer or any chronic illness?
• Have you had a recent blood transfusion?
• Have you received radiation therapy or tissue or organ transplants?
• Do you have any allergies?
• Have you had any surgeries (such as thymectomy or splenectomy)?
• Have you ever been in an accident or suffered injuries?
• What prescription or over-the-counter drugs are you taking?

If the patient can't remember which medications he's taking, find out if he brought them to the hospital. If so, examine the label and contents. Numerous drugs, including corticosteroids, chemotherapeutic agents, and antibiotics, may suppress immune system functioning.

Family history

Because genetic factors have been implicated in many immune disor-

Making the most of your interview time

When conducting a health history interview, you can save time by considering the following tips:
• Use preinterview data to avoid duplication of effort and reduce interview time. Learn as much as you can from secondary sources, such as admission forms, transfer summaries, and the medical history. If necessary, you can ask the patient to clarify specific points. For instance, you might say, "You told Dr. Cohen that you are usually very tired. Can you tell me more about this symptom?"
• Seek assistance where appropriate. Check your hospital's policy regarding who can gather assessment data. A nursing assistant or a licensed practical nurse may be able to collect routine information, such as immunization history and past hospitalizations. Remember, however, that you must review and verify the information.

• Focus on the chief complaint. Begin the interview by asking the patient why he's hospitalized. That way, if the interview is interrupted, you'll still have initial information on which to base a plan of care.
• Follow the assessment form. Organize your information based on your hospital's nursing assessment documentation form.
• During the interview, avoid interrupting the flow of conversation by keeping your notes short. Expand or complete your information as soon as possible after you complete the interview. You can always go back to the patient if you need to clarify information.
• Record your findings in concise, specific phrases and use appropriate abbreviations.

ders, you need to take a thorough family history. Ask if any immediate relatives, such as parents, siblings, and children, have cancer or a chronic disease. If an immediate relative has an immune disorder, inquire about the patient's grandparents, aunts, and uncles.

Lifestyle factors
Assess the patient's dietary habits and cultural and social background. Consider the following questions:
• Does his diet include appropriate amounts of protein, calories, and vitamins?

• Is he suffering from anorexia or weight loss?
• What restrictions and supplements does his diet include?
• Does he react to certain foods? If so, find out which foods and ask him to describe his reactions.
• How would he describe his family and social life?
• Does he use alcohol or illicit drugs? If the patient drinks alcohol, determine the number of drinks he has daily because this may affect specific immunologic treatments.
• Does his work environment expose him to irritating or toxic materials,

radiation, infectious agents, or allergens?

Coping patterns

Assess the patient's ability to cope with stress. If he has an immune disorder, evaluate how illness has affected his life. Consider the following questions:

• In the past 2 years, have you experienced any major changes in your life, such as the death of a loved one, divorce, marriage, or the loss of a job or a job change?

• Is your job or home life stressful?

• How has the illness affected your job, your ability to perform activities of daily living (ADLs), personal relationships, and outside interests?

• Do you feel your coping strategies are helping or hindering your progress?

• Is your family supportive? How do they perceive your illness? If the patient's family doesn't live nearby or if they're not supportive, ask if he has any other support systems.

Use information about the patient's coping patterns to determine his teaching needs. When planning care, take into account his level of knowledge concerning his illness and its management. Also consider his motivation to learn. If the patient isn't ready or willing to accept change, he's unlikely to respond to your teaching.

Physical examination

Your next step is to perform a physical examination, including an assessment of the patient's spleen and lymph nodes. Using a systematic sequence of assessment techniques will help ensure that you don't miss important findings. Because immune disorders have systemic effects, be sure to consider related body systems and organs. Also, note that certain physical assessment skills may require special training.

Assessing overall appearance

When observing the patient's appearance, look for signs of acute illness, such as profuse perspiration, and of chronic illness, such as emaciation and listlessness. Determine whether the patient's appearance reflects his stated age. Chronic disease and nutritional deficiencies related to immune dysfunction may make a patient appear older than his chronologic age.

• Observe the patient's facial features. Note any edema, grimacing, or lack of expression. Nonpitting edema often accompanies myxedema, a severe hypothyroid state.

• Measure the patient's height and weight. Compare the findings with normal values for the patient's age, sex, and bone structure. Weight loss commonly accompanies many immune disorders.

• Check the patient's posture, movements, and gait for abnormalities that may indicate joint, spinal, or neurologic changes caused by an immune disorder.

Assessing mental status

Evaluate the patient's level of consciousness and mental status. Consider the following questions:

• Is your patient alert? Does he respond appropriately to questions and directions?

• Has his mental status changed? A patient with SLE may experience altered mentation, depression, or psychosis. A patient with acquired immunodeficiency syndrome (AIDS) may demonstrate mental status changes due to human immunodeficiency virus (HIV), encephalopathy, or opportunistic diseases affecting the central nervous system.

Timesaving tip: Save time by combining assessment steps. For example, observe the patient's general appearance and mental status as you take the health history. Then confirm your observations quickly at the beginning of the physical examination.

Checking vital signs

Assessment of vital signs should include the patient's temperature, pulse rate, respiratory rate and character, and blood pressure. Fever may indicate infection, a common occurrence in patients with immune disorders. Because other signs of infection or inflammation — such as redness, swelling, and drainage — may be absent in the patient with an immune disorder, fever and accompanying chills may be the only warning signs of a problem.

Assessing skin, hair, and nails

Observe the patient's skin for any color changes. Normally, the skin has a slightly rosy undertone, even in dark-skinned patients.

• Notice any pallor, cyanosis, or jaundice. Check for erythema, which may indicate a local inflammation, and for plethora (red, florid complexion).

• Observe for telangiectasia (reddish blue linear or starlike lesions on the face and trunk), which may be associated with immune disorders such as scleroderma.

• Evaluate skin integrity. Check for signs of inflammation or infection, such as swelling, heat, or tenderness. Also note other signs of infection, such as poor wound healing, wound drainage, induration, or lesions. Pay close attention to sites of recent invasive procedures, such as venipunctures, bone marrow biopsies, or surgery, for evidence of wound healing.

• Check for rashes and note their distribution. For example, a butterfly-shaped rash over the nose and cheeks may indicate SLE.

• Note any palpable, painless, purplish lesions that may indicate Kaposi's sarcoma, an opportunistic cancer common in patients with AIDS.

• Palpate for nodules, especially around joints. You may be able to detect subcutaneous nodules in patients with rheumatoid arthritis (RA).

• Observe hair texture and distribution, noting any alopecia on the arms, legs, or head. Patchy alopecia in these areas and broken hairs above the hairline (lupus hairs) occur with SLE.

• Inspect the color and texture of the patient's nails, which should appear pink, smooth, and slightly convex. Longitudinal striations can indicate anemia. Onycholysis (nail separation from the nail bed) may result from thyroiditis.

Assessing the head and neck

To assess the patient's head and neck, take the following steps:

• Test the patient's eye muscle strength using the six cardinal positions of gaze and the convergence tests. Remember that ocular muscle weakness may accompany disorders such as Graves' disease.

• Inspect the external portion of the eyes. Note any periorbital edema, which may accompany glomerulonephritis or other renal disease, hypothyroidism (which may occur in patients with Hashimoto's thyroiditis), or allergic reactions. Observe the eyelids for signs of infection or inflammation. Eyelid drooping commonly occurs in patients with myasthenia gravis.

• Inspect the color of the patient's conjunctivae (normally pink) and sclerae (normally white). Conjunctival pallor may accompany anemia.

Erythema may signify conjunctivitis, which accompanies allergic reactions and may be seen in patients with AIDS.

• Assess the fundus with an ophthalmoscope. The retina should be light yellow to orange, and the background should be free of exudate, hemorrhages, and aneurysms. Your ophthalmoscopic examination may also reveal hemorrhage or infiltration with vasculitis.

• Inspect the oral mucous membranes. They should be pink, moist, smooth, and without lesions. Fluffy white patches scattered throughout the mouth may indicate candidiasis, a fungal infection. Lacy white plaques on the buccal mucosa may be caused by hairy leukoplakia. Also look for fluid-filled vesicles on any part of the oral mucosa, which may indicate herpes simplex. Such lesions may occur in patients with immunosuppressive disorders or in those who receive chemotherapy.

• Observe the gums. They should be pink, moist, and slightly irregular with no spongy or edematous areas. Gingival swelling, redness, oozing, bleeding, or ulcerations can signal bleeding disorders.

• Inspect the tongue. It should be pink and slightly rough, and fit comfortably into the floor of the mouth. The tongue may appear enlarged in thyroiditis and may lack papillae in pernicious anemia.

• Inspect the neck for an enlarged thyroid gland. Palpate the thyroid gland, noting its size, shape, and consistency. Certain autoimmune disorders, such as Graves' disease and Hashimoto's thyroiditis, can result in diffuse thyroid enlargement.

Assessing the lymph nodes
Use inspection and palpation to assess the patient's superficial lymph nodes, starting with nodes in the head and neck. First inspect the visible lymph nodes. Then palpate those that can't be seen. Apply gentle pressure and rotary motion to feel the underlying nodes without obscuring them by pressing them deeper into soft tissue. (See *Palpating the lymph nodes,* pages 10 to 15.)

If palpation reveals nodal enlargement or other abnormalities, note the location, size, shape, surface, consistency, symmetry, mobility, color, tenderness, temperature, pulsations, and vascularity of the affected nodes. Although lymph nodes aren't commonly palpable in healthy adults, small, discrete, nontender, mobile nodes may sometimes be palpated successfully. Enlarged lymph nodes may result either from an increase in the number and size of lymphocytes and reticuloendothelial cells, which normally line the nodes, or from infiltration by cells not normally part of the nodes, as in metastatic cancers. Tender lymph nodes suggest inflammation, whereas hard or fixed nodes suggest cancer. Nodes covered with red-streaked skin suggest acute lymphadenitis. Generalized lymphadenopathy, involving three or more nodal groups, can indicate an autoimmune disorder, such as SLE, or an infectious or neoplastic disorder. In SLE, nodal enlargement may be localized or generalized.

Assessing the lungs
Observe the patient's respiratory rate, rhythm, and energy expenditure. Does he exhibit dyspnea, tachypnea, or orthopnea? Note whether he changes position to ease breathing. For instance, during an asthma attack, the patient may sit up and use accessory muscles.

(Text continues on page 16.)

Palpating the lymph nodes

When assessing a patient for signs of an immune disorder, you'll need to palpate the superficial lymph nodes of the head and neck and of the axillary, epitrochlear, inguinal, and popliteal areas, using the pads of the index and middle fingers. Normally, lymph nodes aren't palpable, tender, or hot to the touch. However, if superficial lymph nodes are palpable, they should be less than 3 cm in diameter, firm, oval or round, well defined, mobile, nontender, and nonpulsating.

Head and neck lymph nodes
You can palpate the patient's head and neck lymph nodes best when the patient is sitting.

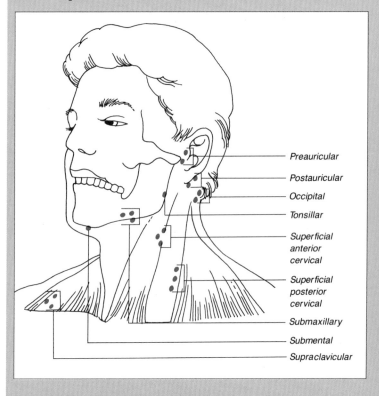

— Preauricular

— Postauricular

— Occipital

— Tonsillar

— Superficial anterior cervical

— Superficial posterior cervical

— Submaxillary

— Submental

— Supraclavicular

To palpate the preauricular lymph nodes, face the patient and place your fingertips over the node site in front of the ear (as shown). Continue to sequentially palpate the postauricular lymph nodes located just behind the ear over the mastoid process, the occipital lymph nodes located behind the ear at the base of the skull, and the tonsillar lymph nodes located at the angle of the mandible.

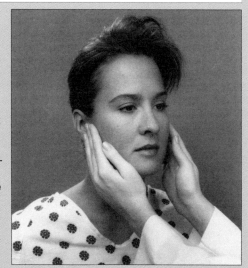

To palpate the submaxillary (submandibular) lymph nodes, flex the patient's head slightly forward and place your fingertips over the node site located between the angle of the mandible and the chin (as shown). Continue to sequentially palpate the submental lymph nodes located just under the chin and the superficial anterior cervical lymph nodes located over the sternocleidomastoid muscle.

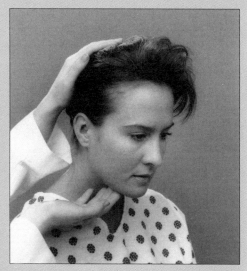

(continued)

Palpating the lymph nodes *(continued)*

Head and neck lymph nodes *(continued)*
To palpate the superficial posterior cervical nodes, place your fingertips along the anterior surface of the trapezius muscle (as shown).

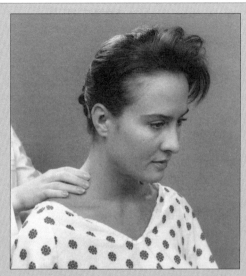

To palpate the supra-clavicular nodes, encourage the patient to relax so that the clavicles drop. Flex the head slightly forward. Then hook your left index finger over the clavicle lateral to the sterno-cleidomastoid muscle (as shown). Rotate your fingers deeply to feel these nodes.

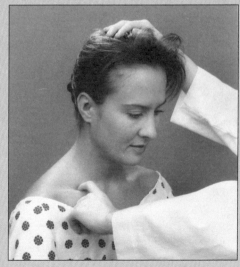

Axillary and epitrochlear lymph nodes

Palpate the axillary and epitrochlear lymph nodes with the patient sitting. You can also palpate the axillary nodes with the patient supine.

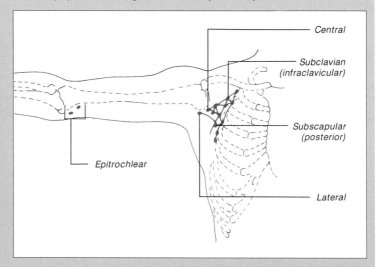

To palpate the axillary lymph nodes, have the patient relax. Then reach as high as you can toward the apex of the axilla. Press your fingers in toward the chest wall, and feel for the central lymph nodes (as shown). Then continue to palpate, feeling for the lateral and subscapular lymph nodes. To palpate the subclavian lymph nodes, palpate below the clavicle.

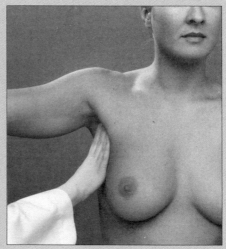

(continued)

Palpating the lymph nodes *(continued)*

Axillary and epitrochlear lymph nodes *(continued)*
To palpate the epitrochlear lymph nodes, place your fingertips in the depression above and posterior to the medial area of the elbow.

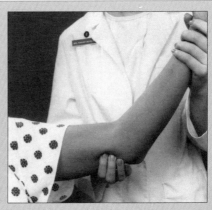

Inguinal and popliteal lymph nodes
Palpate the inguinal and popliteal lymph nodes with the patient in a supine position. You can also palpate the popliteal nodes with the patient sitting or standing.

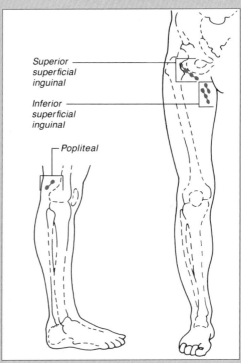

Superior superficial inguinal

Inferior superficial inguinal

Popliteal

To palpate the inferior superficial inguinal lymph nodes, gently press below the junction of the saphenous and femoral veins (as shown).

To palpate the superior superficial inguinal lymph nodes, press along their horizontal course just inferior and parallel to the inguinal ligament (not shown).

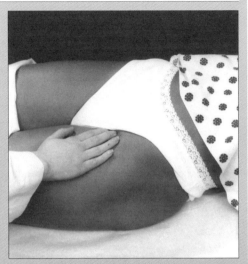

To palpate the popliteal nodes, press gently along the posterior muscles at the back of the knee (as shown).

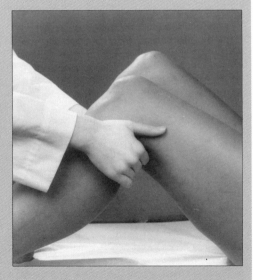

• Percuss the anterior, lateral, and posterior thorax, comparing sides. A dull sound indicates consolidation, which may occur with pneumonia, whereas hyperresonance may indicate trapped air resulting from bronchial asthma.
• Auscultate the lungs to assess for abnormal breath sounds. Wheezing suggests asthma or an allergic response. Crackles may denote a respiratory infection, such as pneumonia, which commonly affects immunocompromised patients. Accompanied by a dry cough, labored breathing, and tachypnea, crackles are a common finding in AIDS patients with *Pneumocystis carinii* pneumonia. Pleural friction rubs may be heard in patients with SLE or RA.

Assessing the heart
Auscultate the patient's heart for rate, rhythm, and abnormal heart sounds. Tachycardia or other arrhythmias may accompany anemia, infection, or Graves' disease. An apical systolic murmur may signify severe anemia, which may occur in patients with autoimmune disorders or immunodeficiencies. A pericardial friction rub may be detected in patients with scleroderma, SLE, or RA.

Assessing the abdomen
Inspect the patient's abdomen for any lesions, nodules, or scars. Auscultate the abdomen for bowel sounds. In autoimmune disorders that cause diarrhea, bowel sounds increase. In scleroderma and in autoimmune disorders that cause constipation, bowel sounds may decrease. Next, percuss abdominal quadrants to detect tympany or dullness. Tympany usually predominates because of gas in the GI tract. Dullness is normally heard over solid organs. Normally, the liver produces a dull sound over a span of 2½″ to 4¾″ (6 to 12 cm). The area of dullness increases when the liver enlarges.

Also palpate the abdomen to detect enlarged organs and tenderness. You may prefer to alternate percussion with palpation when examining the liver, spleen, and other abdominal areas. Note that hepatomegaly may accompany many immune disorders.

To be palpable, the spleen must be enlarged approximately three times its normal size. In patients with immune disorders, splenic tenderness may result from infections. Percussion of the spleen may reveal splenomegaly, which may result from immune disorders that cause cell overproduction or excessive cell destruction. (See *Percussing and palpating the spleen.*)

Assessing the extremities
Assess the patient's peripheral circulation by checking for Raynaud's phenomenon (intermittent arteriolar vasospasm in the fingers, toes, ears, or nose), which can produce blanching in the affected area, followed by cyanosis, pallor, and reddening. Next, palpate the peripheral pulses, which should be symmetrical and regular. Weak, irregular pulses may indicate anemia.

To assess for musculoskeletal involvement, test range of motion of the hand, wrist, and knee. Then palpate the joints to assess for swelling, tenderness, and pain. If appropriate, ask the patient to perform such maneuvers as standing up, walking, and bending over.

Diagnostic test results
The results of diagnostic testing complete the objective data base. Along with the health history and physical examination findings, they form a profile of your patient's condition.

Percussing and palpating the spleen

When assessing the spleen, first use percussion to help estimate its size and to obtain clues about possible enlargement. Then use palpation to detect tenderness and enlargement.

Percussion
Follow these steps to percuss the spleen:
• Percuss the lowest intercostal space in the left anterior axillary line; the percussion notes should be tympanic.
• Ask the patient to take a deep breath, and then percuss this area again. If the spleen is normal in size, the area will remain tympanic. If the tympanic percussion note changes on inspiration to dullness, the spleen is probably enlarged.
• To help estimate spleen size, outline the spleen's edges by percussing in several directions from areas of tympany to areas of dullness.

Palpation
Follow these steps to palpate the spleen:
• Stand on the right side of the supine patient. Reach across her to support the posterior lower left rib cage with your left hand. Then place your right hand below the left costal margin and press inward toward the spleen, as shown below.
• Instruct the patient to take a deep breath. If the spleen is enlarged, you'll feel its rigid border. Note if tenderness is present. Don't overpalpate the spleen; an enlarged spleen may rupture easily.

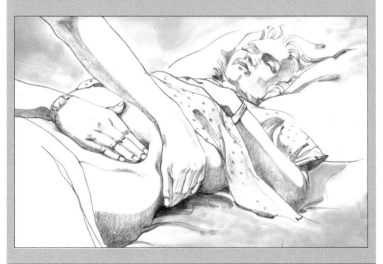

Blood tests are commonly performed on patients with suspected immune disorders. Other tests include serum studies, delayed type hypersensitivity (DTH) tests, bone marrow aspiration and biopsy, and lymph node biopsy.

Blood tests

The following studies help to determine the effectiveness of the immune system.

Tests of cell counts and activity

These tests require uncoagulated blood. Common anticoagulants used include ethylenediaminetetraacetic acid, citrate, and heparin. Blood is usually collected in a lavender top tube, using at least a 20G needle to prevent cell damage. To ensure accurate results, tests are performed within a few hours of drawing blood.

• Total white blood cell (WBC) count (reported as number of cells per microliter [µl] or cubic millimeter [mm³] of blood) can provide a general estimate of bone marrow activity.

• The white blood cell differential provides information regarding the distribution of specific WBCs. This information helps to determine immune function and to assist in the diagnosis of immune or inflammatory disorders. Tests may examine the following WBCs: neutrophils (small phagocytic cells that circulate through the blood in large numbers), monocytes (immature phagocytic cells important in assisting the neutrophils during viral infections), lymphocytes (including T lymphocytes and B lymphocytes), and basophils and eosinophils (small leukocytes that interact with each other). The most commonly measured subsets of lymphocytes are the inducer T cells that express CD4+ and the suppressor T cells that express CD8+. (CD, or cluster of differentiation, describes

a characteristic cell surface marker. The CD4+ T-cell count and the ratio of CD4+ T cells to CD8+ T cells are important laboratory measurements for monitoring HIV-positive patients.)

• Erythrocyte sedimentation rate measures the distance erythrocytes, or red blood cells (RBCs), settle in 1 hour in a tube of 0.9% sodium chloride solution. Erythrocytes normally settle at a specific rate, measured in millimeters (mm). Sedimentation rates increase with illness and with age.

Serum tests

Important serum tests include immunoglobulin levels, complement assay, radioallergosorbent test (RAST), and the antinuclear antibodies (ANA) test.

• Immunoglobulin (Ig) levels measure the five different classes of antibodies (IgA, IgD, IgE, IgG, and IgM) formed in response to a specific antigen. The overall concentration of immunoglobulin levels and the distribution of the various types can reveal information about a patient's immune status.

• Complement assay measures levels of complement and its components. Complement is a collective term for a system of serum proteins that control inflammation. Complement assays are based on complement's ability to destroy sensitized RBCs. Reduced levels may indicate that an autoimmune disorder is consuming available complement and using it to form antibody-antigen complexes. Elevated levels may indicate increased complement production. Complement components are numerically designated as C1 through C9, with C1 having three subcomponents: C1q, C1r, and C1s. (See *Quick review of laboratory findings in immunologic care.*)

Quick review of laboratory findings in immunologic care

Patients with immune disorders generally have detectable increases and decreases of various laboratory test levels. Use the chart below to quickly check the normal adult values and possible causes of increased and decreased values for these tests.

Test	Normal adult values	Possible causes of increased values	Possible causes of decreased values
Total white blood cell (WBC) count	• 4,500 to 10,000/μl	• Acute infection • Inflammation • Dehydration • Leukemia	• Chronic infection • Cancer • Bone marrow failure • Immunosuppression secondary to acquired immunodeficiency syndrome (AIDS), chronic cortisol therapy, myelosuppression, antibiotic use, or chemotherapy
Neutrophils (segs)	• 47.6% to 76.8% of total WBC count • 1,950 to 8,400/μl	• Acute infection	• Chemotherapy • Radiation therapy • Neoplastic invasion of bone marrow • Aplastic anemia • Infections, such as viral hepatitis
Lymphocytes	• 16.2% to 43% of total WBC count • 660 to 4,600/μl	• Dehydration • Leukemia	• Acute infection
T cells	• 60.1% to 88.1% of total lymphocyte count • 644 to 2,201/μl	• Multiple myeloma • Acute lymphocytic leukemia • Occasionally, infectious mononucleosis	• AIDS • Certain congenital T-cell deficiency diseases • B-cell proliferative disorders, such as chronic lymphocytic leukemia
CD4+ T cells	• 34% to 67% of total T-cell count • 493 to 1,191 cells/μl	• Constitutional in allergy-prone individuals	• Immunosuppression • Cancer • AIDS
CD8+ T cells	• 10% to 49.1% of total T-cell count • 182 to 785 cells/μl	• Viral infection	• Systemic lupus erythematosus (SLE)
CD4+ : CD8+ T-cell ratio	• 2:1	• Constitutional in allergy-prone individuals	• Immunosuppression • Cancer • AIDS

(continued)

Quick review of laboratory findings in immunologic care *(continued)*

Test	Normal adult values	Possible causes of increased values	Possible causes of decreased values
B cells	• 3% to 20.8% of total lymphocyte count • 82 to 392 cells/μl	• Chronic lymphocytic leukemia • Multiple myeloma • Waldenström's macroglobulinemia • DiGeorge syndrome	• Acute lymphocytic leukemia • Certain congenital or acquired immunoglobulin deficiency diseases
Monocytes	• 0.6% to 9.6% of total WBC count • 24 to 960/μl	• Mononucleosis • Viral infection	• Immunosuppression
Basophils	• 0.3% to 2% of total WBC count • 12 to 200/μl	• Inflammation	• Bone marrow failure • Immunosuppression
Eosinophils	• 0.3% to 7% of total WBC count • 12 to 760/μl	• Inflammation • Allergic responses • Helminth infestations	• Bone marrow failure • Immunosuppression
Complement assays	• Total complement: 330 to 730 CH_{50} units	• Obstructive jaundice • Thyroiditis • Acute rheumatic fever • Rheumatoid arthritis • Acute myocardial infarction • Ulcerative colitis • Diabetes mellitus	*Decreased total complement:* • SLE • Acute poststreptococcal glomerulonephritis • Acute serum sickness • Advanced cirrhosis • Multiple myeloma • Rapidly rejecting allographs *C1 esterase inhibitor deficiency:* • Hereditary angioedema *C3 deficiency:* • Recurring pyogenic infections *C4 deficiency:* • SLE
Erythrocyte sedimentation rate	• Men: 15 mm/hour • Women: 20 mm/hour • Children: 10 mm/hour	• Infection • Arteritis • Connective tissue disorders, such as rheumatoid arthritis • Cancer	• Iron deficiency anemia • Sickle cell anemia

Quick review of laboratory findings in immunologic care *(continued)*

Test	Normal adult values	Possible causes of increased values	Possible causes of decreased values
Immunoglobulin levels by immunoelectrophoresis			
Immunoglobulin G (IgG)	• 70% of total immunoglobulins • 500 to 1,600 mg/dl	• Infection • Liver disease • Autoimmune disorders • AIDS	• Agammaglobulinemia • Bone marrow failure • Immunosuppression
IgA	• 15% of total immunoglobulins • 90 to 450 mg/dl	• Liver disease • Exercise • Infection	• Congenital or acquired IgA deficiency • Pregnancy • Protein-wasting disorders • Immunosuppression
IgM	• 10% of total immunoglobulins • 60 to 280 mg/dl	• SLE • Autoimmune disorders • Waldenström's macroglobulinemia • Malaria	• Chronic lymphocytic leukemia • Immunosuppression
IgE	• Less than 1% of total immunoglobulins • 0.01 to 0.04 mg/dl	• Asthma • Allergic conditions	• Immunosuppression
IgD	• Less than 1% of total immunoglobulins • 0.5 to 3 mg/dl	• Chronic infections • Connective tissue disorders	• Immunosuppression

• RAST measures the amount of IgE in the serum directed against a specific antigen. It can determine the severity of specific allergies.

• The ANA test measures the number of antibodies directed at the human cell nucleus. Positive findings from serum diluted to a concentration of 1:16 may indicate an autoimmune disorder, most commonly SLE. (See *Detecting autoantibodies in autoimmune disease,* pages 22 and 23.)

Blood and tissue typing

ABO blood typing, Rh typing, crossmatching, and human leukocyte antigen (HLA) tests help classify a patient's blood for transfusion and other purposes.

• ABO blood typing classifies blood according to the presence of the major antigens A and B on RBC surfaces and according to the serum antibodies anti-A and anti-B. Human RBCs are classified as A, B, AB, or O. ABO blood typing is always required before transfusion to prevent a lethal re-

Detecting autoantibodies in autoimmune disease

When the immune system produces autoantibodies against the antigenic determinants on and in cells, an autoimmune disease may result. The chart below lists selected autoimmune diseases, the areas affected, associated antigens and antibodies, and diagnostic tests used to detect autoantibodies.

Disease	Affected area	Antigens	Antibodies	Diagnostic techniques
Hashimoto's thyroiditis	Thyroid gland	Thyroglobulin, second colloid antigens, cytoplasmic microsomes, cell-surface antigens	Antibodies to thyroglobulin and to microsomal antigens	Radioimmunoassay, hemagglutination, complement fixation, immunofluorescence
Pernicious anemia	Hematopoietic system	Intrinsic factor	Antibodies to gastric parietal cells and vitamin B_{12} binding site of intrinsic factor	Immunofluorescence, radioimmunoassay
Pemphigus vulgaris	Skin	Desmosomes between prickle cells in the epidermis	Antibodies to intercellular substances of the skin and mucous membranes	Immunofluorescence
Myasthenia gravis	Neuromuscular system	Acetylcholine receptors of skeletal and heart muscle	Anti-acetylcholine antibody	Immunoprecipitation, radioimmunoassay
Autoimmune hemolytic anemia	Hematopoietic system	Red blood cells (RBCs)	Anti-RBC antibody	Direct and indirect Coombs' test
Primary biliary cirrhosis	Small bile ducts in liver	Mitochondria	Mitochondrial antibody	Immunofluorescence of mitochondrial-rich cells (kidney biopsy)
Rheumatoid arthritis	Joints, blood vessels, skin, muscles, lymph nodes	Immunoglobin G (IgG)	Antigammaglobulin antibody	Sheep RBC agglutination, latex immunoglobulin agglutination, radioimmunoassay, immunofluorescence, immunodiffusion
Goodpasture's syndrome	Lungs and kidneys	Glomerular and lung basement membranes	Anti–basement membrane antibody	Immunofluorescence of kidney biopsy specimen, radioimmunoassay

Detecting autoantibodies in autoimmune disease *(continued)*

Disease	Affected area	Antigens	Antibodies	Diagnostic techniques
Systemic lupus erythematosus	Skin, joints, muscles, lungs, heart, kidneys, brain, eyes	Deoxyribonucleic acid (DNA) nucleoproteins, blood cells, clotting factors, IgG, Wassermann antigens	Antinuclear antibody, anti-DNA antibody, anti-ds-DNA antibody, anti-SS-DNA antibody, antiribonucleoprotein antibody, antigammaglobulin antibody, anti-RBC antibody, antilymphocyte antibody, antiplatelet antibody, antineuronal cell antibody, anti-Sm antibody	Counterelectrophoresis, hemagglutination, radioimmunoassay, immunofluorescence, Coombs' test

action and before allograft transplantation to help prevent graft rejection.

• Rh typing classifies blood by the presence or absence of the Rh_0 (D) antigen on the surface of RBCs. Blood may be typed as Rh-positive, Rh-negative, or Rh-positive D^o. Transfusion may take place only if the donor blood is compatible with the recipient blood.

• Crossmatching establishes the compatibility of the donor's and the recipient's blood. This is the best antibody detection test available for preventing lethal transfusion reactions.

• The HLA test identifies antigens on nucleated cells and lymphocytes. Essential to immunity, these antigens determine the degree of histocompatibility between transplant recipients and donors. The HLA test may also aid in establishing paternity.

Other diagnostic tests

Other diagnostic tests include DTH, anergy panel, and biopsies.

• The DTH test assesses general immune function, with the most common DTH being the intradermal purified protein derivative (PPD) test for tuberculosis (TB). In this test, a small amount of *Mycobacterium tuberculosis* is injected intradermally. If the TB bacillus is or has been present, sensitized T cells and antibodies will react with the PPD within 48 hours. However, if a patient is immunocompromised by drugs, disease, or advanced age, no reaction will occur even if TB is present.

• To confirm whether a patient suspected of having TB, but reacting negatively to the PPD test, may actually have TB, an anergy panel is performed. This panel is a series of intradermal injections using derivatives of common antigens. Such antigens include tetanus toxoid, *Candida*, and *Streptococcus*. If none of the intradermal injections causes a positive skin reaction, the patient is considered to have anergy (inability to mount a proper immune defense). Other conditions related to an anergy response include infections, such as influenza, mumps, measles, typhus, and scarlet fever.

• In bone marrow aspiration and biopsy, a specimen of bone marrow, usually from the posterior iliac crest, is taken and used to diagnose various disorders and cancers, such as leukemia, Hodgkin's disease and other lymphomas, granuloma, aplastic or megaloblastic anemia, and thrombocytopenia.

• In lymph node biopsy, lymph node tissue is taken, usually from the supraclavicular region, by needle aspiration or by surgical excision to confirm possible cancer and to evaluate immune function.

Nursing diagnosis

The next step of the nursing process, nursing diagnosis, describes the patient's actual or potential response to a health problem. The nursing diagnoses reflect your assessment findings and your interpretation of the patient's ability to meet his needs.

To prepare a nursing diagnosis, evaluate the information obtained from your immunologic assessment. Consider such questions as:

• What are the patient's signs and symptoms?

• Which assessment findings are abnormal for this patient?

• How do particular behaviors affect his immunologic health?

• Does the patient understand his illness and its treatment?

• How does his environment affect his health?

• How does the patient respond to his health problem? Is he willing to take steps to improve his health?

• Does he receive adequate support from family and friends?

Chapters 3 through 6 contain common nursing diagnoses for many immune disorders. Keep in mind, however, that since each patient responds to illness and stress differently, you should never allow your nursing diagnoses to become so standardized that they fail to address individual differences and special needs.

For greater accuracy, you should write an etiology, or "related to" statement, for each nursing diagnosis. The etiology should identify conditions that contribute to the development or continuation of that particular nursing diagnosis.

Developing individual nursing diagnoses for each patient can be difficult. You can make this task easier and save time by becoming familiar with the nursing diagnoses most frequently used in immunologic care.

Altered protection

This nursing diagnosis refers to a decrease in the patient's ability to guard himself from internal or external threats such as illness or injury. Defining characteristics include:

• altered clotting
• anorexia
• chills
• cough
• immunodeficiency
• diaphoresis
• disorientation
• dyspnea
• fatigue
• immobility
• impaired healing
• insomnia
• itching

- maladaptive stress response
- neurosensory impairment
- pressure ulcers
- restlessness
- weakness.

Altered protection may be related to extremes of age, inadequate nutrition, abnormal blood profiles, drug therapies (such as immunosuppressants), treatments (such as radiation and organ transplantation), and diseases (such as AIDS). (See *Understanding altered protection,* pages 26 and 27.)

Timesaving tip: To help plan interventions for the patient with numerous nursing diagnoses, consider consolidating multiple nursing diagnoses into a single, encompassing diagnosis. In many cases, the diagnosis *altered protection related to myelosuppression and immunosuppression* may be used to describe a variety of human responses characteristic of an immunocompromised patient: frequent infection, fluid retention, electrolyte disturbances, changes in skin fragility and healing, weakness, and altered nutritional intake. Use this single diagnosis to develop outcomes and interventions.

High risk for infection

This nursing diagnosis describes an accentuated risk of introducing pathogenic microorganisms into the body from either internal or external sources. Consider using this diagnosis whenever the following risk factors are present:
- immobility
- use of an indwelling urinary catheter or an I.V. line
- invasive procedures or use of invasive monitoring devices
- prophylactic antibiotic therapy
- chemotherapy
- hemodialysis
- respiratory treatments

- corticosteroid therapy
- an immune disorder or chronic illness
- suppressed inflammatory response
- immunosuppression
- inadequate immunity
- malnutrition
- lack of understanding of how to avoid exposure to pathogens.

Fatigue

This nursing diagnosis describes an overwhelming sense of exhaustion and decreased capacity for physical and mental work, regardless of adequate sleep. The patient with this diagnosis may exhibit the following characteristics:
- decreased libido
- decreased level of performance
- disinterest in surroundings
- increased irritability.

He may report feeling increasingly introspective, lethargic, or listless. He may be accident-prone as well.

In patients with immune disorders, fatigue may be related to many factors, such as decreased metabolic energy production, altered body chemistry (secondary to chemotherapy, for example), increased energy requirements to perform activities of daily living, overwhelming psychological or emotional demands, and discomfort.

Altered nutrition: Less than body requirements

This nursing diagnosis describes a change in eating patterns that results in decreased body weight. Defining characteristics for this diagnosis include:
- loss of body weight despite adequate food intake
- body weight 20% or more under the ideal weight for height and frame

(Text continues on page 28.)

Understanding altered protection

The nursing diagnosis *altered protection* refers to a decrease in the ability to guard the self from illness. This nursing diagnosis is extremely useful for describing a patient's response to an immunologic problem. Adding a "related to" statement may help you more precisely describe the alterations in protective mechanisms.

Normal immune response
The normal immune response is to recognize a foreign antigen and destroy it.

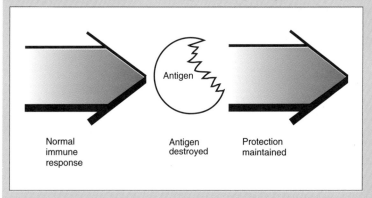

| Normal immune response | Antigen destroyed | Protection maintained |

Altered protection related to immunodeficiency
An immunodeficient patient's immune system is incapable of responding effectively to foreign antigens. As a result, the patient is susceptible to infection or cancer.

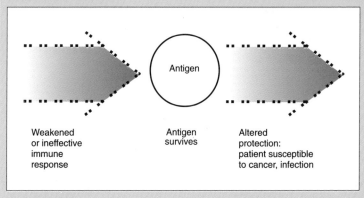

| Weakened or ineffective immune response | Antigen survives | Altered protection: patient susceptible to cancer, infection |

Altered protection related to autoimmunity
In an autoimmune disorder, the immune response fails to differentiate between a self cell and a nonself cell, thereby causing damage to the patient's
own cells and tissues.

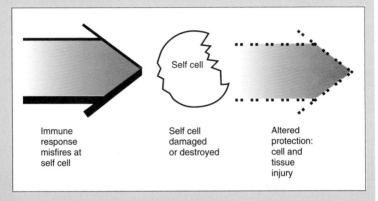

Immune
response
misfires at
self cell

Self cell
damaged
or destroyed

Altered
protection:
cell and
tissue
injury

Altered protection related to hypersensitivity
A hypersensitivity reaction is an exaggerated or inappropriate immune response to an antigen. Rather than destroying invaders, the immune response
leads to damage or disease.

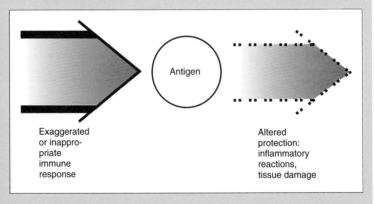

Exaggerated
or inappro-
priate
immune
response

Altered
protection:
inflammatory
reactions,
tissue damage

Identifying common nursing diagnoses in immune disorders

To describe the response patterns of patients with immune disorders, you'll frequently need additional nursing diagnoses. This list identifies and defines these diagnoses.

Activity intolerance • Insufficient physiologic or psychological energy to endure or complete daily activities
Altered oral mucous membrane • Disruption in the tissue layers of the oral cavity
Altered sexuality patterns • Concerns about changes in sexuality
Body image disturbance • Negative or distorted self-perception that impairs healthful functioning
Caregiver role strain • Caregiver's perceived difficulty in providing care

of a family member with significant home care needs
High risk for impaired skin integrity • Accentuated risk for alteration or disruption of skin surface
Impaired physical mobility • Limited ability to move about independently
Ineffective breathing pattern • Inadequate pulmonary inflation or deflation due to faulty inhalation or exhalation
Pain • Severe discomfort or uncomfortable sensations

• abdominal pain (with or without pathologic condition)
• diarrhea or steatorrhea
• hyperactive bowel sounds
• poor muscle tone
• food intake less than recommended daily allowances
• sore, inflamed buccal cavities
• weakness in muscles required for mastication or swallowing.

Altered nutrition in patients with immune disorders may be related to the inability to ingest, digest, or absorb nutrients because of biological or psychological factors. Economic and social factors may also interfere with the patient's ability to obtain adequate food.

Ineffective individual coping
This nursing diagnosis describes an inability to use adaptive behaviors in

response to such difficult life situations as loss of health, a loved one, or a job. Defining characteristics include:
• a change in usual communication patterns
• chronic fatigue
• chronic anxiety
• excessive drinking
• inability to meet role expectations, meet basic needs, or solve problems
• inappropriate use of defense mechanisms
• insomnia
• irritability
• irritable bowel
• muscular tension
• overeating or lack of appetite
• expressing inability to cope
• difficulty asking for help
• verbal manipulation.

Ineffective individual coping by patients with immune disorders can be related to many factors, such as situational crisis, personal vulnerability, inadequate support systems, poor nutrition, unrealistic perceptions, effects of acute or chronic illness, lack of knowledge related to therapeutic regimen or nature of the disease, and his prognosis.

Knowledge deficit

This nursing diagnosis refers to an inadequate understanding of health information or to an inability to practice health-related behaviors. Defining characteristics for this diagnosis include:
• requests for information
• expression of lack of knowledge
• inadequate performance of a skill
• inappropriate or exaggerated behaviors
• failure to take medication or follow instructions.

Knowledge deficit may be associated with a variety of factors, including the following:
• lack of exposure to pertinent information
• misinterpretation of information
• lack of familiarity with information resources
• cognitive impairment
• lack of interest in learning.

Use this diagnosis to document your patient's learning needs.

Additional nursing diagnoses

The patient with an immune disorder may require many nursing diagnoses. Immune disorders may affect any body system as well as the patient's psychosocial well-being, so be prepared to expand the number of diagnoses. (See *Identifying common nursing diagnoses in immune disorders.*)

Planning

In this next step of the nursing process, you'll create a written plan for delivering quality patient care. The plan of care includes relevant nursing diagnoses, patient outcomes, nursing interventions, and evaluation data. It will become a permanent part of the patient's health record. (See *Faster care planning,* page 30.)

When writing your plan, you must assign priorities to nursing diagnoses. Many patients with immune disorders have multiple problems requiring multiple nursing diagnoses. High-priority nursing diagnoses involve the patient's most urgent needs (such as emergency, or immediate, physical needs). Intermediate-priority nursing diagnoses involve nonemergency needs, and low-priority diagnoses involve needs that don't directly relate to the patient's illness or prognosis. (See *Setting priorities among nursing diagnoses,* pages 31 and 32.)

When establishing priorities, always consider the impact on the patient. Maslow's hierarchy of needs can be a useful guide for helping you identify the priorities of the patient's needs. The needs identified by Maslow form five levels: physiologic needs, safety or security, love and belonging, esteem, and self-actualization. This classification of needs is based on the idea that lower-level, physiologic needs must be met before higher-level, more abstract needs.

To encourage compliance, always involve the patient in the planning of his own care. Find out what is most meaningful to him about his care, and explain the need for setting care plan priorities. Encourage the patient to ask questions about his immune disorder and its treatment. Help him un-

Faster care planning

Use the first part of a nursing diagnosis statement (the diagnostic label) to devise outcomes and the second part (the "related to" statement) to develop interventions. For example, suppose your patient has the nursing diagnosis *High risk for infection related to effects of immunosuppressant therapy.*

Writing outcomes
To write outcomes, consider the first part of the diagnosis — *High risk for infection* — then ask yourself, "How will I know that the patient hasn't developed an infection?" Answering this question will help you develop appropriate outcomes; for example:
• The patient will remain free from infection throughout the course of his therapy.
• He will register a normal temperature within 72 hours.

Developing interventions
Look closely at the "related to" statement in the nursing diagnosis. Ask yourself, "What interventions are appropriate for preventing infection in a patient receiving immunosuppressant therapy?" This will help you devise interventions, such as:
• enforcing strict infection-control measures, particularly good handwashing technique
• teaching the patient about the adverse effects of immunosuppressant therapy
• teaching him measures to protect against infection at home
• describing signs and symptoms of infection that must be reported to the doctor and emphasizing the need to report them as quickly as possible.

derstand medical terms by translating them into clear, simple language.

Establishing patient outcomes
You'll need to establish patient outcomes — measurable goals derived from nursing diagnoses that describe behavior or results to be achieved within a specified time. An outcome statement should describe the specific behavior that will show the patient has reached his goal. Include criteria for measuring the behavior, state the conditions under which the behavior should occur, and specify the target date or time frame for achieving the outcome. Because patient outcomes

are the criteria you'll use to evaluate care, you must express them clearly.

For example, if your patient's nursing diagnosis is *Activity intolerance related to chronic illness,* appropriate outcome statements for a patient admitted on 8/15 might include the following:
• The patient will identify risk factors that may lead to activity intolerance by 8/17.
• He will communicate an understanding of the rationale for maintaining his activity level by 8/18.
• He will perform activities of daily living (ADLs) to tolerance level by 8/19.

Setting priorities among nursing diagnoses

Patients with immune disorders typically have multiple problems that must be addressed. When planning care for these patients, you'll need to identify all of the problems, establish appropriate nursing diagnoses, and rank them from highest to lowest priority. To understand how to set these priorities, consider the case history of Dave Morrison, a 33-year-old stockbroker.

Subjective data
Mr. Morrison was brought to the hospital by a friend after experiencing a fever, overwhelming fatigue, and a weight loss of 23 lb (10.5 kg) over the past 3 months. Mr. Morrison complains of feeling "weak and tired all the time." He tells you that he has been diagnosed as positive for the human immunodeficiency virus (HIV) but that until recently he has had only occasional episodes of night sweats and diarrhea. He reports a persistent nonproductive cough and dyspnea with activity.

You learn that Mr. Morrison has been caring for his partner, who has acquired immunodeficiency syndrome (AIDS). Mr. Morrison worries about his ability to care for him if he, too, should become increasingly debilitated. He is also worried about losing his job if his colleagues become aware that he has AIDS.

Objective data
Your examination of Mr. Morrison and your review of his diagnostic test results reveal the following:
• temperature, 101.4° F (39° C); pulse rate, 98 beats/minute and regular; respiratory rate, 28 breaths/minute and shallow; blood pressure, 140/78 mm Hg
• chest X-ray: diffuse, bilateral interstitial infiltrates

• arterial blood gas levels (at rest): partial pressure of oxygen in arterial blood, 70 mm Hg; oxygen saturation, 90%; partial pressure of carbon dioxide in arterial blood, 30 mm Hg; bicarbonate, 24 mEq/liter; pH, 7.46
• complete blood count: hematocrit, 32%; hemoglobin, 11 g/dl; platelet count, 173,000/mm^3; white blood cell count, 13,000/mm^3
• pale, sweaty skin; dry mucous membranes; cracked lips with some bleeding; evidence of diffuse cervical, axillary, and inguinal lymphadenopathy

Identifying problems and setting priorities
Mr. Morrison's fever and abnormal chest X-ray suggest an active pulmonary process requiring a sputum specimen for histologic studies. You suspect that Mr. Morrison may have developed *Pneumocystis carinii* pneumonia. Your first goal is to improve his pulmonary status. You realize that his vital signs and oxygenation status need to be closely monitored. You select as your top-priority nursing diagnosis *Impaired gas exchange related to altered oxygen supply secondary to pulmonary infection.*

(continued)

Setting priorities among nursing diagnoses *(continued)*

Mr. Morrison will require immediate and long-term planning to help him cope with fatigue and weight loss. You select the nursing diagnoses *Activity intolerance related to fatigue* and *Altered nutrition: Less than body requirements, related to reduced intake and nature of the disorder* as your next priorities.

To help Mr. Morrison cope with fatigue, you plan to teach him how to perform daily activities independently or with assistance, to set priorities for daily tasks, to delegate nonessential responsibilities, and to incorporate energy conservation techniques into his daily routine. To improve his nutritional intake, you plan to document his caloric intake, work with the dietitian to develop an appropriate meal plan, and provide patient teaching.

Because his disease has advanced, Mr. Morrison has increased psychosocial needs. His worsening condition may make it difficult for him to continue to act as primary caregiver for his partner. The social stigma associated with AIDS may create anxiety about his professional stand-

ing. To address these needs, you select the diagnoses *Caregiver role strain related to diminished ability to perform caregiving activities* and *Anxiety related to deteriorating condition and social stigma attached to illness.*

By actively listening to Mr. Morrison, you can reassure him that he will be treated respectfully, thereby reducing some of his anxiety. You encourage Mr. Morrison to identify stressful situations and to express his feelings about the stress he feels caring for his partner. You can suggest that he arrange respite periods at designated times. You should also plan to provide him with information about sources of support in the community that will help alleviate the stress and fatigue caused by caring for his sick partner. Consult with your facility's social services department, if available, to discuss available community support.

Once you have prioritized your nursing diagnoses, you can proceed to develop appropriate outcomes, interventions, and evaluation criteria.

• He will perform isometric exercises daily from 8/17 to 8/20.
• He will maintain blood pressure, pulse rate, and respiratory rate within a prescribed range during ADLs or exercise by 8/20.

Developing interventions

After establishing patient outcomes, you'll develop interventions designed to help the patient achieve these out-

comes. Consider such factors as your patient's age, developmental and educational levels, environment, and cultural background. Talk with the patient and his family. The more you know about the patient, the easier it will be to develop appropriate interventions. For example, if your patient has a reading disability and is scheduled for a bone marrow aspiration and biopsy, don't write an intervention for patient teaching that includes sophisticated reading material. Instead, discuss the procedure with the patient or give him a descriptive audiotape.

Timesaving tip: When documenting interventions, clearly state the necessary action. Many interventions must be continued and, possibly, evaluated and modified by other nurses in your absence. Clearly stating the action will prevent needless repetition of effort. If family members are participating in your patient's care, explain interventions to them as well to save teaching time.

When documenting your plan, include how and when to perform the interventions (including supplies or equipment) as well as any special instructions. Examples of clearly stated interventions include the following:

• Assist the patient with a skin care regimen, including maintaining good personal hygiene, using nonirritating (nonalkaline) soap, patting skin dry (rather than rubbing), inspecting skin on a regular basis, and recognizing and reporting the beginnings of skin breakdown (redness, blisters, discoloration).

• Teach the patient diaphragmatic breathing exercises, chest physiotherapy, effective coughing techniques, and proper use of the incentive spirometer, if warranted. Encourage him to practice breathing exercises and effective coughing four times a day (or more) for 8 weeks. Explain that postural drainage, percussion, and vibration help mobilize mucus in the lungs for removal.

• Provide regular mouth care, using 0.9% sodium chloride solution, bicarbonate, or chlorhexidine gluconate mouthwash for daily oral rinsing. Avoid glycerin swabs, which dry the mucous membranes.

Implementation

During this fourth step of the nursing process, you put your plan of care into action. Your activities are directed toward resolving the patient's diagnosis and meeting health care needs. Expect to collaborate with other caregivers, the patient, and his family.

Treatment for the patient with an immune disorder is becoming increasingly sophisticated. The following is a brief review of nursing interventions you may implement in immunologic care.

Therapeutic interventions

These interventions aim to alleviate the effects of the illness or restore optimal function. Examples of therapeutic interventions include:

• administering medications
• maintaining the patient's skin integrity
• ensuring adequate fluid intake
• positioning the patient to ensure maximum comfort
• promoting coughing and deep-breathing exercises to prevent pulmonary stasis
• administering supplemental oxygen
• establishing a regular bowel and bladder routine for an incontinent patient.

Emergency care

You may be called upon to respond to an immunologic emergency. For example, in life-threatening anaphylaxis, emergency care is required to prevent vascular collapse, leading to systemic shock and, possibly, death. If the patient stops breathing, you'll need to initiate cardiopulmonary resuscitation.

Monitoring

Periodic or continuous evaluation of your patient's immune status, response to therapy, and functional abilities is just as important as the initial assessment. Monitoring procedures include reviewing serum studies; assessing respiratory, cardiovascular, and integumentary status; and assessing the spleen and lymph nodes. In addition, you'll monitor vital signs, including temperature, pulse rate, blood pressure, and respirations. You'll also periodically evaluate other indicators of your patient's health, such as skin hydration, intake and output, daily weight, and mental status.

Patient teaching

Teaching may help the patient with an immune disorder live with his disorder and prevent complications. Many of your lessons will focus on providing the patient and his family with information on his disorder, including:
• the nature of his disorder
• risk factors for illness
• signs and symptoms to report to the doctor
• possible complications
• factors that may precipitate an acute immunologic emergency
• techniques that may be used to maintain an adequate baseline condition (for example, breathing, coughing, relaxation).

Teaching is especially important for the discharged patient with an immune disorder because of possible complex home care requirements, such as:
• monitoring for subtle signs and symptoms of infection
• assessing changes in temperature
• reducing exposure to microbes.

Preoperative care

Preoperative nursing care for the patient with an immune disorder may include explaining the procedure, describing special precautions related to his altered immune function, describing the preoperative drug regimen, establishing an I.V. line, recording vital signs, and performing and documenting a complete immunologic assessment to establish a baseline for postoperative evaluation. You may also take special measures to prepare him for preoperative and postoperative procedures — for example, arranging a visit to the intensive care unit to introduce staff members and to explain the equipment.

Postoperative care

Postoperative interventions include monitoring the patient's vital signs and immunologic status and watching carefully for signs of infection or other postoperative complications.

Counseling and emotional support

Expect to plan and implement interventions to enhance your patient's well-being. The patient with an immune disorder needs a trusting, open relationship with health care providers. By providing reassurance, you can help the patient and his family cope with anxiety and the increased demands brought on by the patient's changed condition. By listening openly to the patient's concerns, you can help him combat his feelings of helplessness and loss of control. A trusting relationship also promotes patient compliance with therapeutic interventions. Patients with severe emotional problems may require a referral for psychological counseling.

Preparation for discharge

For many immunocompromised patients, the thought of going home and having to deal with their newly diagnosed immune disorder is overwhelming. By preparing the patient for discharge as far in advance as possible, you can help make this transition smoother and easier for him.

Discharge planning may include:
• instructing the patient to notify the doctor of any signs or symptoms that may signal complications or a deteriorating condition
• reminding him when to return for follow-up appointments
• providing a referral to a home health care agency or a community support organization, as necessary
• making sure that the patient understands the purpose, dosage, and possible adverse effects of all prescribed drugs
• making the patient aware of when he can resume normal activity
• instructing the patient and his family on how to provide required skin care and other home care measures.

Evaluation

In this final stage of the nursing process, you'll judge the effectiveness of your plan of care and gauge your patient's progress in meeting expected outcomes. Evaluate the patient by answering the following questions:
• How would you characterize the patient's overall progress?
• Did he achieve the goals outlined in the plan of care by the target dates specified?
• Are the existing nursing diagnoses still appropriate?
• How did the patient respond to care, including medications, changes in diet or activity, procedures, and patient teaching?
• Does he have any new problems or needs?

Evaluation is an ongoing activity that overlaps other phases of the nursing process. Evaluation findings may trigger a new cycle of assessment, nursing diagnosis, planning, implementation, and further evaluation. (See *Using an evaluation flowchart,* page 36.)

Reassessment

Regularly collect information from all available sources, including the patient, his family, his medical record, and other caregivers. Also include your own observations of the patient and his condition.

Next, compare reassessment data with criteria established in the patient outcomes documented in your plan of care. For example, a patient with vasculitis admitted on 8/15 who has the nursing diagnosis *Altered oral mucous membrane* might have the following patient outcomes:
• reports increased comfort by 8/20
• exhibits improved or healed lesions or wounds by 8/22
• demonstrates oral care routine by 8/24
• discusses feelings about condition by 8/24.

During your reassessment of this patient, check him for mouth lesions and other complications. Ask him if his mouth feels more comfortable than before entering the hospital. Note whether he has discussed his feelings about his condition and whether he can successfully demonstrate oral care.

When evaluating your findings, try to determine if the patient's overall condition is improving or deteriorating. If many problems remain unresolved, determine the factors that are

Using an evaluation flowchart

You can use the flowchart below as a guide throughout the evaluation process.

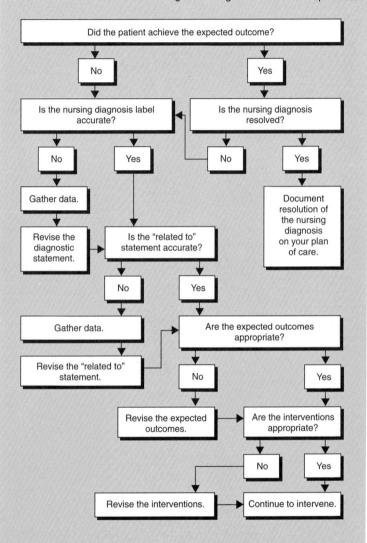

interfering with goal achievement. Consider all possible reasons that a patient may not be able to achieve a desired outcome, such as the following:

• The purpose and goals of the plan of care aren't clear.

• The expected outcomes aren't realistic in light of the patient's condition.

• The plan of care is based on incomplete assessment data.

• The nursing diagnoses are inaccurate.

• The nursing staff experienced conflict with the patient or other members of the health care team.

• Staff members didn't follow the plan of care.

• The patient failed to carry out activities outlined in the plan of care.

• The patient's condition changed.

Reviewing implementation

When trying to determine factors interfering with goal achievement, look closely at the documented interventions and the manner in which they were implemented.

For example, suppose a patient with the nursing diagnosis *Fatigue related to decreased energy and excessive activity* fails to achieve one of his planned outcomes — *patient reports decreased fatigue.* To find out why, consider these questions:

• Were steps taken to conserve the patient's energy through rest, planning, and setting priorities?

• Were activities alternated with periods of rest?

• Were too many demands placed on the patient?

• Was the patient taught techniques for decreasing fatigue?

Answering these questions will help you determine why the patient outcome wasn't achieved.

Writing evaluation statements

Evaluation statements are used to document the patient's response to care. These statements indicate whether expected outcomes were achieved and list the evidence supporting your conclusions. The importance of clearly written evaluation statements cannot be overemphasized: Documentation of patient outcomes is necessary to support the rationales for nursing care and to justify the use of nursing resources. Record your evaluation statements in your progress notes or in the revised plan of care, according to your hospital's documentation policy.

Patient outcome statements in your plan of care can provide a model for writing evaluation statements. When writing each statement, describe the patient's progress by using active verbs, such as "walk," "demonstrate," or "express." Include criteria used to measure the patient's response to care, and describe the conditions under which the response occurred. Write a separate evaluation for each patient response or behavior that you wish to describe, and date the statement.

For example, possible evaluation statements for the nursing diagnosis *Altered protection related to myelosuppression and immunosuppression* may include:

• Patient states that he can walk the length of the hall without fatigue.

• He demonstrates increased strength and resistance.

• He demonstrates a weight gain of 2 lb (0.9 kg) since last week's visit.

• He demonstrates personal cleanliness and maintains a clean environment.

• He reports pain reduced to 1, on a scale of 1 to 10, with analgesia.

• Oral lesions are completely healed.

• Chills, fever, and other signs and symptoms of illness are absent.
• Skin lesions have decreased from 1.5 cm to 1.2 cm in diameter over the last 3 days.

Modifying the plan of care
During the evaluation, you may discover that the plan of care needs to be modified. If the patient outcomes have been achieved, be sure to record this information. Revise other patient outcome statements as necessary. To ensure a successful evaluation, keep an open mind, and never hesitate to consider new patient data or to revise previous judgments. Determine which nursing interventions need to be revised or discontinued. Assess whether changes are needed in priorities assigned to nursing diagnoses.

You may need to document that a nursing diagnosis has been resolved, or you may find that a nursing diagnosis no longer accurately describes the patient's status.

Like all steps of the nursing process, evaluation is ongoing. Continue to assess, diagnose, plan, implement, evaluate, and document for as long as you provide care.

CHAPTER 2

Exploring chief complaints in immune disorders

Fever   40

Fatigue   42

Weight loss   43

Lymphadenopathy   45

Joint pain   46

Rash   48

Several important signs and symptoms — fever, fatigue, weight loss, lymphadenopathy, joint pain, and rash — occur in patients with immune disorders. (Many of these also occur in patients with infectious disorders.) By fully investigating these complaints, you can form a diagnostic impression of your patient's problem and guide your subsequent care.

Fever

Fever is a body temperature above 98.6° F (37° C). Though it is a common sign that may arise from a disorder in virtually any body system, it has little diagnostic value by itself. Cytokines produced by macrophages, especially interleukin-1, alter the thermoregulatory center and represent the ultimate cause of most fevers. (See *Causes of fever.*)

Fever can be classified as low (an oral reading of 99° to 100.4° F, or 37.2° to 38° C), moderate (100.5° to 104° F, or 38.1° to 40° C), or high (above 104° F). Fever above 105° F (40.6° C) constitutes a medical emergency. Fever above 106° F (42.2° C) causes unconsciousness and, if prolonged, brain damage. You should report any fever above 101° F (38.3° C) to the doctor.

If the patient's fever approaches 105° F (40.6° C), take his other vital signs and assess his level of consciousness. Administer antipyretic drugs and begin the following rapid cooling measures: Apply ice packs to the axillae and groin, give tepid sponge baths, and apply a hypothermia blanket. To prevent a rebound hypothermic response, constantly monitor the patient's rectal temperature.

If the patient's fever is low to moderate, proceed with the health history and physical examination according to the guidelines below.

History of the sign
To further explore your patient's fever, consider asking him the following questions:
• How long have you had the fever?
• What was your highest temperature?
• Did the fever begin suddenly or gradually?
• Did it rise steadily or rise, fall, and then rise again?
• Have you been exposed to high environmental temperatures for a prolonged period? If so, how much fluid did you drink?
• Have you recently been exposed to someone with the flu or any other infection?
• In your occupation or leisure activities, do you work with soil?
• Do you have any pets, or have you been exposed to wild animals?
• Have you traveled recently?

Associated findings
Ask the patient if he has experienced any of the following signs or symptoms:
• pain
• changes in level of consciousness (LOC)
• chills, fatigue, or sore throat
• swollen glands
• persistent cough
• morning stiffness
• nocturnal diaphoresis
• skin lesions or open areas that appear inflamed
• pruritus
• diarrhea, anorexia, or weight loss
• oliguria, burning upon urination, or any other urinary changes.

Causes of fever

Fever is often a prominent sign in patients with immune or infectious disorders.

Immune disorders
Fever commonly occurs in hypersensitivity reactions, acquired immunodeficiency syndrome, autoimmune hemolytic anemia, and autoimmune connective tissue diseases such as rheumatoid arthritis, systemic lupus erythematosus, and progressive systemic sclerosis.

Infectious disorders
Fever is the hallmark of infection. All infections, including those caused by bacteria, viruses, fungi, rickettsiae, chlamydiae, mycoplasmas, and parasites, may cause fever. Fever may arise abruptly or insidiously and may be of short or prolonged duration.

Previous conditions and treatments
Consult with the patient, family members, or members of the health care team to determine if the patient has ever had any of the following conditions, treatments, or risk factors:
• surgery or diagnostic testing
• blood transfusion
• bone marrow transplant
• immunizations
• infection
• burns or other trauma
• endocrine dysfunction
• malignant hypertension
• autoimmune disorder
• immunosuppressive treatment, such as chemotherapy or radiotherapy
• immunosuppressive disorder, such as acquired immunodeficiency syndrome
• physical or emotional stress
• allergy
• asthma.

Drug history
Various drugs can cause a hypersensitivity reaction leading to fever. These include:
• penicillins
• procainamide
• sulfonamides.
  Toxic doses of the following may also cause fever:
• salicylates
• amphetamines
• tricyclic antidepressants.
  Inhaled anesthetics and muscle relaxants can trigger malignant hyperthermia in genetically predisposed patients. Chemotherapeutic drugs may also cause fever.

Physical examination
Examine the patient according to the steps described below.
• Assess the patient's vital signs. Check especially for tachycardia and tachypnea.
• Assess LOC and mental status. Be alert for signs of restlessness, irritability, or seizure activity. Also note malaise, fatigue, or anxiety.
• Inspect skin color. Note if the patient's face appears flushed and whether diaphoresis or shivering is present.
• Inspect for signs of dehydration, such as a dry, furrowed tongue.

• Inspect lymph nodes for visible swelling or redness.
• Observe motor activity for possible muscle tremors and twitching.

Let the health history findings guide the remainder of the physical examination.

Fatigue

Fatigue is commonly reported as tiredness, exhaustion, a lack of energy, or a strong desire to rest or sleep. It may be accompanied by weakness, which involves the muscles.

Fatigue may represent a normal response to physical overexertion and sleep deprivation or a nonspecific symptom of psychological or physiologic disorders. It may be acute or chronic and commonly accompanies immune disorders. (See *Causes of fatigue.*)

If your patient complains of fatigue, take his health history and perform a physical examination according to the guidelines below.

History of the symptom
To explore your patient's complaint of fatigue, consider asking him the following questions:
• When did you first feel unusually tired?
• How long have you felt this way?
• How would you rate your fatigue on a scale of 1 (no fatigue) to 10 (extreme fatigue)?
• During what part of the day are you most tired?
• Is your fatigue related to activity?
• Does rest help?
• What makes you feel better? Worse?
• Has fatigue affected your daily activities? If so, how?
• Have you recently experienced unusual stress?
• Has your nutritional intake recently changed?

Associated findings
Ask the patient if he has experienced any of the following signs or symptoms:
• shortness of breath or other respiratory difficulty
• pain or unusual bleeding
• weakness or loss of consciousness
• nocturia
• insomnia
• nausea, vomiting, or diarrhea
• feelings of anxiety or depression
• recent weight changes

Causes of fatigue

Fatigue is a common symptom in patients with immune or infectious disorders.

Immune disorders
Fatigue commonly occurs in acquired immunodeficiency syndromes, rheumatoid arthritis, systemic lupus erythematosus, myasthenia gravis, pernicious anemia, autoimmune hemolytic anemia, Addison's disease, and insulin-dependent diabetes mellitus.

Infectious disorders
In *chronic infection,* fatigue is often the most prominent symptom — and sometimes the only one. In *acute infection,* fatigue is typically brief. Profound fatigue may occur in Lyme disease, viral hepatitis, and mononucleosis caused by cytomegalovirus or Epstein-Barr virus.

- persistent cough
- fever.

Previous conditions and treatments

Consult with the patient, family members, or members of the health care team to determine if the patient has ever had any of the following disorders, risk factors, or treatments:
- cancer
- heart or kidney disease
- chronic obstructive pulmonary disease
- anemia
- diabetes mellitus
- multiple sclerosis
- recent surgery
- rheumatic disease
- mental illness.

Drug history

Obtain a drug history and note past or current use of drugs that may cause fatigue, such as:
- antihypertensives, especially beta blockers
- sedatives
- corticosteroids
- amiodarone
- carbamazepine
- flecainide
- recombinant interferon alfa-2a or alfa-2b, interferon alfa-n3 (derived from human leukocytes), interferon gamma 1-b, or recombinant interleukin-2
- pentamidine isethionate for inhalation
- clomipramine
- dantrolene
- metoclopramide
- etretinate.

Physical examination

Observe the patient's general appearance for signs of depression or organic illness. Note whether he appears pale, unkempt, expressionless, tired, underweight, or otherwise unhealthy.

Assess his mental status, noting especially any of the following characteristics:
- agitation
- poor attention span
- confusion
- psychomotor impairment.

Depending upon the history, you may need to more closely assess a body system or perform a thorough physical examination.

Weight loss

Weight loss may result from decreased food intake, increased metabolic requirements, impaired absorption of nutrients, loss of nutrients in urine or feces, or treatment of fluid retention. Nearly any serious illness can cause weight loss. (See *Causes of weight loss,* page 44.)

If your patient complains of weight loss, take his health history and perform a physical examination according to the guidelines below.

History of the sign

To further understand your patient's weight loss, consider asking him the following questions:
- When did you first notice you were losing weight?
- Has your weight loss stopped or are you still losing weight?
- How much weight have you lost?
- Over how long a period have you been losing weight?
- Was your weight loss intentional?
- Have your eating habits changed? Would you say that you are eating about the same amount, more than usual, or less than usual? If less than usual, do you know why?

Causes of weight loss

Weight loss is common in patients with immune or infectious disorders.

Immune disorders
Weight loss is a major sign in patients with acquired immunodeficiency syndrome and commonly occurs in patients with Crohn's disease, insulin-dependent diabetes mellitus, hyperthyroidism, ulcerative colitis, Addison's disease, rheumatoid arthritis, progressive systemic sclerosis, and other connective tissue disorders, such as ankylosing spondylitis, polymyalgia, rheumatism, and polymyositis with dermatomyositis.

Infectious disorders
Weight loss may occur in occult infections, especially tuberculosis, fungal diseases, amebic abscesses, and bacterial endocarditis.

• Have you recently felt anxious or depressed?
• Do you have any problems obtaining or preparing food? Chewing food?
• How do you feel about your weight loss?

Associated findings
Note whether the patient has experienced any of the following signs or symptoms:
• anorexia, diarrhea, or vomiting
• polyuria or excessive thirst
• steatorrhea
• dysphagia
• fever
• pain
• lymphadenopathy
• fatigue
• stomatitis.

Previous conditions and treatments
Consult with the patient, family members, or members of the health care team to determine if the patient has ever had any of the following conditions, treatments, or risk factors:

• cancer
• alcoholism or drug abuse
• diabetes mellitus or other endocrine diseases
• gastrointestinal disease
• recent surgery
• trauma
• psychosocial factors, such as poverty or social isolation
• human immunodeficiency virus infection, high-risk sexual activity, I.V. drug abuse, or blood transfusions between 1977 and 1988.

Drug history
Ask the patient about past or current use of the drugs listed below:
• diuretics
• appetite suppressants
• thyroid preparations
• laxatives
• chemotherapeutic drugs
• interferon gamma 1-b, recombinant interferon alpha-2a, or interleukin-2
• alprazolam
• guanadrel
• tolmetin
• bupropion.

Physical examination

Carefully check the patient's height and weight and vital signs, including temperature, blood pressure, respiratory rate and depth, and pulse rate and rhythm. Assess his general appearance. Be sure to note any of the following findings:

• evidence of malnourishment or overly loose clothing
• signs of muscle wasting
• skin turgor and abnormal pigmentation, especially around the joints
• jaundice or pallor
• sparse and dry hair
• signs of infection or irritation on the roof of the mouth
• swelling in the neck or ankles.

Palpate the patient's liver for enlargement and tenderness. Let the health history guide the remainder of the physical examination.

Lymphadenopathy

Normally, lymph nodes are discrete, mobile, nontender, and nonpalpable, ranging in size from 0.5 to 2.5 cm. Presence of nodes larger than 3 cm indicates lymphadenopathy and is cause for concern. Lymph nodes may be tender and erythematous, suggesting a draining lesion, or hard and fixed, tender or nontender.

Enlargement of one or more lymph nodes may be generalized or localized. Generalized lymphadenopathy (involving three or more node groups) may stem from connective tissue disease, an endocrine disorder, a neoplasm, or an inflammatory process, such as bacterial or viral infection. Localized lymphadenopathy (involving one or two node groups) commonly results from infection or trauma affecting the drained area. (See *Causes of lymphadenopathy*.)

Causes of lymphadenopathy

Lymphadenopathy often appears in patients with immune disorders or infectious disorders, including local infections.

Immune disorders
Lymphadenopathy commonly occurs in acquired immunodeficiency syndrome and in other immunodeficiency disorders in association with opportunistic infections. It also occurs in rheumatoid arthritis, Sjögren's syndrome, systemic lupus erythematosus, serum sickness, and sarcoidosis.

Infectious disorders
Lymphadenopathy commonly occurs in infections such as streptococcal infection, rubella, rubeola, varicella infection, cat-scratch fever, gingivitis, glossitis, dental infections, sexually transmitted diseases, infectious mononucleosis, cytomegalovirus infection, bacterial endocarditis, tuberculous lymphadenitis, nontuberculous mycobacterial disease, brucellosis, and fungal infection.

If your patient reports swollen lymph nodes, take his health history and perform a physical examination according to the guidelines that follow.

History of the sign

To further explore your patient's swollen lymph nodes, consider asking the following questions:
• When did you first notice the swelling?

• Are the swollen areas painful?
• Have you recently had a cold, a virus, or any other health problems?

Associated findings

Note whether the patient has experienced any of the following signs or symptoms:
• fever
• pain
• fatigue
• weight loss
• night sweats
• purulent drainage.

Previous conditions and treatments

Consult with the patient, family members, or members of the health care team to determine if the patient has ever had any of the following disorders, risk factors, or treatments:
• valvular heart disease
• cancer
• trauma
• biopsy or surgery
• sexually transmitted disease or other infection, including human immunodeficiency virus infection
• high-risk sexual activity
• I.V. drug abuse
• blood transfusion between 1977 and 1988.

Drug history

Ask the patient about past and current use of the following drugs:
• phenytoin
• hydrazaline
• allopurinol
• typhoid vaccine.

Physical examination

Assess the patient's height, weight, and vital signs, including temperature, blood pressure, respiratory rate and depth, and pulse rate and rhythm. Then examine him according to the steps that follow.

Inspection

• Note if the patient appears tired, cachectic, flushed, or in distress.
• Inspect his mouth and pharynx for redness, swelling, and exudation.
• Note needle tracks or wounds of any type.

Palpation

• Palpate all lymph nodes to determine the extent of lymphadenopathy and to detect any other areas of local enlargement.
• Use the pads of your index and middle fingers to move the skin over underlying tissues at the nodal area. Note the location and extent of enlarged lymph nodes.
• Record the size of enlarged nodes in centimeters and note if they're fixed or mobile, tender or nontender, pale or reddened. Is the node discrete or does the area feel matted?
• If you detect tender, hot nodes, check the area drained by them for signs of infection, such as erythema and swelling.

Let the patient's history and lymph node assessment guide the remainder of the physical examination.

Joint pain

Any disorder involving inflammation or degeneration of joints or surrounding structures may cause pain. Joint pain may also stem from joint overuse or trauma. It may restrict range of motion and interfere with the ability to perform daily activities.

In certain disorders, pain may affect one joint (for example, bursitis, tendinitis, or injury); other disorders, such as rheumatoid arthritis, may affect many joints. Pain may be progressive, as in ankylosing spondylitis, or the patient may experience simultaneous inflammation in multiple joints, as in rheumatic fever. Arthralgia — joint pain unaccompanied by heat, redness, and swelling — is a common vague complaint in many infections. (See *Causes of joint pain*.)

If your patient complains of joint pain, take his health history and perform a physical examination according to the guidelines that follow.

History of the symptom
To further explore your patient's joint pain, consider asking him the following questions:
- When did you first feel joint pain?
- Did the pain occur suddenly? Or did it develop over weeks or months?
- Does the pain involve one joint or several? Have the patient locate the affected joints.
- If several, has the pain spread to other joints while remaining in the initial one? Or has it disappeared from the original site?
- How would you describe the type of pain? How would you rate its intensity on a scale of 1 (least severe) to 10 (most severe)?
- At what time of day is your pain worst?
- What makes the pain worse? What helps to relieve it?
- How does the pain affect your ability to carry out daily activities?
- Does it affect your sleep?
- Does it affect your emotional well-being?

Associated findings
Note whether the patient has experienced any of the following signs and symptoms:
- joint stiffness or deformity
- joint warmth, redness, and swelling
- limitation of movement
- fever with or without chills
- fatigue
- anorexia

Causes of joint pain

Joint pain may occur in many immune or infectious disorders.

Immune disorders
Joint pain commonly occurs in rheumatoid arthritis, systemic lupus erythematosus, progressive systemic sclerosis, inflammatory bowel disease, and acute rheumatic fever. Other autoimmune rheumatic disorders that cause joint pain include polymyositis with dermatomyositis, ankylosing spondylitis, Reiter's syndrome, Behçet's syndrome, and mixed connective tissue disease.

Infectious disorders
Joint pain is a prominent symptom in patients with nongonococcal septic arthritis, gonococcal arthritis, and Lyme disease. It may also occur in patients with mycobacterial and fungal infections.

- weight loss
- muscle weakness
- lymphadenopathy
- skin lesions
- sore throat
- diarrhea
- abdominal pain
- urinary burning, frequency, or urgency.

Previous conditions and treatments
Consult with the patient, family members, or members of the health care team to determine if the patient has

ever had any of the following disorders, risk factors, or treatments:
• trauma
• excessive use of joints
• infection, especially gonorrhea or Lyme disease
• rheumatic disease
• arthroscopy
• joint surgery, including joint replacement.

Drug history

Note past or current use of any of the drugs listed below.

The following drugs may cause drug-induced arthralgia:
• isotretinoin
• interferon alfa-n3 (derived from human leukocytes)
• lymphocyte immune globulin, antithymocyte globulin (equine)
• epoetin alfa
• nicotine transdermal systems
• etretinate
• naltrexone.

The following may cause drug-induced lupus syndrome with arthralgia:
• hydrazaline
• procainamide
• methyldopa
• isoniazid
• cephalosporins
• phenytoin
• quinidine
• sulfonamides
• bleomycin
• oral contraceptives.

Physical examination

Examine the patient according to the steps described below.
• Check the patient's height, weight, and vital signs, including temperature, blood pressure, respiratory rate and depth, and pulse rate and rhythm.
• Note the patient's general appearance and mobility.

• Inspect for signs of joint inflammation, including swelling around the joint and redness of the overlying skin.
• Note the presence of joint deformities, and check for symmetrical involvement. Observe the surrounding area for abnormalities, such as subcutaneous nodules and muscle atrophy.
• Firmly palpate each joint, noting any thickening, swelling, laxity, tenderness, or crepitus.
• Note any limitation in the normal range of joint motion.
• Test strength of surrounding muscles, noting any weakness.

Let the patient's history and musculoskeletal assessment findings guide the remainder of the physical examination.

Rash

Rashes and skin lesions are classified as follows:
• Macular lesions, such as petechiae, are less than 1 cm and are circumscribed and flat.
• A patch is similar to a macular lesion but larger.
• Papules are palpably elevated solid lesions up to 0.5 cm.
• Plaque is similar to papules but larger.
• Wheals are irregular, transient, superficial areas of localized skin edema, such as hives.
• Vesicles, which occur in herpes simplex, are circumscribed, superficial, fluid-filled elevations up to 0.5 cm.
• Bullae, which occur in bullous pemphigoid, are circumscribed superficial elevations greater than 0.5 cm filled with serous fluid.

Causes of rash

Rash is a prominent sign in many patients with immune or infectious disorders.

Immune disorders
Rash commonly occurs in acquired immunodeficiency syndrome, histoplasmosis, infection caused by *Mycobacterium haemophilum,* cutaneous T-cell lymphoma, molluscum contagiosum, systemic lupus erythematosus, polymyositis with dermatomyositis, acute rheumatic fever, progressive systemic sclerosis, pemphigus vulgaris, and bullous pemphigoid. Rash also occurs in hypersensitivity reactions, such as serum sickness, allergic reaction to insect bites, ana-phylaxis, allergic dermatitis, contact dermatitis, and atopic dermatitis.

Infectious disorders
Rash may occur in herpes simplex viral infections, herpes zoster, infectious mononucleosis, staphylococcal scalded skin syndrome, toxic shock syndrome, impetigo contagiosa, secondary syphilis, gonococcemia, Lyme disease, blastomycosis, scabies, chicken pox, rubeola infection, and rubella infection.

• Pustules, which occur in acne, are circumscribed superficial elevations filled with pus.

Outbreak of a rash may be accompanied by pruritus and discomfort. A rash may profoundly affect the patient's body image. (See *Causes of rash.*)

If your patient complains of rash, take his health history and perform a physical examination according to the guidelines that follow.

History of the sign
To further explore the patient's complaint of rash, consider asking the following questions:
• When did the rash erupt? What did it look like? What parts of your body did it affect?
• Has the rash spread or changed in any way? If so, when and how did it spread?
• Does the rash itch or burn? Is it painful or tender?

• Have you recently been bitten by an insect or a rodent?
• Have you had direct skin contact with known allergens, such as detergents or foods?
• Have you recently been exposed to anyone with an infectious disease?
• Which medications have you recently taken?
• Have you applied any topical agents to the rash and, if so, when was the last application? Were any of them effective?
• What childhood diseases have you had?
• What immunizations have you had?
• How do you feel about the appearance of the rash?

Associated findings
Note if the patient has experienced any of the following signs or symptoms:
• headache
• fever

- cough
- fatigue
- joint pain
- lymphadenopathy
- diarrhea
- urinary burning or frequency
- difficulty breathing, stridor, or wheezing
- unusual bleeding or bruising.

Previous conditions and treatments
Consult with the patient, family members, or members of the health care team to determine if the patient has ever had any of the following disorders, treatments, or risk factors:
- allergies
- recent diagnostic studies using contrast agents
- immunosuppressive therapy
- other skin disorders
- sexually transmitted disease or other infection
- connective tissue disease
- cancer
- trauma.

Drug history
Obtain a drug history. Many drugs can cause rashes; some of the most common include:
- penicillins
- sulfonamides
- aspirin
- barbiturates
- gold compounds
- glucocorticoids
- oral contraceptives
- thiazides
- tetracyclines
- phenylbutazone
- captopril
- enalaprilat
- enalapril maleate
- isocarboxazid
- bleomycin
- lymphocyte immune globulin, antithymocyte globulin (equine)
- allopurinol
- methyldopa
- phenytoin.

Physical examination
Check the patient's height, weight, and vital signs, including temperature, blood pressure, respiratory rate and depth, and pulse rate and rhythm. Then examine the patient according to the steps described below.

Inspection
- Observe the patient's general appearance. Note if he appears in distress and if he's scratching the lesion. Does he appear cachectic, lethargic, listless, or restless and anxious?
- Inspect the patient's skin, noting whether it's dry or oily. Note the anatomic location, general distribution and arrangement, color, shape, and size of the lesions.
- Check for crusts, macules, papules, vesicles, scales, scars, and wheals. Note if the outer layer of epidermis separates easily from the basal layer.

Palpation
- Feel the temperature of the patient's skin, using the back of your fingers. Compare affected and unaffected areas, noting whether they feel cool or hot.
- Palpate vesicles or bullae to determine whether they're flaccid or tense.

Let the patient's history and dermatologic assessment findings guide the rest of the physical examination.

CHAPTER 3

Caring for patients with immunodeficiency disorders

Acquired immunodeficiency syndrome   52

*Immunodeficiency caused by cancer
and its treatment*   71

Immunodeficiency refers to an inadequate number or function of any immune system component. Immunodeficiency disorders are commonly classified according to the deficient component. They include:

• humoral (B-cell) immunodeficiency
• cell-mediated (T-cell) immunodeficiency
• combined B-cell and T-cell immunodeficiency
• phagocytic dysfunction
• complement deficiency.

In immunodeficiencies, the immune system can't properly recognize or respond to antigens, leaving the patient vulnerable to infections, cancers, and other disorders. Some immunodeficiencies result from genetic transmission. (See *Primary congenital immunodeficiencies.*) Most, however, result from malnutrition, stress, injury, disease, or iatrogenic factors.

Malnutrition
Malnutrition hinders lymphocyte production, particularly by reducing T-cell number and function. It may be the most common cause of immunodeficiency today.

Stress
Severe or chronic stress can result in temporary or long-standing immunosuppression. It's associated with atrophy of the lymphoid organs, lymphopenia, and decreased resistance to infection and disease.

Injury
Trauma, especially involving burns or hemorrhage, results in massive protein and tissue loss as well as damage to skin and other first-line defenses. Loss of blood, tissue, and cellular components leaves the trauma victim with a low neutrophil count and low immunoglobulin levels.

Disease
Autoimmune disorders, sickle cell disease, acute viral infections, and diabetes mellitus are all associated with secondary immunodeficiencies. Malignant tumors can suppress the production of lymphocytes and neutrophils. Lymphomas and leukemias cause abnormal production or function of immature or pathologic immune components.

Iatrogenic factors
Improved treatments, although often lifesaving, may cause immunosuppression. Sometimes this immunosuppression is desired, as in prevention of organ transplant rejection or treatment of certain autoimmune or hyperinflammatory conditions. In other cases it's an undesired complication, as in cancer therapy or treatment with certain antimicrobial drugs.

Multiple factors
In many patients, secondary immunodeficiencies have multiple causes. For example, in a patient with cancer, immunodeficiency may result from the tumor and its treatment as well as from the accompanying stress and malnutrition.

Acquired immunodeficiency syndrome

Acquired immunodeficiency syndrome (AIDS) represents one of the most serious health challenges of our time. It's marked by a gradual destruction of CD4+ T cells by the human immunodeficiency virus (HIV).

Primary congenital immunodeficiencies

Disorder	Clinical findings	Pathologic findings
Humoral		
Bruton's hypogammaglobulinemia	Recurrent pyogenic infections, especially pneumonia, sinusitis, otitis, furunculosis, meningitis, sepsis, panhypogammaglobulinemia, arthritis of the large joints	Absence of plasma cells, decreased B-cell count, failure of pre–B cells to secrete immunoglobulin (decreased IgA, IgG, IgM levels)
Transient hypogammaglobulinemia of infancy	Recurrent respiratory tract infections beginning 5 to 6 months after birth, with recovery in 1 to 2 years	Uncertain cause, decreased IgG level, low or normal IgA and IgM levels
Selective IgA deficiency	Bacterial infections of respiratory, GI, and genitourinary tracts; diarrhea; malabsorption; frequently associated with autoimmune disease	IgA synthesis but not secretion, possibly high levels of circulating anti-IgA antibody
Common variable immune deficiency (may be acquired)	Recurrent pyogenic infections (similar to Bruton's), malabsorption, diarrhea, giardiasis, autoimmune disease, lymphoreticular malignancy	Normal B-cell count; low immunoglobulin levels, suggesting diminished synthesis or secretion
Cell-mediated		
DiGeorge syndrome	Thymic hypoplasia, hypocalcemia, parathyroid hypoplasia, otitis, tuberculosis, *Candida albicans,* abnormal facies, congenital cardiac anomalies, chronic diarrhea, failure to thrive, esophageal atresia	Thymic and parathyroid hypoplasia, deficient T-cell count, often increased B-cell count
Chronic mucocutaneous candidiasis	Chronic, resistant *C. albicans* infections of skin, nails, and mucous membranes; rarely life-threatening; possibly some endocrine abnormalities	Normal T-cell count, but failure of lymphokine production in the clone responsive to *Candida* antigen
Combined		
Severe combined immunodeficiency	Multiple, severe infections (bacterial, fungal, and viral); graft-versus-host disease; diarrhea; extreme wasting	Decreased T- and B-cell counts; few or no antibodies

(continued)

Primary congenital immunodeficiencies *(continued)*

Disorder	Clinical findings	Pathologic findings
Combined *(continued)*		
Immunodeficiency with ataxia-telangiectasia	Progressive cerebellar ataxia, multiple telangiectasia of skin and ocular mucosa, recurrent sinopulmonary infections, endocrine abnormalities, lymphomas	Possible decreased T-cell counts, impaired T-cell function, decreased IgA and IgE levels in some patients
Wiskott-Aldrich syndrome	Thrombocytopenia with hemorrhagic tendency, eczema, recurrent infections, lymphoreticular malignancy	Possible hypercatabolism of immunoglobulin, decreased IgM and IgG levels, increased IgA and IgE levels, decreased T-cell count

Virtually any cell that has the CD4+ molecule on its surface may be infected by HIV. These include monocytes, macrophages, bone marrow progenitors, and glial, gut, and epithelial cells. The resulting immunodeficiency predisposes the patient to opportunistic infections, unusual cancers, and other health problems.

Definition
The Centers for Disease Control and Prevention (CDC) defines AIDS as an illness characterized by laboratory evidence of HIV infection and severe immunosuppression coexisting with one or more indicator conditions. In 1993, the CDC expanded its definition for AIDS. (See *Classifying HIV infection and AIDS,* opposite, and *Key points about AIDS,* page 57.)

Prevalence
The exact prevalence of HIV infection is unknown. The World Health Organization estimates that 1 million people in North America carry the vi-

rus and that, by December 1993, close to 436,000 people had developed AIDS. The average length of time between HIV exposure and diagnosis is 8 to 10 years, although this period can vary.

Disease course
The course of AIDS can vary, but the syndrome usually results in death from opportunistic infections. Antiretroviral therapy and prophylaxis and treatment for common opportunistic infections can prolong and improve life but can't stop the syndrome's progression. Most experts believe that virtually everyone infected with HIV will develop AIDS. As a result, prevention of HIV infection remains the most effective strategy for controlling AIDS.

Causes
A human retrovirus, classified as either HIV-1 or HIV-2, causes AIDS. HIV-1 is the more common cause throughout the world. HIV-2 has

Classifying HIV infection and AIDS

In 1993, the Centers for Disease Control and Prevention (CDC) revised its classification system for human immunodeficiency virus (HIV) infection and expanded its definition of acquired immunodeficiency syndrome (AIDS). The new classification groups HIV-infected patients according to CD4+ T-cell count and disease category. The following chart shows the nine possible subgroups.

CD4+ T-cell counts	Disease categories		
	A Asymptomatic, acute (primary) HIV, or PGL	B Symptomatic, but not A or C conditions	C AIDS-indicator conditions
Greater than or equal to 500/μl	A1	B1	C1
200 to 499/μl	A2	B2	C2
Less than 200/μl	A3	B3	C3

CD4+ T-cell categories

These CD4+ T-cell ranges are considered positive markers for HIV infection:
• *Category 1:* 500 or more cells/μl of blood
• *Category 2:* 200 to 499 cells/μl of blood
• *Category 3:* less than 200 cells/μl of blood.

Disease categories

The CDC defines three related disease categories as described below.

Category A

This category includes patients with persistent generalized lymphadenopathy (PGL) or acute (primary) HIV infection but without symptoms or B- or C-category conditions.

Category B

This category consists of HIV-infected patients with symptoms or diseases not included in category C, such as:
• bacillary angiomatosis
• oropharyngeal or persistent vulvovaginal candidiasis
• fever or diarrhea lasting over 1 month
• idiopathic thrombocytopenic purpura
• pelvic inflammatory disease (particularly if complicated by tubo-ovarian abscess)
• peripheral neuropathy.

Category C

This category includes HIV-infected patients with disorders defined by the CDC as AIDS-indicator conditions, such as:
• candidiasis of the bronchi, trachea, or lungs
• candidiasis of the esophagus
• cervical cancer, invasive
• coccidioidomycosis, disseminated or extrapulmonary
• cryptococcosis, extrapulmonary

(continued)

Classifying HIV infection and AIDS (continued)

- cryptosporidiosis, chronic intestinal (persisting over 1 month)
- cytomegalovirus (CMV) disease affecting organs other than the liver, spleen, or lymph nodes
- CMV retinitis with vision loss
- encephalopathy related to HIV
- herpes simplex, involving chronic ulcers (persisting over 1 month) or herpetic bronchitis, pneumonitis, or esophagitis
- histoplasmosis, disseminated or extrapulmonary
- isosporiasis persisting more than 1 month
- Kaposi's sarcoma
- lymphoma, Burkitt's (or its equivalent)

- lymphoma, immunoblastic (or its equivalent)
- lymphoma of the brain, primary
- *Mycobacterium avium* complex or *M. kansasii,* disseminated or extrapulmonary
- *M. tuberculosis* at any site, pulmonary or extrapulmonary
- *Mycobacterium,* any other species, disseminated or extrapulmonary
- *Pneumocystis carinii* pneumonia
- pneumonia, recurrent
- progressive multifocal leukoencephalopathy
- *Salmonella* septicemia, recurrent
- toxoplasmosis of the brain
- wasting syndrome caused by HIV.

been predominantly identified in western Africa and is thought to be less pathogenic than HIV-1. Both viruses destroy CD4+ T cells, the essential regulators and effectors of the normal immune response. (See *Understanding HIV infection and immunodeficiency,* pages 58 and 59.)

Transmission of HIV infection occurs through contact with infected blood or body fluids. Common routes of transmission include contact with semen or vaginal secretions during intercourse, contact with contaminated blood during transfusion or sharing of contaminated needles during I.V. drug abuse, and placental exchange between an infected mother and the fetus. Other as yet unidentified routes may exist as well. HIV has been recovered in tears, urine, saliva, cerebrospinal fluid, and alveolar flu-

id; however, *there is no evidence* to suggest that these fluids transmit the virus.

ASSESSMENT

Your assessment should include a careful consideration of the patient's health history (including a sexual history), physical examination findings, and diagnostic test results.

Health history
The patient's history may indicate exposure to HIV — most often through sharing I.V. needles or engaging in unprotected sexual relations with an infected partner.

Timesaving tip: When investigating high-risk behaviors, ask direct questions in a nonjudgmental way. You'll save time, elicit honest answers, and make the patient more comfortable. For example, instead of asking the patient if he abuses I.V. drugs, ask, "Have you ever injected drugs?" Instead of asking if the patient is homosexual or bisexual, ask, "Are you sexually active with both men and women?"

Patient complaints

Acute infection usually occurs about 3 to 6 weeks following primary infection. The patient may report fever, rigors, arthralgia, myalgia, maculopapular rash, urticaria, abdominal cramps, and diarrhea. Symptoms of aseptic meningitis, such as a severe headache and a stiff neck, may also occur.

Following acute infection, the patient is asymptomatic for a variable period. Some patients, otherwise asymptomatic, develop lymphadenopathy at two or more extrainguinal sites that persist for more than 3 months.

As the syndrome progresses, the patient may report generalized symptoms, such as fatigue, weight loss, night sweats, and fever. He may also report symptoms of HIV encephalopathy, opportunistic infection, or cancer. (See *Opportunistic diseases associated with AIDS,* pages 60 to 65.)

Pediatric findings

A child's signs and symptoms resemble those of an adult, except that children are more likely to have a history of bacterial infections, such as otitis media, pneumonias other than that caused by *Pneumocystis carinii,* sepsis, chronic salivary gland enlargement, and lymphoid interstitial pneumonia.

Complications

Your patient may report signs and symptoms of complications directly

FactFinder

Key points about AIDS

• *Most commonly affected groups:* These include homosexual and bisexual men, I.V. drug users, neonates of HIV-infected mothers, recipients of contaminated blood or blood products (although the risk of receiving contaminated blood has been significantly reduced since 1985), and partners of those in high-risk groups.

• *Disturbing trend:* AIDS is the sixth leading cause of death nationwide for women ages 25 to 44. Incidence is rising more rapidly in women than in any other group. HIV infection strikes women more severely than men. Women also survive a shorter time, perhaps because of delayed diagnosis.

• *Reassuring findings:* Prior to 1986 and the use of zidovudine, the median survival time for AIDS patients was less than 1 year. With current therapies, survival time has more than doubled and will probably continue to increase. In addition, evidence shows that casual contact, vaccines, and insects can't transmit HIV.

• *Progression rate:* HIV infection usually progresses more rapidly in neonates and children and in adults infected after age 40.

• *Key indicator:* The initial sign of AIDS strongly predicts the length of survival. Kaposi's sarcoma is associated with the longest survival; *Pneumocystis carinii* pneumonia, the second longest; central nervous system lymphoma, cryptococcal infection, and *Mycobacterium avium* complex, the shortest.

Understanding HIV infection and immunodeficiency

In order to replicate, human immunodeficiency virus (HIV) invades the human cell and uses the cell machinery to reproduce. The illustration below depicts the process of HIV infection at the cellular level.

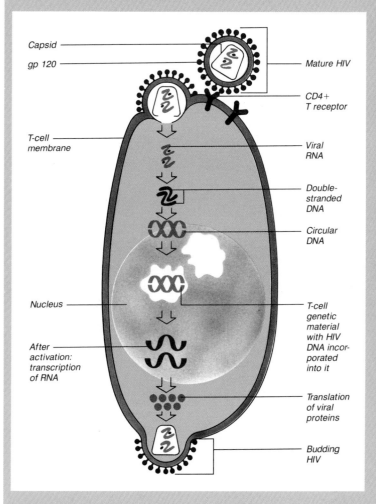

The infection process
HIV consists of ribonucleic acid (RNA) wrapped in a capsid and encased in a lipid envelope. To enter a human cell, the envelope's main glycoprotein, gp 120, attaches to a cell surface receptor, most likely the CD4+ antigen but, possibly, the recently discovered CD34. After binding, the virus fuses with the cell membrane, sheds its coat, and injects its RNA into the cell.

Enzymes known as reverse transcriptase help transcribe viral RNA into double-stranded deoxyribonucleic acid (DNA),which forms a circle and travels to the cell nucleus. Here, the viral DNA is integrated into the cell chromosomal DNA, now known as proviral DNA.

The infected cell may be activated or remain in a latent state in which replication of HIV is restricted — a possible explanation for the infection's long incubation period.

Activation results in transcription of RNA and translation of viral proteins used in packaging and budding of progeny viral particles. This leads to the production of huge numbers of new HIV particles.

The results of infection
The majority of cells infected by HIV are T4 lymphocytes, which affect almost every other human immune response. Their destruction causes widespread immunodeficiency, leaving the patient vulnerable to numerous opportunistic infections.

associated with HIV infection, including:
- AIDS dementia complex (a dementia that occurs in 40% to 60% of all patients)
- a wasting syndrome involving a loss of 10% or more of body weight and including persistent diarrhea, weakness, or fever
- widely varying opportunistic infections and cancers, most commonly *Pneumocystis carinii* pneumonia and Kaposi's sarcoma.

Physical examination
Perform a thorough examination. Inspect the skin for lesions, discoloration, drainage, dryness, alopecia, and edema. Check the oral mucosa for lesions, plaques, exudates, and discoloration.

Assess the patient for altered level of consciousness; for deficits in cognitive function, cranial nerve function, motor and sensory function, cerebellar function, and reflexes; and for signs of meningeal irritation, such as nuchal rigidity, Kernig's sign, and Brudzinski's sign. Ask friends or family members about the patient's mental status (subtle changes may go unnoticed by the patient).

During funduscopic examination, assess the patient's vision noting any cotton-wool patches or similar manifestations, retinal hemorrhages, or papilledema. Also assess for visual field deficits.

Auscultate for breath sounds, noting tachypnea, dyspnea, dullness on percussion, decreased breath sounds, crackles, or wheezes. Auscultate for heart sounds, noting any arrhythmias, pericardial friction rub, or decreased peripheral pulses.

During your abdominal examination, auscultate for hyperactive bowel sounds and palpate for masses, ten-

(Text continues on page 65.)

Opportunistic diseases associated with AIDS

The following chart describes some common infections, their characteristic signs and symptoms, and their treatments.

Infection	Signs and symptoms	Treatment
Bacterial		
Mycobacterium tuberculosis		
An aerobic, acid-fast bacillus spread through inhalation of droplet nuclei that are aerosolized by coughing, sneezing, or talking	Fever, weight loss, night sweats, and fatigue, followed by dyspnea, chills, hemoptysis, and chest pain	Isoniazid, rifampin, pyrazinamide, and ethambutol or streptomycin during the first 2 months of therapy, followed by rifampin and isoniazid for a minimum of 9 months and for at least 6 months after culture is negative for bacteria
***Mycobacterium avium* complex**		
A primary infection acquired by oral ingestion or inhalation; can infect the bone marrow, liver, spleen, GI tract, lymph nodes, lungs, skin, brain, adrenal glands, and kidneys; is chronic and may be both localized and disseminated in its course of infection	Multiple, nonspecific symptoms consistent with systemic illness: fever, fatigue, weight loss, anorexia, night sweats, abdominal pain, and chronic diarrhea. *Physical examination findings:* emaciation, generalized lymphadenopathy, diffuse tenderness, jaundice, and hepatosplenomegaly. *Laboratory findings:* anemia, leukopenia, and thrombocytopenia	Treatment regimens vary and can include two to six drugs. The Centers for Disease Control and Prevention currently recommends that every patient take either azithromycin or clarithromycin. Many experts prefer ethambutol as a second drug. Additional drugs include clofazimine, rifabutin, rifampin, ciprofloxacin, and sometimes amikacin. Isoniazid and pyrazinamide are not useful.
Salmonellosis		
Usually acquired by ingestion of contaminated food or water but also linked to snake powders, pet turtles, and domestic turkeys; also can be spread by contaminated medications or diagnostic agents, direct fecal-oral transmission (especially during sexual activity), transfusion of contaminated blood products, and inadequately sterilized fiber-optic instruments used in upper GI endoscopic procedures	Nonspecific signs and symptoms, including fever, chills, sweats, weight loss, diarrhea, and anorexia	Although treatment of nontyphoid salmonellosis is usually unnecessary in immunocompetent individuals, it is required in persons with human immunodeficiency virus (HIV) disease. Antibiotic selection depends on drug sensitivities. However, treatment may include cotrimoxazole, amoxicillin, fluoroquinolones, ampicillin, or third-generation cephalosporins.

Opportunistic diseases associated with AIDS *(continued)*

Infection	Signs and symptoms	Treatment
Fungal		
Coccidioides		
Mold that grows in soil in arid regions in the southwestern United States, Mexico, Central America, and South America	Influenza-like illness (malaise, fever, backache, headache, cough, arthralgia), periarticular swelling in knees and ankles, meningitis, bony lesions, skin findings, genitourinary (GU) involvement	Fluconazole, itraconazole, amphotericin B
Candidiasis		
Yeasts that exist in unicellular forms on teeth, gingivae, and skin and in the oropharynx, vagina, and large intestine; majority of infections endogenous and related to interruption of normal defense mechanisms; possible human-to-human transmission, including congenital transmission in neonates, in whom thrush develops after vaginal delivery	*Thrush, the most prevalent form in HIV-infected individuals:* creamy, curdlike, yellowish patches, surrounded by an erythematous base, found on buccal membrane and tongue surfaces. *Nail infection:* inflammation and tenderness of tissue surrounding the nails or the nail itself. *Vaginitis:* intense pruritus of the vulva and curdlike vaginal discharge	Nystatin suspension and clotrimazole troches for thrush; nystatin suspension or pastilles, clotrimazole troches, or oral ketoconazole, fluconazole, or itraconazole for esophagitis; topical clotrimazole, miconazole, or ketoconazole for cutaneous candidiasis; topical imidazole or oral fluconazole, ketoconazole, or both for candidiasis of nails; topical clotrimazole or miconazole or oral ketoconazole for vaginitis
Cryptococcosis		
Yeastlike fungus, found in nature, that can be aerosolized and inhaled; settles in the lungs, where it can remain dormant or spread to other parts of the body, particularly the central nervous system (CNS); responsible for three forms of infection: pulmonary, CNS, and disseminated; most pulmonary cases found serendipitously	*Pulmonary cryptococcosis:* fever, cough, dyspnea, and pleuritic chest pain. *CNS cryptococcosis:* fever, malaise, headaches, stiff neck, nausea and vomiting, and altered mentation. *Disseminated cryptococcosis:* lymphadenopathy, multifocal cutaneous lesions. *Other clinical symptoms:* macules, papules, skin lesions, oral lesions, placental infection, myocarditis, prostatic infection, optic neuropathy, rectal abscess, and peripheral and mediastinal lymph node infection	Primary therapy for initial infection: amphotericin B administered I.V. for 6 to 8 weeks; sometimes amphotericin B and flucytosine combination therapy; fluconazole and itraconazole also used

(continued)

Opportunistic diseases associated with AIDS *(continued)*

Infection	Signs and symptoms	Treatment
Fungal *(continued)*		
Histoplasmosis		
Fungus that exists in nature, is readily airborne, and can reach the bronchioles and alveoli when inhaled	*Most common:* fever, weight loss, hepatomegaly, splenomegaly, and pancytopenia. *Less common:* diarrhea, cerebritis, chorioretinitis, meningitis, oral and cutaneous lesions, and GI mucosal lesions causing bleeding	Drug of choice: amphotericin B, used as lifelong suppressive therapy, not a cure. Under investigation: itraconazole
Protozoan		
***Pneumocystis carinii* pneumonia**		
Also has properties of fungal infection, exists in human lungs, and is transmitted by airborne exposure; the most common life-threatening opportunistic infection in individuals with AIDS	Fever, fatigue, and weight loss for several weeks to months before respiratory symptoms develop. *Respiratory symptoms:* dyspnea, usually noted initially on exertion, later at rest; and cough, usually starting out dry and nonproductive and later becoming productive	Co-trimoxazole orally or I.V. (about 20% of AIDS patients are hypersensitive to sulfa drugs), or I.V. pentamidine isethionate (many adverse effects, including permanent diabetes mellitus). *Also used:* dapsone with trimethoprim, clindamycin, primaquine, atovaquone, or corticosteroids. *Prophylaxis following treatment:* co-trimoxazole, aerosolized pentamidine isethionate or dapsone
Cryptosporidiosis		
An intestinal infection by the protozoan *Cryptosporidium;* transmitted by person-to-person contact, water, food contaminants, and airborne exposure; most common site: small intestine	Profuse watery diarrhea, abdominal cramping, flatulence, weight loss, anorexia, malaise, fever, nausea, vomiting, and myalgia	No effective therapy. Most medical therapy is palliative and directed toward symptom control, focusing on fluid replacement, occasionally total parenteral nutrition, correction of electrolyte imbalances, and analgesic, antidiarrheal, and antiperistaltic agents. Paromomycin, spiramycin, and eflornithine are used.

Opportunistic diseases associated with AIDS *(continued)*

Infection	Signs and symptoms	Treatment
Protozoan *(continued)*		
Toxoplasmosis		
Caused in humans by *Toxoplasma gondii*, an obligate protozoan; major means of transmission through ingestion of undercooked meats and vegetables containing oocysts; causes focal or diffuse meningoencephalitis with cellular necrosis and progresses unchecked to the lungs, heart, and skeletal muscle	Localized neurologic deficits, fever, headache, altered mental status, and seizures	Sulfadiazine or clindamycin with pyrimethamine (however, about 20% of AIDS patients are hypersensitive to sulfa drugs); folinic acid to prevent marrow toxicity from pyrimethamine
Isosporiasis		
Caused by coccidian protozoan parasite *Isospora belli;* after ingestion, infects the small intestine and results in malabsorption and diarrhea	Watery, nonbloody diarrhea; crampy abdominal pain; nausea; anorexia; weight loss; weakness; occasional vomiting; and a low-grade fever	Co-trimoxazole for 10 days
Viral		
Herpes simplex virus (HSV)		
Chronic infection caused by a herpes virus; often a reactivation of an earlier herpes infection	Red, blisterlike lesions occurring in oral, anal, and genital areas; may also be found on the esophageal and tracheobronchial mucosa in AIDS patients; pain, bleeding, and discharge	Acyclovir is the primary therapy for HSV and is available in I.V., oral, and topical preparations. Vidarabine or foscarnet is used in acyclovir-resistant HSV.
Cytomegalovirus (CMV)		
Herpes virus that may result in serious, widespread infection in AIDS patients; most common sites: lungs, adrenal glands, eyes, CNS, GI tract, male GU tract, and blood	Unexplained fever, malaise, GI ulcers, diarrhea, weight loss, swollen lymph nodes, hepatomegaly, splenomegaly, blurred vision, floaters, dyspnea (especially on exertion), and dry, nonproductive cough; vision changes leading to blindness not uncommon in patients with ocular infection	Foscarnet is the drug of choice for CMV retinitis, because it lacks the hematologic toxicity of the old standard, gancyclovir, and has shown some anti-HIV properties.

(continued)

Opportunistic diseases associated with AIDS *(continued)*

Infection	Signs and symptoms	Treatment
Viral *(continued)*		
Progressive multifocal leukoencephalopathy (PML)		
Progressive demyelinating disorder caused by hyperactivation of a papovavirus that leads to gradual brain degeneration	Progressive dementia, memory loss, headache, confusion, and weakness. Possible other neurologic complications, such as seizures	No form of therapy for PML has been effective, but attempted therapies include prednisone, acyclovir, and adenine arabinoside administered both I.V. and intrathecally.
Varicella zoster		
Also known as herpes zoster and shingles; acute infection caused by reactivation of the chicken pox virus	Small clusters of painful, reddened papules that follow the route of inflamed nerves; may be disseminated, involving two or more dermatomes	Varicella zoster is most often treated with oral acyclovir capsules until healed. Treatment may have to continue at lower doses indefinitely to prevent recurrence. I.V. acyclovir has been effective in treating disseminated varicella zoster lesions in some patients. Medications may be used to relieve pain associated with the infection and postherpetic neuropathies.
Neoplasms		
Kaposi's sarcoma		
A generalized disease with characteristic lesions involving all skin surfaces, including the face (tip of the nose, eyelids), head, upper and lower limbs, soles of the feet, palms of the hands, conjunctivae, sclerae, pharynx, larynx, trachea, hard palate, stomach, liver, small and large intestines, and glans penis	Manifested cutaneously and subcutaneously; usually painless, nonpruritic tumor nodules that are pigmented and violaceous (red to blue), nonblanching and palpable; patchy lesions appearing early and possibly mistaken for bruises, purpura, or diffuse cutaneous hemorrhages	Treatment isn't indicated for all individuals. Indications include cosmetically offensive, painful, or obstructive lesions or rapidly progressing disease. Systemic chemotherapy using single or multiple drugs may be given to alleviate symptoms. Radiation therapy may be used to treat lesions. Intralesional therapy with vinblastine may be given for cosmetic purposes to treat small cutaneous lesions, and laser therapy and cryotherapy to treat small isolated lesions. Interferon alfa-2a and interferon alfa-2b are also used.

Opportunistic diseases associated with AIDS *(continued)*

Infection	Signs and symptoms	Treatment
Neoplasms *(continued)*		
Malignant lymphomas		
Immune system cancer in which lymph tissue cells begin growing abnormally and spread to other organs; incidence in persons with AIDS: about 4% to 10%; diagnosed in HIV-infected individuals as widespread disease involving extranodal sites, most commonly in the GI tract, CNS, bone marrow, and liver	Unexplained fever, night sweats, or weight loss greater than 10% of patient's total body weight; signs and symptoms often confined to one body system: CNS (confusion, lethargy, and memory loss) or GI tract (pain, obstruction, changes in bowel habits, bleeding, and fever)	Individualized therapy; modified combination of methotrexate, bleomycin, doxorubicin, cyclophosphamide, vincristine, and dexamethasone; radiation therapy, not chemotherapy, to treat primary CNS lymphoma
Cervical neoplasm		
Emerging as a significant opportunistic complication of HIV infection as more women become infected with HIV and live longer with illness because of antiretroviral prophylaxis and treatment	*Possible indicators of early invasive disease:* abnormal vaginal bleeding, persistent vaginal discharge, or postcoital pain and bleeding. *Possible indicators of advanced disease:* pelvic pain, vaginal leakage of urine and feces from a fistula, anorexia, weight loss, and fatigue	Treatment tailored to disease stage. Preinvasive lesions: possible total excisional biopsy, cryosurgery, laser destruction, conization (and frequent Papanicolaou test follow-up); rarely, hysterectomy. Invasive squamous cell carcinoma: possible radical hysterectomy and radiation therapy

derness, hepatomegaly, and splenomegaly. Examine the patient's genitalia and perianal area for lesions and discharge. In addition, check for lymphadenopathy and note any pain when assessing range of motion.

Diagnostic test results
The following tests are used for patients age 13 or older:
• enzyme-linked immunoabsorbent assay (ELISA) for the HIV-1 antibody, with supplemental identification of the HIV-1 antibody by Western blot and immunofluorescence assay
• virus isolation
• antigen detection
• detection of HIV genetic material (DNA or RNA) by polymerase chain reaction (rarely performed).

A CD4+ T-cell count measures the extent of immunosuppression in an HIV-positive patient. An absolute

CD4+ T-cell count under 200 cells/µl indicates severe immunosuppression. If the absolute count is unavailable, you may substitute the percentage of CD4+ cells in total T cells: Less than 15% indicates severe immunosuppression.

Other markers of immune status may be useful in evaluating individual patients, including:
• serum neopterin
• beta-2 microglobulin
• HIV p24 antigen
• soluble interleukin-2 receptors
• immunoglobulin A
• delayed hypersensitivity skin tests.

However, these tests are not strong predictors of disease progression or as specific for HIV-related immunosuppression as CD4+ T-cell counts. Delayed hypersensitivity skin tests are often used with the Mantoux test to evaluate HIV-infected patients for tuberculosis and anergy.

Because many opportunistic infections are reactivations of previous infections, the patient may be tested for syphilis, hepatitis B, tuberculosis, toxoplasmosis, and histoplasmosis (in some geographic areas).

NURSING DIAGNOSIS

Common nursing diagnoses for an AIDS patient include:
• Anticipatory grieving related to the incurable, progressive nature of the syndrome
• High risk for infection related to immunodeficiency
• Social isolation related to progression of HIV infection, fear of AIDS transmission, and social stigma
• Fatigue related to the syndrome's effects, such as opportunistic infection, cancer, anemia, and malnutrition

• Diarrhea related to GI infection, adverse drug reaction, or intolerance to concentrated dietary supplements
• Impaired skin integrity related to opportunistic infection, cancer, or malnutrition
• Altered thought processes related to HIV infection or opportunistic disease
• High risk for caregiver role strain related to chronic debilitating disease and lack of respite.

PLANNING

Based on the nursing diagnosis *anticipatory grieving,* develop appropriate patient outcomes. For example, your patient will:
• identify, express, and accept his feelings about progressive disability and death
• use appropriate coping mechanisms and support groups to deal with his prognosis.

Based on the nursing diagnosis *high risk for infection,* develop appropriate patient outcomes. For example, your patient will:
• identify signs of opportunistic infection and notify the doctor if they occur
• adhere to prescribed prophylactic regimen
• keep medical appointments.

Based on the nursing diagnosis *social isolation,* develop appropriate patient outcomes. For example, your patient will:
• participate in social activity, as his health permits
• express his feelings of isolation and identify specific ways to lessen this feeling
• contact available resources to establish supportive relationships.

Based on the nursing diagnosis *fatigue,* develop appropriate patient outcomes. For example, your patient will:

• perform daily activities independently or with assistance, as tolerated
• set priorities for daily tasks
• delegate nonessential responsibilities
• incorporate energy conservation techniques into daily routine.

Based on the nursing diagnosis *diarrhea,* develop appropriate patient outcomes. For example, your patient will:

• report fewer episodes of diarrhea
• avoid complications of excessive diarrhea, such as fluid and electrolyte imbalance and skin breakdown
• identify and avoid foods that aggravate diarrhea.

Based on the nursing diagnosis *impaired skin integrity,* develop appropriate patient outcomes. For example, your patient will:

• implement strategies to prevent skin breakdown
• exhibit no evidence of skin breakdown.

Based on the nursing diagnosis *altered thought processes,* develop appropriate patient outcomes. For example, your patient will:

• identify and report signs of central nervous system infection
• participate in daily activities, as tolerated
• initiate and execute advance directives and durable power of attorney.

Based on the nursing diagnosis *high risk for caregiver role strain,* develop appropriate outcomes. For example, the caregiver will:

• identify stressful situations and express feelings about stress
• arrange respite periods at designated times
• seek assistance from community resources during high-stress periods.

IMPLEMENTATION

Focus your care on attending to the patient's physical and psychological needs, helping to minimize disabilities, and improving his quality of life. Because the course of the syndrome can vary greatly, expect to tailor your nursing care to meet the patient's individual needs. (See *Medical care of the patient with AIDS,* page 68.)

Nursing interventions

• Follow universal precautions when caring for the patient.
• Monitor the patient for fever, noting any pattern.
• Look for signs of infection, for example, skin breakdown, frequent or burning urination, headache, nuchal rigidity, photophobia, cough, sore throat, and diarrhea.
• Palpate for swollen, tender lymph nodes.
• Review laboratory test results regularly.
• Assess the patient's mental and neurologic status.
• If the patient develops Kaposi's sarcoma, monitor the progression of lesions.
• Treat infections as prescribed.
• Provide the patient with a diluted solution of sodium chloride, bicarbonate, or other prescribed mouthwash for daily oral rinsing. Avoid using glycerin swabs, which dry the mucous membranes.
• Record the patient's caloric intake and weight. Encourage a high-protein, high-calorie diet. Offer frequent, small meals.
• Ensure adequate intake of fluids during episodes of diarrhea.
• Provide meticulous skin care, especially for the debilitated patient.

Timesaving tip: Save time by combining nursing care activities. For example, while provid-

Treatments

Medical care of the patient with AIDS

Acquired immunodeficiency syndrome (AIDS) has no cure. However, several antiretroviral treatments can slow the progression of human immunodeficiency virus (HIV) infection or temporarily inactivate the virus.

Antiretroviral therapy

Zidovudine, the most commonly used antiretroviral drug, effectively slows the progress of HIV infection, decreasing the number of opportunistic infections and curbing the progress of associated dementia. However, the drug often produces severe adverse effects. Zidovudine is recommended for asymptomatic or symptomatic patients with CD4+ T-cells counts of 500 cells/µl or less.

Didanosine (formerly ddl), another antiretroviral drug, treats advanced HIV infection in adult patients and in pediatric patients over age 6 months. Initially, the drug was limited to patients who couldn't tolerate zidovudine or whose condition had deteriorated during zidovudine therapy. Currently, it can also be used in adult patients with advanced HIV infection who have already received prolonged treatment with zidovudine.

Zalcitabine (formerly ddC) is currently approved for use in combination with zidovudine to treat patients with CD4+ T-cell counts of 300/µl or less.

Combating opportunistic infections

Anti-infective and antineoplastic drugs combat opportunistic infections and associated cancers. Some anti-infectives are also used to prevent opportunistic infections. New protocols combine two or more of these drugs to produce the maximum benefit with the fewest adverse effects.

Although many opportunistic infections respond to anti-infective drugs, they tend to recur after treatment. Because of this, the patient usually requires continued suppressive therapy until the drug loses its effectiveness or can no longer be tolerated.

Supportive treatment

Supportive treatment helps maintain adequate nutrition and relieve pain and other distressing symptoms.

ing skin care, you can teach the patient skin care techniques, explain how to combat diarrhea, and note any changes in his signs and symptoms.

• Encourage the patient to participate in as much physical activity as he can tolerate. Make sure that his schedule includes time for both exercise and rest.

• If neurologic disease is evident, provide a safe environment, reorient the patient frequently, assist with daily activities, and initiate seizure precautions.

• Recognize that a diagnosis of AIDS has a devastating impact on the patient, his socioeconomic status, and his family relationships. Help him cope with an altered body image, the emotional burden of serious illness, and the threat of death. (See *Providing psychosocial support for AIDS patients.*)

Patient teaching

• Evaluate your patient's level of knowledge. He may already be familiar with some aspects of care.

• Teach the patient and his family members, sexual partners, and friends about the syndrome and its transmission. Explain that the patient should not share his toothbrush, razor, or other items possibly contaminated with blood.

• Urge the patient to inform potential sexual partners and health care workers that he is infected with HIV.

• If the patient injects drugs, caution him not to share needles.

• Teach the patient about high-risk sexual practices — those that exchange body fluids — for example, vaginal or anal intercourse without a condom. Discuss safe sexual practices, such as hugging, touching, or mutual masturbation. If the patient chooses to engage in sexual intercourse, teach him the proper use of a latex condom. Also, discuss new products, such as the lubricant nonoxynal 9 and the female condom.

• If the patient is female, explain the need to avoid pregnancy. Explain that an infant may become infected before birth, during delivery, or during breast-feeding.

• Teach the patient the signs of infection and cancer, and stress the importance of seeking immediate medical attention if any of the signs appear.

• Explain all prescribed medications, including any possible adverse effects and drug interactions.

• Explain all self-care or assisted-care measures, such as nutritional guidelines and skin and mouth care.

Providing psychosocial support for AIDS patients

The patient with acquired immunodeficiency syndrome (AIDS) and his sexual partner, family, and friends all experience major psychosocial stresses associated with the diagnosis. To enhance psychosocial support, consider the following measures:

• Accept, value, and do not judge the patient.

• Become knowledgeable about transmission of AIDS and infection-control measures so that you don't fear the patient.

• Support the patient's need for hope, independence, and control.

• Become educated about the major psychosocial issues associated with a diagnosis of AIDS so that you can effectively intervene or refer the patient.

• Provide accurate, current information about AIDS prevention, treatment, and related care.

• Encourage the patient and significant others to verbalize feelings.

• Become familiar with community mental health, social, political, spiritual, and financial resources and sources of support. Refer the patient and significant others.

Support at the end stage of illness

Follow the patient's advanced directives concerning life-sustaining measures, and reassure the patient that his wishes will be honored. Help him and his significant others cope with grief.

Discharge TimeSaver

Ensuring continued care for the patient with AIDS

Review the following teaching topics, referrals, and follow-up appointments to make sure that your patient is adequately prepared for discharge.

Teaching topics
Make sure that the following topics have been covered and that your patient's learning has been evaluated:
☐ how human immunodeficiency virus is transmitted
☐ preventive measures, including safe sexual and contraceptive practices; safe I.V. needle use, if applicable; and avoidance of complications, such as diarrhea and impaired skin integrity
☐ medications
☐ dietary guidelines
☐ balanced rest and activity
☐ symptom management
☐ signs and symptoms of infection
☐ need to report symptoms promptly
☐ infection-control measures in the home
☐ sources of support.

Referrals (for patient and care provider)
Make sure that the patient and principal care provider have been provided with necessary referrals to:
☐ support groups
☐ respite services
☐ community resources
☐ psychological counseling
☐ dietitian
☐ social services
☐ home health care services
☐ hospice services
☐ acquired immunodeficiency syndrome (AIDS) organizations
☐ physical therapist
☐ occupational therapist
☐ day care program.

Follow-up appointments
Make sure that the necessary follow-up appointments have been scheduled and that the patient has been notified:
☐ doctor
☐ further diagnostic tests.

• Explain the proper use of assistive devices, when appropriate, to ease ambulation and promote independence.
• Help the patient plan alternating daily periods of activity and rest to help him cope with fatigue. Teach energy conservation techniques. Encourage the patient to set priorities, accept the help of others, and delegate nonessential tasks.

• Teach the patient how to cope with diarrhea, including skin care of the perianal area. Explain that a low residue diet that is high in protein and calories will help. Advise drinking up to 3 liters of noncarbonated, caffeine-free fluids a day, for example, Gatorade or diluted fruit juices. Encourage the proper use of antidiarrheal agents.

• If the patient's prognosis is poor (less than 6 months to live), suggest immediate hospice care.

• Explain the benefits of initiating and executing advance directives and a durable power of attorney.

• Teach family members and companions about infection-control precautions they should adopt at home. Discuss coping strategies, including their need for respite. (See *Ensuring continued care for the patient with AIDS*.)

EVALUATION

When evaluating the patient's response to your nursing care, gather reassessment data and compare this information with the patient outcomes specified in your plan of care.

Teaching and counseling
Begin by determining the effectiveness of your teaching. Consider the following questions:

• Has the patient expressed feelings of loss? Has he accepted these feelings and the need for changes in his behavior?

• Has he identified effective coping mechanisms that help him deal with his sense of loss?

• Does he socialize as much as his health permits?

• Is he willing to seek medical intervention if he notes signs of infection or cancer?

• Does he acknowledge the importance of prophylactic drugs? Does he follow the prescribed regimen?

• Has he contacted resource groups to establish supportive relationships?

• Does he perform daily activities independently or does he require assistance?

• Has he set priorities for daily tasks and delegated nonessential tasks to friends and family members?

• Does he demonstrate energy-conserving techniques in his daily activities?

You'll also need to evaluate your effectiveness in conveying directions, advice, and support for the caregiver. Consider the following questions:

• Have the patient's family and friends expressed their feelings of stress? Are they using effective stress reduction techniques?

• Have they planned regular respite periods at designated times?

• Have they sought assistance from community-based support groups?

Physical condition
A physical examination and diagnostic tests will provide additional information. Note whether the following outcomes have been achieved:

• absence of complications associated with excessive diarrhea

• no evidence of impaired skin integrity

• absence of complications associated with confusion and disorientation.

Immunodeficiency caused by cancer and its treatment

Cancer and its treatments — surgery, chemotherapy, radiation therapy, and bone marrow transplantation — can lead to a dangerous secondary immunodeficiency. In many cases, the patient's neutrophil count is lowered, resulting in neutropenia and a heightened risk for infection. (See *Reviewing hematopoiesis,* page 72, and *Understanding neutropenia,* page 73.)

Causes
A combination of factors usually causes immunosuppression in cancer patients.

(Text continues on page 74.)

Reviewing hematopoiesis

All blood cells initially begin as stem cells in the bone marrow. By various pathways, the stem cells eventually differentiate into one of the three major types of mature blood cells: leukocytes (white blood cells), thrombocytes (platelets), or erythrocytes (red blood cells). The leukocyte line is responsible for carrying out inflammatory and immune responses; its significant subgroups are illustrated and described below:

• Neutrophils are considered the body's first line of defense. Through phagocytosis, they neutralize foreign invaders, especially bacteria.

• Eosinophils defend mainly against parasites and release vasoactive amines during allergic reactions. They also perform some phagocytic activity.

• Basophils release histamine and heparin into areas of tissue damage, functioning mainly in acute inflammatory reactions.

• Monocytes are responsible for destroying bacteria and removing dead or damaged cells and debris from circulation. They mature into macrophages.

• Lymphocytes commit to either the B-cell or T-cell lines. B lymphocytes secrete antibodies and are involved in antibody-mediated (humoral) immunity. T lymphocytes fill a variety of roles in cell-mediated immunity.

All of these cells work together to provide protection against effects of tissue injury or foreign invasion.

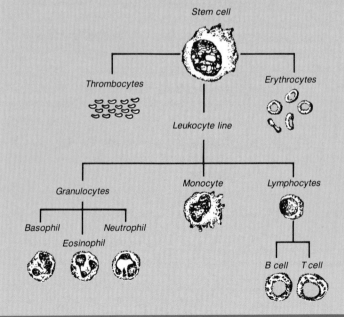

Understanding neutropenia

Neutrophils function as a first line of defense in the inflammatory process. They offer nonspecific protection by carrying out immediate phagocytosis of invading microorganisms. To accomplish their task, neutrophils must be produced in appropriate numbers; they must be mature and segmented; and they must arrive at the site of inflammation.

Gauging infection risk
Neutropenia, a deficiency in the number of mature neutrophils, is the most common immune system deficiency. Knowing the absolute neutrophil count (ANC) — the percentage and actual number of circulating mature neutrophils — enables you to gauge the patient's vulnerability to infection. Infections are most likely to develop if the ANC falls below 1,000/µl. Common infections that occur secondary to neutropenia include aerobic gram-negative bacilli and *Staphylococcus aureus,* and certain fungal infections, such as candidiasis and aspergillosis.

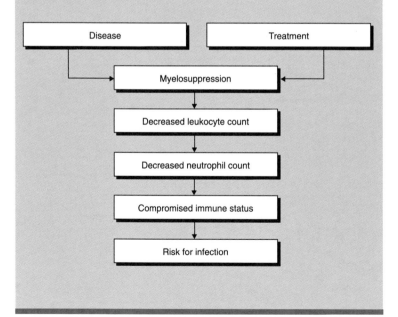

Cancer's effects

Patients with acute lymphoblastic leukemia, acute or chronic myelogenous leukemia, or multiple myeloma may experience abnormalities in granulocytes. Tumors that invade the bone marrow, such as metastatic breast, prostate, and lung cancers, as well as leukemia and lymphoma, can alter and decrease the development of leukocytes. Tumors that invade lymph organs, such as the spleen or lymph nodes, may interrupt the flow of lymphatic fluid or cause tissue and organ breakdown by direct growth and extension.

Iatrogenic effects

Treatment of cancer may involve surgery, chemotherapy, radiation therapy, and bone marrow transplantation.

Surgery

Invasive procedures may provoke stress and the release of glucocorticoids, specifically cortisol. Cortisol can inhibit many immune-system functions, compromising the patient. In addition, surgical removal of lymph tissue can impair the transport of lymph, leading to lymphadenopathy and predisposing the patient to infection. The removal of any immune-system organ, such as the spleen, can alter immunocompetence.

Chemotherapy

Chemotherapeutic drugs cause myelosuppression by inhibiting proliferation of cells in the bone marrow. Myelosuppression places the patient at risk for leukopenia, thrombocytopenia, and anemia. Immunosuppression primarily involves leukocytes that replicate rapidly, such as granulocytes — more specifically, neutrophils.

Most chemotherapeutic drugs produce some degree of myelosuppression and neutropenia. The extent of immunosuppression is determined by the specific drug, dose, and frequency of administration. (See *Quick review of chemotherapeutic drugs.*)

The period of lowest blood count, called the nadir, occurs at a specific time after administration of chemotherapy. During the nadir period, the risk for complications, especially infection, is greatest. Depending on the drug used, the nadir may occur anytime from days to weeks after administration. Usually, it's within 14 days of treatment.

Radiation therapy

The dose and site of radiation therapy affect the extent of myelosuppression. If the radiation fields include sites of bone marrow production, the white blood cell (WBC) count may decline sharply. Neutrophils are most affected, leaving the patient vulnerable to infection. Neutropenia usually resolves within 6 months of completing therapy.

Bone marrow transplantation

In this procedure, the patient is given ablative doses of chemotherapy or chemotherapy plus radiation therapy followed by infusion of bone marrow. During the period following the ablative regimen, the patient produces no erythrocytes, platelets, or leukocytes and is extremely anemic, thrombocytopenic, and immunosuppressed. The inflammatory response and the humoral and cell-mediated immune responses are all deficient, leaving him susceptible to infections.

ASSESSMENT

Your assessment should include a careful consideration of the patient's

Quick review of chemotherapeutic drugs

Use this list of chemotherapeutic drugs as a quick reference. Note drugs that are severely myelosuppressive.

Alkylating agents
- Busulfan (Myleran)*†
- Carboplatin (Paraplatin)
- Chlorambucil (Leukeran)†
- Cisplatin (Platinol)
- Cyclophosphamide (Cytoxan)*
- Dacarbazine (DTIC-Dome)
- Ifosfamide (Ifex)
- Mechlorethamine (Mustargen)*
- Melphalan (Alkeran)
- Thiotepa (Thiotepa)

Antimetabolites
- Cytarabine, ara-C (Cytosar-U)
- Floxuridine (FUDR)
- Fluorouracil, 5-FU (Adrucil)
- Hydroxyurea (Hydrea)
- Mercaptopurine (Purinethol)
- Methotrexate sodium (Folex)
- Thioguanine (Lanvis)

Antitumor antibiotics
- Bleomycin (Blenoxane)
- Dactinomycin (Cosmegen)*
- Daunorubicin (Cerubidine)
- Doxorubicin (Adriamycin)*
- Idarubicin (Idamycin)
- Mitomycin (Mutamycin)†
- Mitoxantrone (Novantrone)
- Pentostatin (Nipent)
- Plicamycin (Mithracin)

Hormonal agents
- Corticosteroids

Nitrosoureas
- Carmustine (BiCNU)†
- Lomustine (CeeNU)†
- Streptozocin (Zanosar)

Plant alkaloids
- Etoposide (VePesid)*
- Vinblastine (Velban)
- Vincristine (Oncovin)

* indicates severely myelosuppressive
† indicates prolonged nadir

health history, physical examination findings, and diagnostic test results.

Health history
If the patient has received chemotherapy, determine which drugs were used and ask about administration dates and dosages. If he has received radiation therapy, ask about dates and sites. If he has received other cancer therapy, ask him about the clinical course.

Be alert for complaints that may indicate infection, such as fever, chills, fatigue, headache, and difficulty swallowing. Ask about abdominal pain, pain on defecation, and pain at any vascular access sites. The patient may also report shortness of breath, productive or nonproductive cough, frequent or burning urination, or vaginal discharge.

Quickly calculating ANC

Depending on the health care setting, the white blood cell (WBC) differential may not identify the absolute neutrophil count (ANC). To quickly assess your patient's risk for infection, you can calculate an ANC using the following formula. Note that segmented neutrophils (segs) and bands must be expressed as percentages.

ANC = total WBC × (segs + bands)

An example

If the patient has a total WBC count of 400/μl, the segmented (fully mature) neutrophils are 20%, and the bands (less mature neutrophils) are 16%, calculate as follows:

400 × (20% + 16%) =
400 × 36% =
400 × .36 = 144/μl ANC

This finding indicates the patient is extremely neutropenic and at severe risk for infection.

Physical examination

Be alert for signs of infection. However, keep in mind that an immunocompromised patient may not exhibit the usual signs and symptoms of infection. He may, for example, only report pain at the infection site.

In a neutropenic patient, the most reliable physical finding may be fever. If present, fever indicates an emergency. Progression of the infection to sepsis can be rapid and life-threatening. The neutropenic patient may exhibit other signs of infection, depending on the site. Sites of infec-tion may include the following:

• mouth, as evidenced by ulcers or white patches
• lungs, as evidenced by crackles or tachypnea
• urinary tract and perineal or perirectal areas, as evidenced by breakdown, tenderness, redness, or discharge
• skin, as evidenced by breakdown, lesions, or rashes, especially in the skin folds
• wounds or vascular access sites, as evidenced by redness, swelling, or discharge.

Diagnostic test results

The complete blood count with differential provides essential information concerning the extent of immunosuppression.

The absolute neutrophil count (ANC) is more important than the total leukocyte count in assessing the patient's risk for infection. (See *Quickly calculating ANC.*) Note the significance of different ANC levels:

• 3,000 to 6,000/μl: normal
• 1,500 to 3,000/μl: no serious risk for infection
• 1,200 to 1,500/μl: minimal risk for infection
• 500 to 1,200/μl: moderate risk for infection
• less than 500/μl: severe risk for infection.

Also, with myelosuppression, you'll see:

• a platelet count below 50,000/mm^3 (normal is 130,000 to 370,000), indicating a risk for bleeding. Spontaneous bleeding may occur when platelet counts are less than 20,000/mm^3.
• hemoglobin level under 8 g/dl and signs of anemia.

If fever occurs, blood and urine cultures, possibly chest X-ray, and other diagnostic tests may help identify the infection.

Treatments
Medical care of the patient with cancer-related immunosuppression

Treatment seeks to address neutropenia and, if necessary, to eliminate infection. Administration of granulocyte colony-stimulating factor (G-CSF) is the primary method of preventing and managing neutropenia.

Antimicrobial therapy
If fever or other signs of infection occur, broad-spectrum antibiotic therapy should be initiated as soon as possible to help prevent life-threatening sepsis. If methicillin-resistant *Staphylococcus aureus* is suspected as a causative agent, vancomycin may be added to the regimen. Some clinicians immediately prescribe vancomycin, especially for patients with venous access devices.

If fever persists for 7 days, amphotericin B may be administered to treat a possible fungal infection.

NURSING DIAGNOSIS

Common nursing diagnoses for a patient with secondary immunodeficiency caused by cancer and its treatment include:
• Altered protection (leukopenia, thrombocytopenia, or anemia) related to cancer and its treatment
• Fear related to threat of death from cancer and possible severe effects of treatment.

PLANNING

Based on the nursing diagnosis *altered protection,* develop appropriate patient outcomes. For example, the patient will:
• identify signs and symptoms of infection, anemia, and bleeding
• implement measures to reduce risk of infection
• learn ways to reduce risk of bleeding
• learn to control fatigue associated with anemia

• express the importance of reporting fever or other signs of complications to his doctor
• state his intention to have blood studies performed at prescribed periods
• show no signs of infection, especially fever.

Based on the nursing diagnosis *fear,* develop appropriate patient outcomes. For example, the patient will:
• show less fear by discussing his feelings
• use effective coping mechanisms.

IMPLEMENTATION

Focus your nursing care on careful monitoring of vital signs and WBC count to detect and prevent infection. (See *Medical care of the patient with cancer-related immunosuppression.*)

Nursing interventions
⬛ **Timesaving tip:** Having a neutropenia regimen printed and available for all staff members cuts down on time lost investigating

appropriate care measures. It also helps ensure safe, consistent care.
• Arrange a private room for the patient, if possible. Prevent contact with any person who is ill, including all visitors and nonessential hospital staff.
• Monitor WBC count with differential daily.
• Monitor vital signs every 4 hours. Notify the doctor of changes in vital signs, especially a temperature greater than 101° F (38.3° C). Keep in mind that chills may indicate an upcoming temperature spike in the neutropenic patient.
• Observe good hand-washing precautions.
• Assess the oral cavity using a penlight and tongue blade, paying close attention to any lesions or white patches.
• Encourage the patient to perform frequent mouth care with a soft toothbrush or Toothette and to rinse with sodium chloride or sodium bicarbonate solution.
• Inspect the skin of all body sites, including the axillae, groin, perineum, buttocks, beneath breasts, rectal area, I.V. sites, and vascular access device sites, noting any erythema, pain, swelling, or discharge.
• Encourage the patient to prevent skin breakdown by showering daily.
• Avoid invasive procedures, such as subcutaneous and intramuscular injections and insertion of peripheral venous or other invasive lines. Also avoid urinary catheters, enemas, suppositories, rectal thermometers, rectal examinations, and douching.
• If the patient had a vascular access device before myelosuppression, provide regular care using aseptic technique, according to hospital policy.
• Assess for changes in the patient's respiratory rate and breath sounds,

and for a productive or nonproductive cough.
• Encourage mobility, coughing, and deep breathing.
• Assess for changes in urine volume, color, and odor as well as the presence of hematuria or glycosuria.
• Assess for signs of rectal abscess.
• Administer stool softeners to prevent trauma to the rectal mucosa, which can serve as an entry point for bacteria.
• Assess for vaginal discharge.
• Assess for changes in LOC.
• Avoid letting water stagnate in denture cups, vases, soap dishes, plant pots, and respiratory equipment. Stagnant water serves as a medium for bacteria.
• Encourage a well-balanced diet, including high-calorie and high-protein foods. Make sure that all the patient's food, including fruits and vegetables, is thoroughly cooked.
• Encourage the patient to drink 3,000 ml of fluid over 24 hours if not contraindicated.
• Encourage frequent rest periods to help conserve energy.
• If ordered, administer colony-stimulating factors.
• Avoid using antipyretics, which can mask the signs of infection. If fever or other signs of infection occur, notify the doctor at once. Immediately obtain blood, urine, sputum, or wound cultures as ordered. Expect to administer antimicrobial therapy *promptly* (a potentially lifesaving intervention). Obtain other diagnostic studies as ordered, such as a chest X-ray. Keep in mind that slight infiltrates may be the only indication of severe pneumonia. Continue to monitor the patient and his complete blood count closely.

Patient teaching

Timesaving tip: Provide the patient with handouts that describe adverse effects of chemotherapy and methods of avoiding or minimizing them. This will provide necessary background information and, thereby, shorten teaching time. The handouts also serve as a good reference after discharge.

Include the following in your teaching program:

• Explain to the patient the reason he's at increased risk for infection and possibly bleeding and anemia.

• Explain that fever may be a life-threatening event, and instruct him to call the doctor *immediately* if fever occurs.

• Explain the need to avoid contact with ill people.

• Teach good personal hygiene (hand washing and daily bathing). Instruct a female patient to perform perineal care, cleaning from front to back.

• Encourage good oral hygiene using a soft toothbrush and sodium chloride or sodium bicarbonate rinses every 4 hours.

• Teach the patient how to assess his skin for signs of infection or bleeding, and encourage him to report changes to the doctor.

• Also instruct the patient to report changes in respiratory function, such as shortness of breath and a productive or nonproductive cough, and in urinary or bowel function.

• Assist the patient in planning uninterrupted rest periods.

• Explain the proper care of a vascular access device, including reporting signs of infection, such as pain or redness at the access site.

• If the patient is at risk for thrombocytopenia, instruct him to avoid tight-fitting clothes, strenuous exercise, and sharp objects. Suggest that he wear gloves when doing yard work or similar chores, and that he use an electric razor rather than a razor blade. Instruct the patient not to take aspirin or over-the-counter products containing aspirin because they may promote bleeding. Remind him that "salicylate" in a list of ingredients on a medication label may mean aspirin.

• If appropriate, tell the patient to report signs and symptoms of anemia, such as severe fatigue and shortness of breath. In some cases, a transfusion of packed red blood cells may be necessary.

• Help the patient plan meals that are high in calories and protein.

• Consult with the doctor concerning appropriate forms of sexual expression for your patient. If the patient seems to avoid discussing sexuality, you can explain that many patients ask whether sexual activity is permitted during periods of immunosuppression. Then ask if he has similar questions or concerns. (See *Ensuring continued care for the patient with cancer-related immunosuppression,* page 80.)

EVALUATION

When evaluating the patient's response to your nursing care, gather reassessment data and compare this information with the patient outcomes specified in your plan of care.

Teaching and counseling

Begin by determining the effectiveness of your teaching and counseling. Consider the following questions:

• Can the patient identify signs and symptoms of infection, anemia, and bleeding?

• Has he implemented measures to reduce the risk of infection and bleeding?

Discharge TimeSaver
Ensuring continued care for the patient with cancer-related immunosuppression

Review the following teaching topics, referrals, and follow-up appointments to make sure that your patient is adequately prepared for discharge.

Teaching topics
Make sure that the following topics have been covered and that your patient's learning has been evaluated:
☐ meaning of immunosuppression
☐ signs and symptoms of infection
☐ reasons to call doctor
☐ strategies for preventing infection
☐ strategies for preventing bleeding, if appropriate
☐ dietary guidelines
☐ activity guidelines.

Referrals
Make sure that the patient has been provided with necessary referrals to:
☐ social services
☐ home health care.

Follow-up appointments
Make sure that the necessary follow-up appointments have been scheduled and that the patient has been notified:
☐ blood tests
☐ doctor.

• Can he control fatigue associated with anemia?
• Is he aware of the importance of reporting fever or other signs of complications to his doctor?
• Has he stated his intent to receive blood tests at prescribed periods?
• Does he report feeling less fearful?

Physical condition
A physical examination and diagnostic tests will provide additional information. If treatment has been successful, the patient should be free of signs and symptoms of infection, especially fever. Also note the presence or absence of the following:
• fever
• chills
• headache
• difficulty swallowing
• abdominal pain
• pain on defecation
• shortness of breath
• productive or nonproductive cough

• urinary frequency or urgency
• dysuria
• vaginal discharge
• ulcers or white patches in mouth
• skin lesions or rashes
• crackles or tachypnea
• redness, swelling, or discharge at vascular access sites.

Caring for patients with hypersensitivity disorders

Anaphylaxis   *82*

Atopic dermatitis   *88*

Asthma   *92*

Blood transfusion reaction   *102*

Hypersensitivity is an exaggerated or inappropriate immune response occurring after exposure to an antigen. Varying widely from person to person, hypersensitivity often causes inflammation and tissue damage. Severe hypersensitivity can even cause death.

Hypersensitivity reactions are classified into four types based on the speed of the reaction and the immunologic pathogenesis, with Type I being the most rapid. Antibodies mediate Types I, II, and III reactions, whereas T cells and macrophages mediate Type IV reactions.

Type I hypersensitivity reactions generally develop immediately after contact with an antigen or allergen; reactions are mediated almost exclusively by immunoglobulin E (IgE) antibodies. Examples include anaphylaxis, extrinsic asthma, atopic allergies such as allergic rhinitis, and allergies to dust, mold, medications, foods, and stinging insects.

In Type II cytotoxic hypersensitivity reactions, antibodies act against a cell surface or tissue antigen, resulting in the destruction of the body's own cells. Examples of Type II hypersensitivity disorders include hemolytic transfusion reactions, hemolytic disease of the newborn, autoimmune hemolytic anemia, hyperacute graft rejection, Goodpasture's syndrome, and myasthenia gravis.

Type III immune complex–mediated hypersensitivity reactions usually occur when excess antigens are created. Examples of Type III hypersensitivity include systemic lupus erythematosus, rheumatoid arthritis, glomerulonephritis, and polymyositis and dermatomyositis. Also, repeated inhalation of allergens such as molds, pollen, animal dander, and other plant and animal products can cause immune complex formation in the lungs or at other body surfaces.

Type IV delayed hypersensitivity reactions occur when antigens that are trapped in macrophages can't be cleared. Examples of Type IV hypersensitivity disorders include contact dermatitis, acute allograft rejection, tuberculosis, and sarcoidosis.

Keep in mind that hypersensitivity can sometimes result from other reactions. For the most part, however, the hypersensitivity reactions you'll see will be Types I and IV.

Anaphylaxis

A dramatic, acute atopic reaction, anaphylaxis is marked by the sudden onset of rapidly progressive urticaria and respiratory distress. A severe reaction may initiate vascular collapse, leading to systemic shock and, possibly, death.

After initial exposure to an antigen, the immune system activates a series of cellular reactions that, if left unchecked, will lead to rapid vascular collapse and, ultimately, hemorrhage, disseminated intravascular coagulation, respiratory obstruction, and cardiopulmonary arrest. Potentially fatal complications may occur within minutes or hours after the first symptoms appear. A delayed or persistent reaction, however, may last up to 24 hours. (See *How anaphylaxis progresses.*)

Causes
Anaphylaxis results from systemic exposure to sensitizing drugs or other specific antigens or, rarely, a ruptured hydatid cyst. (See *What triggers anaphylaxis?* page 84.)

How anaphylaxis progresses

When a hypersensitive patient is exposed to an allergen, his immune system produces immunoglobulin E (IgE) antibodies. On subsequent exposures to the allergen, the previously sensitized plasma cells manufacture and release huge quantities of IgE.

The IgE molecules immediately attach to mast cells or basophils, which then release their granular contents into the extracellular fluid (degranulation).

Degranulation releases potent chemical mediators including histamine, enzymes, chemotactic factors, heparin, prostaglandins, and leukotrienes.

Vasodilation, increased capillary permeability, and smooth-muscle contraction occur, leading to anaphylaxis, which affects major body systems. Severe manifestations can occur within seconds.

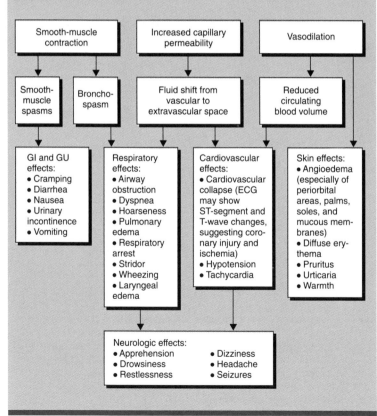

Smooth-muscle contraction

Increased capillary permeability

Vasodilation

Smooth-muscle spasms

Broncho-spasm

Fluid shift from vascular to extravascular space

Reduced circulating blood volume

GI and GU effects:
• Cramping
• Diarrhea
• Nausea
• Urinary incontinence
• Vomiting

Respiratory effects:
• Airway obstruction
• Dyspnea
• Hoarseness
• Pulmonary edema
• Respiratory arrest
• Stridor
• Wheezing
• Laryngeal edema

Cardiovascular effects:
• Cardiovascular collapse (ECG may show ST-segment and T-wave changes, suggesting coronary injury and ischemia)
• Hypotension
• Tachycardia

Skin effects:
• Angioedema (especially of periorbital areas, palms, soles, and mucous membranes)
• Diffuse erythema
• Pruritus
• Urticaria
• Warmth

Neurologic effects:
• Apprehension
• Drowsiness
• Restlessness
• Dizziness
• Headache
• Seizures

What triggers anaphylaxis?

Various drugs, foods, and other substances can trigger anaphylaxis or anaphylactoid reactions.

Local anesthetics
- Lidocaine
- Procaine

Antibiotics
- Aminoglycosides
- Amphotericin B
- Cephalosporins
- Nitrofurantoin
- Penicillins
- Sulfonamides
- Tetracyclines

Diagnostic agents
- Contrast media

Other drugs
- Barbiturates
- Diazepam
- Iron dextran
- Phenytoin
- Protamine
- Salicylates

Enzymes
- Chymopapain
- Chymotrypsin
- Penicillinase
- Trypsin
- L-asparaginase

Food additives
- Bisulfites

Foods
- Beans
- Chocolate
- Cottonseed oil
- Eggs
- Fruits
- Grains
- Nuts
- Shellfish

Hormones
- Adrenocorticotropic hormone
- Estradiol
- Insulin
- Parathyroid hormone
- Vasopressin

Pollens
- Grass
- Ragweed

Proteins
- Horse and rabbit serum

Venoms
- Hymenoptera (bees, wasps, hornets)
- Fire ants
- Snakes

ASSESSMENT

Your assessment should include a careful consideration of the patient's health history and physical examination findings. Note that other conditions may mimic anaphylaxis; you'll need to rule out these disorders.

Health history

The patient or a family member or companion may report the patient's exposure to an antigen. Immediately after exposure, the patient may complain of a feeling of impending doom or fright, weakness, sweating, sneezing, nasal pruritus, and urticaria. Angioedema may cause him to complain of a "lump" in his throat. Complaints of wheezing, dyspnea, and chest tightness suggest bronchial obstruction. These are early signs of impending, potentially fatal respiratory failure.

Other effects may follow rapidly. The patient may report GI and genitourinary effects, including severe abdominal cramps, nausea, diarrhea, and urinary urgency and incontinence. Neurologic effects include dizziness, drowsiness, headache, restlessness, and seizures. The patient may appear extremely anxious. The sooner symptoms begin after exposure to the antigen, the more severe the anaphylaxis.

Physical examination

The patient's skin may display well-circumscribed, discrete cutaneous wheals with erythematous, raised, serpiginous borders and blanched centers. They may coalesce to form giant hives. You may observe signs of respiratory distress and detect audible stridor and wheezing. Upon auscultation, you may detect crackles, wheezing and, possibly, decreased breath sounds. Cardiovascular effects include hypotension and a rapid, weak pulse accompanied by diaphoresis. Shock and cardiac arrhythmias can occur within minutes and may precipitate vascular collapse. The patient's level of consciousness may deteriorate quickly.

Timesaving tip: Be prepared to respond immediately to suspected anaphylaxis. Do not leave the patient unattended; anxiety can quicken vascular collapse. Call for help using the patient's telephone, call light, or emergency bathroom light, and initiate a code. Start an I.V. line before vascular collapse, administer emergency oxygen, and request a crash cart.

Diagnostic test results

No tests are required to identify anaphylaxis. The patient's history and symptoms establish the diagnosis. If symptoms occur without a known allergic stimulus, other possible causes of shock, such as acute myocardial infarction, status asthmaticus, or congestive heart failure, must be considered and ruled out.

NURSING DIAGNOSIS

Common nursing diagnoses for a patient with anaphylaxis include:
• Anxiety related to rapid deterioration of body functions and a feeling of impending doom
• Inability to sustain spontaneous ventilation related to airway obstruction brought on by laryngospasm or bronchoconstriction
• Decreased cardiac output related to arrhythmias and decreased circulating blood volume brought on by vascular collapse
• Knowledge deficit related to the causes of anaphylaxis and the prevention and management of subsequent exposure.

PLANNING

Based on the nursing diagnosis *anxiety,* develop appropriate patient outcomes. For example, your patient will:

- express feelings of anxiety
- exhibit diminished symptoms of anxiety following treatment.

Based on the nursing diagnosis *inability to sustain spontaneous ventilation,* develop appropriate patient outcomes. For example, your patient will:

- maintain adequate ventilation with a respiratory rate between 20 and 28 breaths/minute, clear breath sounds, and arterial blood gas levels (ABG) within normal limits
- experience relief of respiratory symptoms.

Based on the nursing diagnosis *decreased cardiac output,* develop appropriate patient outcomes. For example, your patient will:

- demonstrate hemodynamic stability
- maintain normal cardiac rate and rhythm.

Based on the nursing diagnosis *knowledge deficit,* develop appropriate patient outcomes. For example, your patient will:

- try to identify the offending allergen
- prevent exposure to the offending allergen, when known
- state the importance of wearing a medical identification bracelet and carrying an anaphylaxis treatment kit
- describe how to manage exposure to the allergen.

IMPLEMENTATION

Maintaining a patent airway is a key goal of treatment. Watch for early signs of laryngeal edema (stridor, hoarseness, and dyspnea), and be prepared to assist with endotracheal tube insertion or a tracheotomy. (See *Medical care of the patient with anaphylaxis.*)

Nursing interventions

- If the patient's airway is patent, provide supplemental oxygen via nasal cannula or face mask, and observe the patient's response by monitoring his respiratory rate and ABG results and auscultating his breath sounds.

Timesaving tip: Place the patient on continuous pulse oximetry to monitor his degree of hypoxia quickly and to measure his ABG levels.

- As soon as possible, administer epinephrine 1:1,000 aqueous solution, 0.1 to 0.5 ml S.C., as ordered. Expect to repeat the dose every 3 to 20 minutes as directed. In severe reactions, when the adult patient is unconscious and hypotensive, administer epinephrine 1:10,000 aqueous solution, 3 to 5 ml I.V., as ordered.
- Monitor the patient's mental status for restlessness or confusion, which could indicate cerebral hypoxia.
- Monitor the patient's vital signs at least every 15 minutes.
- Observe the patient's heart rate and rhythm on the cardiac monitor because arrhythmias can result from anaphylaxis and its treatment.
- Insert a large-gauge peripheral I.V. line to allow administration of emergency drugs and volume expanders. Give 0.9% sodium chloride solution rapidly, and be prepared to administer other volume expanders (plasma, plasma protein fraction, and albumin) as ordered.
- If needed, give I.V. vasopressors, such as norepinephrine, phenylephrine, and dopamine, as prescribed, to stabilize blood pressure.
- Monitor the patient's blood pressure, central venous pressure, and urine output.
- Administer other prescribed medications and monitor for therapeutic effects and any adverse reactions.

Treatments

Medical care of the patient with anaphylaxis

Treatment seeks to maintain a patent airway and adequate respirations. The patient may require supplemental oxygen. If he exhibits signs of laryngeal edema, he may require endotracheal intubation or a tracheotomy and mechanical ventilation. If the causative allergen can be identified, it should be removed immediately. For example, if the patient is receiving I.V. penicillin, the drug should be discontinued promptly.

Drug therapy
In severe anaphylactic reactions, when the adult patient is unconscious and hypotensive, give epinephrine 1:1,000 aqueous solution S.C. or 1:10,000 I.V., as ordered.

Aminophylline may be prescribed in severe bronchospasm. Antihistamines may block histamine's effects on the bronchioles, GI tract, and blood vessels. Corticosteroids may inhibit mast cell degranulation and serve as an anti-inflammatory. Other useful drugs include isoproterenol and ephedrine for their bronchodilating and vasoconstrictive effects.

To maintain circulatory volume, the doctor may order I.V. volume expanders (plasma, plasma expanders, 0.9% sodium chloride solution, and albumin). In severely decompensated patients, norepinephrine, phenylephrine, and dopamine may be given to raise blood pressure and increase cardiac output.

• Stay with the patient and continually reassure him. Speak calmly to him so as not to convey any anxiety. If necessary, reorient him to his situation and surroundings. After his anxiety has diminished, explain all tests and treatments, answer his questions, and address any concerns.

Patient teaching
• Explain how anaphylaxis occurs.
• Teach the patient to avoid exposure to known allergens. Instruct him not to consume offending foods or drugs in any form. If he's allergic to insect stings, he should avoid open fields and wooded areas during seasons when insects are prevalent.
• If exposure to a known allergen occurs, explain what actions to take, including how to use prescribed emergency drugs.
• If appropriate, emphasize the importance of carrying an emergency anaphylaxis treatment kit and teach him how to use it.
• Instruct him to always wear a medical identification bracelet. (See *Ensuring continued care for the patient with anaphylaxis,* page 88.)

EVALUATION

When evaluating the patient's response to nursing care, gather reassessment data and compare this information with the patient outcomes specified in your plan of care.

Discharge TimeSaver
Ensuring continued care for the patient with anaphylaxis

Review the following teaching topics, referrals, and follow-up appointments to make sure that your patient is adequately prepared for discharge.

Teaching topics
Make sure that the following topics have been covered and that your patient's learning has been evaluated:
☐ the allergic process — how it arises and its associated risks
☐ known allergens
☐ how to assemble and use an anaphylaxis kit
☐ how to recognize and respond to early signs of anaphylaxis
☐ the need to wear a medical identification bracelet.

Referrals
Make sure that the patient has been provided with necessary referrals to:
☐ dietitian (if food or additives are the known allergen)
☐ allergist.

Follow-up appointments
Make sure that the necessary follow-up appointment has been scheduled and that the patient has been notified:
☐ doctor.

Teaching and counseling
Talk to the patient to determine the effectiveness of your teaching and counseling. Consider the following questions:
• Can the patient discuss his anxiety?
• Does he demonstrate reduced signs of anxiety?
• Can he state how to avoid known triggers of anaphylaxis?
• Does he understand he must wear a medical identification bracelet and carry an anaphylaxis treatment kit?
• Can he identify early symptoms of anaphylaxis?
• Can he explain appropriate management of subsequent exposure to the allergen?

Physical condition
Consider the following questions:
• Is the patient maintaining a patent airway and adequate ventilation as evidenced by a respiratory rate between 20 and 28 breaths/minute,

clear breath sounds, and normal ABG levels?
• Are his vital signs normal?
• Does his electrocardiogram show a normal cardiac rhythm and rate?

Atopic dermatitis

A Type I immediate hypersensitivity reaction, atopic dermatitis is a chronic skin disorder marked by superficial inflammation and intense itching. This disorder usually occurs during infancy or early childhood and resolves itself by adolescence. However, recurrences sometimes occur in adulthood. Complications may include secondary bacterial or fungal infections, and viral infections such as herpes simplex.

Causes

This disorder occurs in people genetically predisposed to respond to certain allergens. A patient often has a personal or family history of associated atopic reactions. As many as 70% of patients with atopic dermatitis have a family history of asthma or hay fever, and parents who have had atopic dermatitis have a 50% to 75% chance of having children who experience atopic reactions.

Although the condition is linked to genetic hypersensitivity, its precise etiology is unknown. Infections, commonly from *Staphylococcus aureus*, and food allergens (such as soybeans, fish, and nuts) may exacerbate the condition. Infants may be exposed to food allergens through breast milk. The disorder hasn't been definitively linked to inhaled allergens, such as house dust and animal dander.

ASSESSMENT

Your assessment should include a careful consideration of the patient's health history, physical examination findings, and diagnostic test results.

Health history

The patient may report severe itching, which leads to uncontrolled scratching. It may occur on a daily, weekly, or seasonal basis. Scratching may cause the patient's skin to become inflamed and may expose nerve endings.

He may also report bacterial, fungal, and viral skin infections or ocular complications. Depending on the extent and appearance of the skin lesions, the patient or his family may report that changes in his appearance interfere with his social life.

Physical examination

The skin appears dry and erythematous. Lesions in adults appear scaly and lichenified and usually occur in areas of flexion and extension such as the neck, antecubital fossa, and popliteal folds. The face, upper chest, and region behind the ears may also be affected. You may see weeping lesions caused by scratching. Fever usually signals secondary infection.

Diagnostic test results

Serum analysis done during an episode of atopic dermatitis may reveal eosinophilia and elevated immunoglobulin E (IgE) levels. Additional testing may identify the allergen.

NURSING DIAGNOSIS

Common nursing diagnoses for a patient with atopic dermatitis include:
• Impaired skin integrity related to scratching
• High risk for infection (secondary) related to open, weeping skin lesions
• Body image disturbance related to recurrent skin lesions
• Social isolation related to a perceived negative response to skin lesions
• Knowledge deficit related to offending allergens and prevention and management of subsequent exposure.

PLANNING

Based on the nursing diagnosis *impaired skin integrity,* develop appropriate patient outcomes. For example, your patient will:
• exhibit healing of skin lesions.

Based on the nursing diagnosis *high risk for infection,* develop appropriate patient outcomes. For example, your patient will:

Medical care of atopic dermatitis

Drug therapy typically consists of topical corticosteroids and anti-pruritics. Topical corticosteroids (fluocinolone acetonide and flurandrenolide) should be used immediately after bathing for optimal skin penetration.

Antipruritic drugs may include:
• oral antihistamines (hydroxyzine)
• phenothiazine derivatives (methdilazine and trimeprazine).

Additionally, if secondary infection occurs, therapy may include antibiotics.

• remain free from secondary infections during exacerbation of skin lesions.

Based on the nursing diagnosis *body image disturbance,* develop appropriate patient outcomes. For example, your patient will:
• discuss feelings about the effects of his disease
• speak positively about himself and his abilities.

Based on the nursing diagnosis *social isolation,* develop appropriate patient outcomes. For example, your patient will:
• initiate conversation with family members, friends, and acquaintances throughout the acute exacerbation of his illness
• express his intention to maintain social contacts.

Based on the nursing diagnosis *knowledge deficit,* develop appropriate patient outcomes. For example, your patient will:
• describe his disease

• explain proposed treatment and describe patient and family participation
• identify factors precipitating acute exacerbations
• describe strategies to manage exacerbations.

IMPLEMENTATION

Care for atopic dermatitis consists of drug therapy and supportive measures. (See *Medical care of atopic dermatitis.*)

Nursing interventions
• Provide meticulous skin care. Because dry skin aggravates itchiness, frequently apply nonirritating, water-based topical lubricants, especially after the patient has bathed or showered. Because creams and ointments tend to seal in body heat, aggravating the dermatitis, use moisturizing lotions, which may be better tolerated.

Timesaving tip: Provide the patient with a supply of moisturizer, and encourage him to apply it liberally to affected areas. Teach him to use disposable gloves while applying lotion — if he uses an ungloved hand during application, he is much more likely to scratch and pick at lesions. Fill gloves with ice and instruct patient to apply for 5 minutes to itchy areas for relief, instead of scratching or rubbing.
• Inspect the skin for signs of secondary infection in areas that have been scratched.
• Reduce or minimize environmental exposure to offending allergens and irritants, such as wools and harsh detergent residues. To discover the allergens, tell the patient or his family to record activities and ingested foods.

• Monitor the patient's compliance with drug therapy.

• Encourage the patient to discuss his illness. Offer support as the patient learns to cope. If the patient's disorder poses a severe strain on family and social relationships, refer him for appropriate counseling.

Patient teaching
• Teach the patient and his family about the disorder. Explain the importance of avoiding known irritants.
• Emphasize the importance of performing a regular personal hygiene regimen, using warm, not hot, water. Suggest bathing with hypoallergenic soap, and advise the patient to avoid bubble baths.
• Advise the patient to use laundry detergents sparingly. Tell him to avoid additives, such as bleach and fabric softeners. Suggest rinsing clothes twice to remove all the detergent from the clothing.

• Explain measures to alleviate dry skin, such as taking a 30-minute bath two to three times a day, with oil or colloidal oatmeal. The bath should be followed immediately with the application of a lanolin-based cream or water-in-oil-based cream. Instruct the patient to avoid alcohol-based cleansers.

• Teach the patient and his family ways to identify secondary infection, such as pain, erythema, induration, increased warmth, purulent drainage, or fever. (See *Ensuring continued care for the patient with atopic dermatitis.*)

• Explain how to monitor nutritional status. Provide a list of foods to replace nutrients lost by avoiding the offending foods.

Timesaving tip: Involve the dietitian early when food allergens are known or suspected. The di-

etitian can assist in identifying the offending food or food additive, as well as teach diet modification and follow up, saving you time.
• Demonstrate how to apply topical corticosteroids and review the patient's application schedule.
• Encourage the patient to express his feelings about his illness. Discuss its effect on his social relationships. Show him how to use positive coping mechanisms. If problems persist or worsen, suggest counseling.

EVALUATION

When evaluating the patient's response to nursing care, gather reassessment data and compare this information with the patient outcomes specified in your plan of care.

Teaching and counseling
Talk to the patient to determine the effectiveness of your teaching and counseling. Consider the following questions:
• Does the patient describe himself and his abilities in a positive manner?
• Has he maintained social interactions?
• Can he describe the disease, skin care regimen, and medications?
• Are major precipitants of his dermatitis known? If so, can he describe them? Does he know to avoid them?
• Can he identify signs of skin infection?

Physical condition
Consider the following questions:
• Did the skin lesions disappear with treatment?
• Is the patient free from secondary infection?

Asthma

A chronic reactive airway disorder, asthma causes bronchoconstriction, increased mucus secretions, and mucosal edema that lead to episodic, reversible airway obstruction. Signs of asthma include paroxysmal dyspnea, wheezing, and coughing. Life-threatening complications include status asthmaticus and respiratory failure.

Causes
Several factors may contribute to bronchoconstriction. These include hereditary predisposition and sensitivity to allergens or irritants such as pollutants, viral infections, tartrazine (a yellow food dye), psychological stress, cold air, exercise, and aspirin, beta blockers, nonsteroidal anti-inflammatory drugs, and other drugs.

Extrinsic, or atopic, asthma may result from sensitivity to specific external allergens such as pollen, animal dander, house dust or mold, kapok or feather pillows, and food additives containing sulfites. Extrinsic asthma begins in childhood and is commonly accompanied by other manifestations of atopy, such as eczema and allergic rhinitis. (See *Understanding ABPA.*)

Internal, nonallergenic factors cause intrinsic, or nonatopic, asthma. Most episodes follow a respiratory tract infection, especially in adults. Irritants, emotional stress, fatigue, endocrine changes, temperature and humidity variations, and exposure to noxious fumes may aggravate intrinsic asthma attacks. In many asthmatics, especially children, intrinsic and extrinsic asthma coexist. (See *What happens in asthma,* pages 94 and 95.)

ASSESSMENT

Your assessment should include consideration of the patient's health history, physical examination findings, and diagnostic test results.

Health history

Typically, the patient reports exposure to a particular allergen followed by a sudden onset of dyspnea and wheezing. He may describe a feeling of tightness in his chest, a cough that produces thick, clear or yellow sputum, and a feeling of suffocation. He may report that the attack began dramatically, with simultaneous onset of severe, multiple symptoms, or insidiously, with gradually increasing respiratory distress.

Ask about smoking, allergies, home environment, occupation, hobbies, and other possible precipitating factors such as cold air, exercise, and upper respiratory tract infection. Also inquire about sleep patterns and obtain a family history.

Physical examination

The patient may be visibly anxious, dyspneic, and able to speak only a few words before pausing to catch his breath. He may use accessory respiratory muscles to breathe. You may observe him sweating profusely, and may note an increased anteroposterior thoracic diameter.

Percussion may produce hyperresonance, and palpation may reveal vocal fremitus. Auscultation may disclose tachycardia, mild systolic hypertension, pulsus paradoxus, harsh respirations with both inspiratory and expiratory wheezes, a prolonged expiratory phase of respiration, and diminished breath sounds.

Cyanosis, confusion, absence of breath sounds, and lethargy indicate

Understanding ABPA

Allergic bronchopulmonary aspergillosis (ABPA) may trigger extrinsic asthma. ABPA is one of five pulmonary diseases caused by *Aspergillus*. Suspect ABPA in asthmatic patients with:

• an eosinophil count above 1,000/mm^3
• positive immediate or late-phase reaction to a skin test for *Aspergillus* antigen
• immunoglobulin G antibodies to *Aspergillus* antigens
• presence of *Aspergillus* in sputum
• elevated serum immunoglobulin E levels
• pulmonary infiltrates, often transitory
• central, saccular bronchiectasis
• expectorated golden-brown mucus plugs or mucus tinged with golden-brown specks.

the onset of life-threatening impending respiratory failure.

Diagnostic test results

• Pulmonary function studies reveal evidence of airway obstruction: decreased flow rates and forced expiratory volume in 1 second (FEV$_1$), low-normal or decreased vital capacity, and increased total lung and residual capacities. However, pulmonary function may be normal between attacks.
• Typically, arterial blood gas (ABG) analysis reveals normal partial pressure of oxygen and decreased partial pressure of carbon dioxide in arterial blood (PaCO$_2$). However, in severe

What happens in asthma

The following illustrations show what happens in asthma.

1. When the patient inhales a substance to which he's hypersensitive, this triggers immunoglobulin E – sensitized mast cells in the lung interstitium to release both histamine (H) and the slow-reacting substance of anaphylaxis (SRS-A). *At this stage, the patient has no detectable signs or symptoms.*

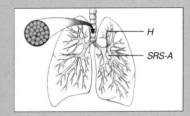

2. Histamine attaches to receptor sites in the larger bronchi, where it causes swelling in smooth muscles. Mucous membranes become inflamed, irritated, and swollen. *The patient may experience dyspnea, prolonged expiration, and an increased respiratory rate.*

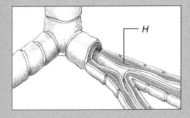

3. SRS-A attaches to receptor sites in the smaller bronchi and causes swelling of smooth muscle there. It also causes fatty acids called prostaglandins to travel in the bloodstream to the lungs, where they enhance histamine's effects. *Listen to the patient's cough for wheezing. The higher the pitch, the narrower the bronchial lumen.*

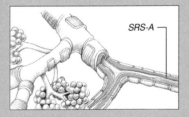

asthma, $PaCO_2$ may be normal or increased, indicating severe bronchial obstruction. In fact, FEV_1 will probably be less than 25% of the predicted value. Treatment tends to improve the airflow. However, even when the asthma attack appears controlled, the spirometric values (FEV_1 and forced expiratory flow) remain abnormal, necessitating frequent ABG analyses.
• Monitoring of serum immunoglobulin E (IgE) levels may reveal a rise due to an allergic reaction.

4. Histamine stimulates the mucous membranes to secrete excessive mucus, further narrowing the bronchial lumen (see top right of illustration). Goblet cells secrete a viscous mucus that's difficult to cough up. *Listen for coughing, rhonchi, high-pitched wheezing, and increased respiratory distress.*

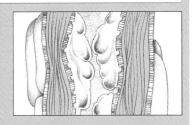

5. On inhalation, the narrowed bronchial lumen can still expand slightly, allowing air to reach the alveoli. On exhalation, increased intrathoracic pressure closes the bronchial lumen completely. Air can get in, but not out. *Assess for hyperresonance to percussion and cessation of wheezing.*

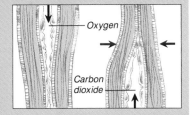

6. Mucus fills the lung bases, inhibiting alveolar ventilation. Blood, shunted to alveoli in other lung parts, still can't compensate for diminished ventilation. Respiratory acidosis results. *Look for signs of hypoxemia: reduced partial pressure of oxygen in arterial blood (despite increased fraction of inspired oxygen), elevated partial pressure of carbon dioxide in arterial blood, and decreased serum pH.*

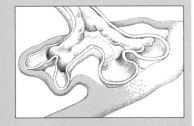

- Complete blood count with differential may reveal increased eosinophil count.
- Chest X-rays may show hyperinflation with areas of focal atelectasis.

NURSING DIAGNOSIS

Common nursing diagnoses for a patient with asthma include:
- Ineffective airway clearance related to retained viscous secretions, fatigue, and anxiety

• Impaired gas exchange related to bronchoconstriction and mucosal edema
• Anxiety related to dyspnea and feeling of impending doom
• Knowledge deficit related to the disease, its precipitating factors, its treatment, and management of acute episodes.

PLANNING

Based on the nursing diagnosis *ineffective airway clearance,* develop appropriate patient outcomes. For example, your patient will:
• cough and deep breathe adequately to expectorate secretions
• exhibit clear breath sounds bilaterally
• maintain a patent airway.

Based on the nursing diagnosis *impaired gas exchange,* develop appropriate patient outcomes. For example, your patient will:
• demonstrate normal gas exchange
• recover from an acute asthma attack without experiencing residual lung damage.

Based on the nursing diagnosis *anxiety,* develop appropriate patient outcomes. For example, your patient will:
• discuss feelings of anxiety
• demonstrate reduced symptoms of anxiety following treatment.

Based on the nursing diagnosis *knowledge deficit,* develop appropriate patient outcomes. For example, your patient will:
• describe the disease
• identify factors that precipitate acute asthma, and discuss strategies to manage them
• explain proposed treatment and describe patient and family participation
• list steps to follow during an acute asthma attack.

IMPLEMENTATION

To control his asthma, the patient must adhere to a medical regimen and avoid triggering factors. (See *Medical care of the patient with asthma.*)

Nursing interventions
• Control exercise-induced asthma by having the patient sit down, rest, and use diaphragmatic and pursed-lip breathing until shortness of breath subsides.
• In an acute attack, find out if the patient has used an inhaler; the patient should have access to an albuterol or metaproterenol inhaler at all times. (See *How to use an inhaler,* pages 98 and 99.)
• Reassure the patient and stay with him. Place him in semi-Fowler's position and encourage diaphragmatic breathing. Help him to relax.
• As ordered, administer humidified oxygen by nasal cannula at 2 liters/minute to ease breathing and to increase arterial oxygen saturation (SaO_2) during an acute attack. Later, adjust oxygen according to the patient's vital functions and ABG measurements.

Timesaving tip: Place the patient on continuous pulse oximetry. That way you can reassure yourself that he is breathing effectively without awakening him unnecessarily.

• Administer drugs and I.V. fluids as ordered. Continue epinephrine, subcutaneously or by inhalation, for a patient experiencing an acute attack. Give aminophylline I.V. as a loading dose. Follow with an I.V. drip, as ordered. When possible, use an infusion pump. Don't administer I.V. aminophylline any faster than 25 mg/minute. Simultaneously, give a loading

Treatments

Medical care of the patient with asthma

The best treatment for asthma is prevention: identifying and avoiding precipitating factors, such as environmental allergens or irritants. Usually, such stimuli can't be removed entirely. Desensitization to specific antigens may be more helpful in children than in adults with bronchial asthma.

Drug therapy

Usually including bronchodilators, drug therapy proves most effective when begun soon after the onset of symptoms. Commonly used drugs include:
• rapid-acting epinephrine
• terbutaline
• aminophylline
• theophylline and theophylline-containing oral preparations
• oral sympathomimetics
• corticosteroids
• aerosolized sympathomimetics, such as metaproterenol and albuterol.

Other treatments

These measures may include:

• arterial blood gas (ABG) determinations, to help evaluate the severity of an asthma attack and the patient's response to treatment
• low-flow oxygen
• antibiotics
• fluid replacement.

Treatment for status asthmaticus

Status asthmaticus must be treated promptly to prevent fatal respiratory failure. The patient with increasingly severe asthma that doesn't respond to drug therapy is usually admitted to the intensive care unit for treatment with:
• corticosteroids
• epinephrine
• sympathomimetic aerosol sprays
• I.V. aminophylline.

He'll need frequent ABG analysis and pulse oximetry to assess respiratory status, particularly after ventilator therapy or a change in oxygen concentration. He may require endotracheal intubation and mechanical ventilation if his partial pressure of carbon dioxide in arterial blood rises.

---

dose of a corticosteroid I.V. or I.M., as ordered.
• Watch serum theophylline levels closely to be sure they're in the therapeutic range. Observe for signs of toxicity, such as vomiting, diarrhea, and headache, and for signs of subtherapeutic dosage, such as respiratory distress and increased wheezing.
• If the patient is taking systemic corticosteroids, observe for adverse reactions, such as hyperglycemia, gas-

tritis, mental status changes, or fluid overload.
• If the patient is taking corticosteroids by inhaler, watch for signs of infection in the mouth and pharynx, such as white plaques on the buccal mucosa, tongue, or palate.
• Note the frequency and severity of the patient's coughs, and whether the cough is productive. Then auscultate the lungs, noting adventitious sounds

(Text continues on page 100.)

Teaching TimeSaver

How to use an inhaler

Be sure that your patient knows how to use his inhaler by reviewing these instructions with him.

Preparing the inhaler
• Make sure that the canister is fully and firmly inserted into the plastic shell or actuator.
• Press the canister firmly into the actuator and rotate back and forth several times without firing the aerosol.
• Remove the cap from the mouthpiece and check for foreign objects.
• Shake the inhaler well.

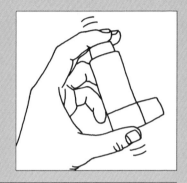

Administering the dose
• Breathe out fully through the mouth, expelling as much air from your lungs as possible. Place the mouthpiece fully into the mouth, holding the inhaler upright and closing the lips tightly around the mouthpiece.

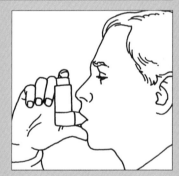

• Release the dose by depressing the top of the metal canister between your forefinger and thumb. At the same time, breathe in deeply and slowly through the mouth.

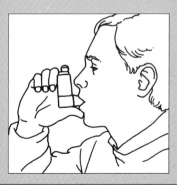

• Continue inhaling to make sure that the spray reaches deeply into your lungs. Hold your breath for as long as possible.

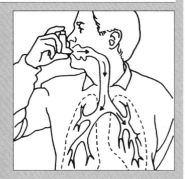

• Breathe out gently, wait 1 minute (or as long as directed), and repeat the procedure for a second puff. Remember to shake the canister again.

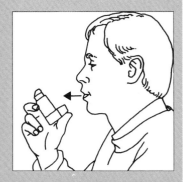

Instruct the patient to take no more than three puffs every 4 hours. If he needs the inhaler again before 4 hours elapse, however, allow him to use it and have him call the doctor for further instruction. Excessive use can progressively weaken the patient's response, mask underlying inflammation and, in rare cases, even lead to cardiac arrest and death.

Teaching TimeSaver

How to prevent recurring attacks

• Show the patient how to breathe deeply.
• Instruct him to cough up secretions accumulated overnight. Teach him to inhale fully and gently, then bend over, crossing his arms over his abdomen or splinting it with a pillow, and then cough.
• Explain that he has to allow time for medications to work.
• Urge him to drink at least six 8-oz glasses of water daily to help loosen secretions and maintain hydration.
• Encourage a well-balanced diet to prevent respiratory infection and fatigue. Teach him to identify and avoid foods that trigger an attack.
• Teach the patient and his family to avoid known allergens and irritants, such as aerosol sprays, smoke, and automobile exhaust.
• Refer the patient to community resources, such as the American Lung Association and the Asthma and Allergy Foundation of America.

• Combat dehydration with I.V. fluids until the patient can tolerate oral fluids.
• Keep the room temperature comfortable. Use an air conditioner in hot, humid weather.
• Continue to monitor the patient's respiratory status to detect baseline changes, assess response to treatment, and detect complications.
• Auscultate the lungs frequently, noting the degree of wheezing and quality of air movement.
• Monitor vital signs. Keep in mind that developing or worsening tachypnea can mean worsening asthma. Tachycardia may indicate worsening disease or drug toxicity. Blood pressure readings may reveal pulsus paradoxus, indicating severe asthma, or hypertension, indicating asthma-related hypoxia or complications.
• Review ABG levels, pulmonary function test results, and SaO_2 readings.
• If the patient's breathing fails to maintain sufficient gas exchange because of respiratory arrest, progressive hypercapnia with respiratory acidosis, or progressive hypoxia with mental status deterioration, anticipate intubation and mechanical ventilation.
• Monitor the patient's anxiety level. Keep in mind that measures that reduce hypoxia and breathlessness should help relieve anxiety. Encourage him to express his fears and concerns. Answer his questions honestly. Offer reassurance, and relaxation techniques, such as massage and soothing music.

Patient teaching
If the patient has a history of asthma, assess his knowledge of the disorder before initiating teaching. (See *How to prevent recurring attacks.*)

or absent sounds. If the cough isn't productive and rhonchi are present, teach effective coughing techniques. Also perform postural drainage and chest percussion to clear secretions if the patient can tolerate these procedures. Suction the intubated patient as needed.
• If the airway obstruction doesn't improve with conservative treatment, anticipate bronchoscopy or bronchial lavage if the area of collapse is a lobe or larger.

Discharge TimeSaver

Ensuring continued care for the patient with asthma

Review the following teaching topics, referrals, and follow-up appointments to make sure that your patient is adequately prepared for discharge.

Teaching topics
Make sure that the following topics have been covered and that your patient's learning has been evaluated:
☐ asthma disease process and complications
☐ avoidance of triggering factors
☐ warning signs and symptoms
☐ medications
☐ exercise and activity guidelines
☐ breathing and coughing techniques
☐ relaxation techniques
☐ chest physiotherapy
☐ use and cleaning of equipment, such as an inhaler or peak flow meter
☐ importance of follow-up care.

Referrals
Make sure that the patient has been provided with necessary referrals to:
☐ pulmonologist
☐ allergist
☐ social services for financial consultation regarding equipment and medications.

Follow-up appointments
Make sure that the necessary follow-up appointments have been scheduled and that the patient has been notified:
☐ doctor
☐ further diagnostic tests.

• Teach him and his family about diaphragmatic and pursed-lip breathing. Encourage him to perform relaxation exercises as needed.
• Teach him how to use an oral inhaler or a turbo-inhaler. The addition of spacer devices may help optimize drug delivery.
• Discuss the possible adverse effects of his medications and the need to notify his doctor if these occur. Provide written cards or sheets for each drug. (See *Ensuring continued care for the patient with asthma.*)

EVALUATION

When evaluating the patient's response to nursing care, gather reassessment data and compare this information with the patient outcomes specified in your plan of care. (See *Assessing failure to respond to asthma therapy,* page 102.)

Teaching and counseling
Talk to the patient to determine the effectiveness of your teaching and counseling. Consider the following questions:
• Does the patient express feelings of anxiety during an attack?
• Have signs of anxiety diminished?
• Can he describe asthma and its effects and treatment?
• Can he demonstrate proper use of an inhaler?
• Can he identify factors that trigger an attack and explain strategies to manage them?
• Can he list actions to take if an acute attack occurs?

Evaluation TimeSaver

Assessing failure to respond to asthma therapy

If your patient fails to respond to treatment, refer to this checklist to help evaluate the underlying causes. Consult with the patient and his family for help in your evaluation. Review the patient's drug therapy with his doctor.

Factors interfering with compliance
☐ Inability to understand the disorder
☐ Inadequate patient teaching
☐ Inability to afford medication
☐ Language barrier
☐ Lack of clear, written instructions
☐ Memory impairment
☐ Inability to tolerate adverse drug effects

Factors interfering with drug therapy
☐ Failure to use inhaler correctly
☐ Improper drug dosage
☐ Improper drugs or drug combinations
☐ Failure of patient to report for tests of theophylline blood levels

☐ Failure of health care provider to monitor theophylline blood levels

Environmental factors
☐ Environmental pollutants and allergens (pollen, dust, animal dander)
☐ Smoke
☐ Cold air
☐ Humidity
☐ Occupational exposures

Other factors
☐ Drug therapy (beta blockers, aspirin, nonsteroidal anti-inflammatory agents)
☐ Exercise
☐ Diet
☐ Stress

Physical condition
Consider the following questions:
• Does the patient maintain a patent airway?
• Does he demonstrate normal gas exchange?
• Following an acute asthma attack, is residual lung damage absent?

Blood transfusion reaction

A transfusion reaction may occur during administration of blood and blood components or several hours or days later. Its severity varies. Depending on the amount of blood transfused, the type of reaction, and his general health, the patient may experience fever and chills, acute renal failure, bronchospasm (possibly leading to acute respiratory failure), anaphylactic shock, vascular collapse, or disseminated intravascular coagulation (DIC).

Causes
Blood transfusion reactions have varying immune-related causes. Rh incompatibility may result in an acute or a delayed hemolytic reaction. Transfusion with Rh-incompatible

blood usually triggers a less serious hemolytic reaction than ABO incompatibility, known as Rh isoimmunization. ABO incompatibility usually leads to rapid intravascular hemolysis.

Multiple transfusions may cause a patient to become sensitized to white blood cells and lead to febrile nonhemolytic transfusion reactions, whereas patients who have a history of allergies may have allergic transfusion reactions. Minor red blood cell antigens may also be implicated in hemolytic transfusion reactions.

ASSESSMENT

Your assessment should include a careful consideration of the patient's health history, physical examination findings, and diagnostic test results.

Health history

The immediate effects of an acute hemolytic transfusion reaction develop within a few minutes or hours after the transfusion begins. The patient may report chills followed by fever, nausea, vomiting, chest tightness, and chest and back pain. He may experience a sense of impending doom. In a delayed hemolytic reaction, symptoms are usually milder. The patient may report malaise and fever.

If the patient experiences a febrile nonhemolytic transfusion reaction, he may complain of chills followed by fever and possibly nausea, vomiting, and headache. If he experiences an allergic transfusion reaction, he may first report hives (urticaria) and itching. Signs and symptoms may occur during the transfusion or up to 24 hours later. With anaphylactic reactions, the patient may report severe dyspnea and substernal pain.

Physical examination

An acute hemolytic reaction may lead to fever, tachycardia, tachypnea, and hypotension. The patient may appear dyspneic and apprehensive. The patient's urine output may fall, and cyanosis may be present. His level of consciousness (LOC) may deteriorate. A delayed hemolytic transfusion reaction that occurs several weeks after the transfusion may produce milder signs such as fever and jaundice. Mild to severe fever is the hallmark of a febrile nonhemolytic transfusion reaction.

Inspection may reveal urticaria and angioedema in an allergic reaction. Auscultation may reveal wheezing if bronchospasm occurs. Stridor may occur with laryngeal edema. Anaphylaxis may result in signs of shock.

Timesaving tip: The most severe reactions occur rapidly. Therefore, plan your patient's care so that you can spend the first 15 minutes of each transfusion in his room, and be sure to teach him what symptoms he should report to you immediately.

Diagnostic test results

The patient suspected of having a transfusion reaction should have his blood retyped and crossmatched with the donor's blood. Proof of blood incompatibility and evidence of hemolysis include:
• hemoglobinuria
• anti-A or anti-B antibodies in serum
• low serum hemoglobin level
• elevated bilirubin level.

After a hemolytic transfusion reaction, laboratory test results show:
• increased indirect bilirubin level
• decreased hemoglobin level
• decreased haptoglobin level
• hemoglobinuria.

Treatments

Medical care of the patient with blood transfusion reaction

Treatment depends on the type of transfusion reaction.

Hemolytic reaction

A hemolytic transfusion reaction requires immediate cessation of the transfusion. If the patient is oliguric, osmotic or loop diuretics may be administered. Symptomatic treatments may include:
• I.V. vasopressors and 0.9% sodium chloride solution to combat shock
• epinephrine and oxygen to relieve dyspnea and wheezing
• hemodialysis, if renal failure occurs.
  The patient should also be monitored for signs of disseminated intravascular coagulation.

Febrile nonhemolytic reaction

A febrile nonhemolytic transfusion reaction is treated with antipyretics.

Allergic reaction

In an allergic transfusion reaction, drug therapy may include diphenhydramine to combat cellular histamine released from mast cells, corticosteroids to reduce inflammation, and administration of vasopressors and epinephrine. To treat shock, the doctor may order I.V. fluids. Respiratory therapy may be necessary as well.

Preventing future reactions

A patient with a history of transfusion reactions may require specific interventions to prevent future reactions. If a severe transfusion reaction resulted from immunoglobulin A (IgA) antibodies, the doctor may order blood that lacks IgA. When an IgA-negative donor isn't available, a special filter may be used to remove IgA.
  Patients with antibodies to white blood cells can receive washed cells—packed red blood cells (RBCs) from which leukocytes are removed. Some centers use frozen and thawed RBCs.

As the reaction progresses, tests may show signs of DIC, such as:
• thrombocytopenia
• prolonged prothrombin time
• decreased fibrinogen level and increased fibrin split products.
  Laboratory test results may also show signs of acute tubular necrosis, such as:
• elevated blood urea nitrogen level
• increased creatinine level.

NURSING DIAGNOSIS

Common nursing diagnoses for a patient with blood transfusion reaction include:
• Anxiety related to the severe symptoms and a feeling of impending doom
• Decreased cardiac output related to arrhythmias, and decreased circulating blood volume brought on by vascular collapse
• Hyperthermia related to hemolytic or febrile nonhemolytic transfusion reaction.

PLANNING

Based on the nursing diagnosis *anxiety,* develop appropriate patient outcomes. For example, your patient will:

• demonstrate fewer symptoms of anxiety following treatment.

Based on the nursing diagnosis *decreased cardiac output,* develop appropriate patient outcomes. For example, your patient will:

• exhibit hemodynamic stability

• resume normal cardiac rate and rhythm.

Based on the nursing diagnosis *hyperthermia,* develop appropriate patient outcomes. For example, your patient will:

• have a normal temperature and no complications of hyperthermia.

IMPLEMENTATION

Blood transfusion reactions require prompt intervention. If a reaction occurs during a transfusion, stop the transfusion and notify the doctor at once. (See *Medical care of the patient with blood transfusion reaction,* opposite page, and *Administering safe transfusions.*)

Nursing interventions

• Try to alleviate the patient's anxiety by keeping him informed throughout treatments.

• Don't remove the needle. Keep the vein open with a solution such as 0.9% sodium chloride if allowed.

• Send a fresh sample of the patient's blood to the laboratory so it can be observed for hemolysis. Also return the donor blood for a repeat crossmatch.

• Monitor the patient's vital signs every 15 to 30 minutes; if signs of shock are present, administer medications as ordered.

Administering safe transfusions

Follow these directions to help ensure safe transfusions.

• Check the doctor's order and, with another nurse, identify the patient, matching the name and number on his identification band with those on the blood component tag.

• Check the blood bag label, the attached tag, and the laboratory requisition slip to ensure that ABO and Rh types are identical.

• Check the bag's expiration date and check that the type of blood component is correct.

• Check to be sure the blood bag is intact, and observe for clumping or extraneous material.

• Obtain the patient's baseline vital signs, including temperature, before the transfusion.

• Wear gloves when you set up the transfusion.

• Monitor the patient closely during the first 15 minutes of the transfusion. Check his vital signs every 5 minutes for the first 15 minutes, then at least every 30 minutes, depending on his condition.

• Observe the patient for chills, flushing, itching, dyspnea, rash, hives, and other signs of transfusion reactions.

• Flush the I.V. line with 0.9% sodium chloride solution after the transfusion.

• If fever is present, take the patient's temperature at least every hour. Initiate cooling measures for fever over 101° F (38.3° C).

Discharge TimeSaver

Ensuring continued care for the patient with transfusion reaction

Review the following teaching topics, referrals, and follow-up appointments to make sure that your patient is adequately prepared for discharge.

Teaching topics
Make sure that the following topics have been covered and that your patient's learning has been evaluated:
☐ an explanation of how reactions occur
☐ an explanation of the patient's type of reaction
☐ any precautions before future transfusions.

Referrals
No referrals are necessary.

Follow-up appointments
Make sure that the necessary follow-up appointment has been scheduled and that the patient has been notified:
☐ doctor, if warranted.

• Provide supplemental oxygen if the patient is dyspneic.
• If he has a severe hemolytic reaction, insert an indwelling urinary catheter. Monitor intake and output. Report output of less than 30 ml/hour.
• Afterward, fully document the transfusion reaction on the patient's chart, including all interventions. Note the duration of the transfusion and the amount of blood absorbed.

Patient teaching
• Explain transfusion reactions and the need for treatment.
• Tell the patient who has experienced a transfusion reaction to make this known before he receives any subsequent transfusions. (See *Ensuring continued care for the patient with transfusion reaction*.)

EVALUATION
When evaluating the patient's response to nursing care, gather reassessment data and compare this in-

formation with the patient outcomes specified in your plan of care.

Teaching and counseling
Talk to the patient to determine the effectiveness of your teaching and counseling. Consider the following questions:
• Does the patient feel less anxious?
• Does he understand what caused his reaction?

Physical condition
Consider the following questions:
• Are the patient's vital signs, including temperature, normal?
• Is his cardiac rate and rhythm normal?
• Does he maintain a urine output of at least 30 ml/hour?
• Is his LOC at baseline?

Caring for patients with autoimmune disorders

Rheumatoid arthritis　　　108

Systemic lupus erythematosus　　　119

Systemic sclerosis　　　127

Autoimmune thrombocytopenic purpura　　　134

Hashimoto's disease　　　141

Autoimmune disorders occur when the immune system produces antibodies that act on normal endogenous tissue. Depending on the severity of the autoimmune response, these autoantibodies can cause tissue damage ranging from minor local effects to potentially life-threatening systemic complications.

Just why autoimmunity occurs isn't known. It's thought to result from a combination of immunologic, genetic, hormonal, virologic, and other factors.

Autoimmune disorders may be classified as organ-specific or systemic (organ-nonspecific). Organ-specific disorders, such as Hashimoto's disease (which affects the thyroid gland), involve autoimmune responses in a specific organ. Systemic autoimmune disorders, such as systemic lupus erythematosus, involve widespread autoimmune responses to cells, tissues, or both. In these systemic disorders, immune complexes are deposited throughout the body, especially in the kidneys, joints, and skin.

Although few confirmed autoimmune disorders exist, many disorders are strongly thought to have an autoimmune component. This chapter discusses several suspected or confirmed autoimmune disorders. (See *Suspected autoimmune disorders.*)

Rheumatoid arthritis

A chronic, progressive, inflammatory disease, rheumatoid arthritis (RA) primarily attacks peripheral joints and surrounding muscles, tendons, ligaments, and blood vessels and causes similar inflammatory responses in any organ system connected by tissue. Patients usually require life-long treatment and, sometimes, surgery. (See *Key points about rheumatoid arthritis,* page 110.)

If left untreated, RA's inflammation and joint damage can result in peripheral neuropathy, permanent joint deformities, muscle wasting and atrophy, secondary osteoporosis and bone fractures, carpal tunnel syndrome, and spinal cord compression. Other possible complications include vasculitis, pericarditis, myocarditis, anemia, and scleritis. Renal insufficiency, pleural effusion, pneumonitis, pulmonary interstitial fibrosis, or pulmonary hypertension, as well as Sjögren's, Felty's, or Caplan's syndromes, may also develop.

Causes

The cause of RA's chronic inflammation is unknown. The immune complex hypothesis speculates that a genetically susceptible patient's natural immunoglobin G (IgG) antibodies are altered after exposure to an antigen. Not recognizing the altered IgG antibodies, the body generates another antibody, called rheumatoid factor, to fight the altered IgG. As rheumatoid factors accumulate, inflammation and cartilage damage result, triggering further immune responses and ultimately joint destruction.

A family history of RA increases a person's risk two to three times. Also, up to 70% of affected patients carry the human leukocyte antigen D4 (HLA-D4) and HLA-DR4 genes.

Hormonal influence may be a contributing factor. RA strikes women approximately three times more often than it strikes men, although this difference disappears with age.

The autoimmune response may also be triggered by either viral or bacterial infection, such as Epstein-Barr virus or rubella.

Suspected autoimmune disorders

Organ-specific disorders	Autoantibody target
Addison's disease	Adrenal cells
Agranulocytosis (idiopathic neutropenia)	Neutrophils
Autoimmune hemolytic anemia	Erythrocytes
Bullous pemphigoid	Skin basement membrane
Glomerulonephritis	Glomerular basement membrane
Graves' disease	Thyroid-stimulating-hormone receptor
Myasthenia gravis	Acetylcholine
Pernicious anemia	Intrinsic factor, vitamin B_{12}, and gastric parietal cell
Premature ovarian failure	Corpus luteum cells and interstitial cells
Primary biliary cirrhosis	Mitochondria
Rheumatic fever	Myocardial cells
Type I diabetes mellitus (insulin-dependent)	Pancreatic beta cells
Uveitis	Uvea
Systemic disorders	**Autoantibody target**
Goodpasture's syndrome	Basement membranes of renal glomeruli, renal tubules, and pulmonary alveoli
Mixed connective tissue disease	Ribonucleoprotein
Sjögren's syndrome	Salivary duct and other antigens

Although not yet considered a cause of RA, stress — both emotional and physical — is linked to exacerbations.

ASSESSMENT

Your assessment should include a careful consideration of the patient's health history, physical examination findings, and diagnostic test results.

Health history

Begin by asking about the patient's chief complaint, which is commonly bilateral, symmetrical joint pain and stiffness. Usually, the proximal interphalangeal and metacarpophalangeal joints of the hands are affected at first. As the disease progresses, any joint may become inflamed. Consider asking the patient the following questions:

• When did your symptoms first appear?
• Did they appear suddenly or gradually?
• How often do they occur?
• How long do they last?

FactFinder

Key points about rheumatoid arthritis

- *Incidence:* The second most common connective tissue disorder and a major cause of disability, rheumatoid arthritis (RA) usually strikes adults between ages 20 and 50 and affects three times as many women as men. However, women who take oral contraceptives are at a reduced risk.
- *Prognosis:* Spontaneous remissions and unpredictable exacerbations mark the course of this potentially crippling disease.
- *Diagnostic methods:* No test confirms RA, but imaging tests and blood studies provide diagnostic support.
- *Treatment:* Medical care consists primarily of drugs, supportive care, and physical therapy.

- Do they become more or less severe over time, or remain constant?

The patient often reports pain and stiffness that are worse in the morning but subside during the day. She may also complain of joints being tender and painful when moved or, later in the disease, even at rest. Other complaints may include stiff, weak, or painful muscles and paresthesia in the hands or feet.

Timesaving tip: Have your patient rate her pain or discomfort on a scale of 1 to 10. Record her response to help you understand her perception of pain and to use for comparison during subsequent episodes.

Ask about a family history of RA to help confirm the patient's diagnosis and to determine how the condition of family members may affect her.

Be alert for a history of emotional and physical exhaustion from overwork, worry, or acute infection. As RA progresses, the patient may reveal an increasing inability to work or to perform normal household duties or activities of daily living (ADLs) independently.

In assessing psychosocial status, determine if physical limitations have diminished the patient's sexual activity or socialization. Note any feelings of poor body image, altered role performance, financial concern, embarrassment, or depression. Be sure to assess the patient's coping mechanisms and sources of support.

Physical examination

In acute RA, inspection of joints may reveal redness and swelling, with the skin appearing thin and shiny. Later manifestations may include joint deformities, often in the hands. Inspection and palpation of pressure areas, such as the elbows, may reveal subcutaneous, round, hard masses (rheumatoid nodules). In acute and subacute (but perhaps not chronic) RA, palpation may also reveal joints that are painful, boggy, and hot to the touch; crepitus, indicating loss of cartilage; splenomegaly; and lymphadenopathy.

Assess range of motion (ROM) and guarded movement, especially in the elbows, wrists, and shoulders. Check for reduced muscle strength, including a weak grip and the inability to make a tight fist.

Conclude by performing a thorough baseline examination, noting extra-articular findings related to systemic involvement, such as lesions and leg ulcers in vasculitis or eye redness in scleritis or episcleritis.

Diagnostic test results

Although no test confirms RA, the following ones support the diagnosis:

• X-rays show bone demineralization and soft-tissue swelling in the early stages of RA. Later, they show the extent of cartilage and bone destruction, erosion, subluxation, and deformity and typical symmetrical involvement.

• Magnetic resonance imaging may aid early detection of carpal tunnel inflammation and avascular necrosis of the hip.

• Computed tomography can determine the presence of synovial cysts or the degree of cervical spine involvement.

• Rheumatoid factor (RF) test measures the presence of unusual IgG and IgM antibodies. This test is positive in 75% to 80% of patients, as indicated by a titer of 1:80 or higher. Although the presence of RF doesn't confirm RA, it helps determine the prognosis. A patient with a high titer usually has a more severe and progressive case of the disease, with corresponding extra-articular manifestations.

• Serum protein electrophoresis may show elevated serum globulin levels.

• Erythrocyte sedimentation rate (ESR), elevated in 85% to 90% of patients, can confirm inflammation or infection in any organ system. Although not specific, it helps monitor the response to therapy because an elevation often parallels disease activity.

• Complete blood count usually shows moderate anemia and slight leukocytosis.

• Synovial fluid analysis shows increased volume and turbidity, but decreased viscosity and complement (C3 and C4) levels. The white blood cell count often ranges from 5,000 to 20,000/mm³, of which 75% are polymorphonuclear neutrophils. RF may be present.

• C-reactive protein (CRP) test, an antigen-antibody test, helps evaluate inflammation. A positive titer is significant whether it's 1:2 or 1:64. CRP tends to increase before the ESR does.

NURSING DIAGNOSIS

Common nursing diagnoses for a patient with RA include:

• Altered role performance related to the crippling effects of RA

• Impaired physical mobility related to joint deformities

• Pain related to joint inflammation

• Activity intolerance related to joint immobility and pain

• Fatigue related to chronic disease and anemia.

PLANNING

Based on the nursing diagnosis *altered role performance,* develop appropriate patient outcomes. For example, your patient will:

• recognize the limitations imposed by RA

• make decisions about the treatment and management of her illness

• function in her usual role within the recognized limitations.

Based on the nursing diagnosis *impaired physical mobility,* develop appropriate patient outcomes. For example, your patient will:

• maintain her maximum muscle strength and ROM

• remain free of complications, such as contractures, skin breakdown, or venous stasis.

Based on the nursing diagnosis *pain,* develop appropriate patient outcomes. For example, your patient will:

• identify pain-relief measures, including appropriate application of heat and cold

• inform you of pain reduction or relief
• exercise to relieve stiffness and pain
• avoid activities that cause or increase joint pain.

Based on the nursing diagnosis *activity intolerance,* develop appropriate patient outcomes. For example, your patient will:
• identify symptoms of activity intolerance
• plan to balance rest with activity
• perform ADLs more independently within limitations, using assistive devices as needed.

Based on the nursing diagnosis *fatigue,* develop appropriate patient outcomes. For example, your patient will:
• verbalize less fatigue
• verbalize the ability to sleep uninterrupted for a minimum of 6 hours. (See *Determining the patient's care needs.*)

IMPLEMENTATION

Make sure your patient understands the importance of complying with her medication and physical rehabilitation programs. (See *Medical care of the patient with rheumatoid arthritis,* page 115.)

Nursing interventions
Adjust your nursing interventions to suit the patient's condition.
• Relieve pain in affected joints with prescribed drugs, heat or cold packs, warm tub baths, or whirlpool baths. Hypnosis, music therapy, and other relaxation techniques may also help.
• Administer medications, as prescribed, and watch for adverse reactions. Monitor therapeutic effectiveness by assessing pain relief and reduced signs of joint inflammation.
• Monitor the duration of morning stiffness.

• Encourage the patient with inflamed knees and hips to rest until the acute episode improves. If her arms are affected, tell her to avoid overuse. This may require you to provide extensive assistance in performing ADLs.
• Implement measures to help prevent flexion contractures, including the use of resting splints. Assist with ROM exercises. Ensure proper body alignment.
• Provide meticulous skin care. Monitor the patient for pressure ulcers and skin breakdown, especially if she's in traction or wearing splints. Use lotion or cleansing oil — not soap — on dry skin.
• As the patient's condition moves to the subacute phase, encourage her to participate in activities. Consult with the physical therapist for recommended exercises. Provide balance between rest and activity.

Timesaving tip: Ask when the patient can best participate in her personal care. Usually, it's later in the morning after stiffness subsides. Also, don't schedule nursing care, exercise, or physical or occupational therapy too closely together because this will exhaust the patient and interfere with her independent participation in activities.
• Encourage a well-balanced diet high in protein, iron, and vitamin C. For a patient with chewing and swallowing limitations, suggest nutrient-dense foods to maximize intake.

Before serving a meal tray, open cartons, remove metal lids, and unwrap utensils. When possible, provide lightweight cups and utensils. Allow sufficient time to eat. If the patient has trouble grasping utensils (as well as pens, toothbrushes, and other thin-handled items), wrap the handles with padding and tape. Ask the

Determining the patient's care needs

After establishing nursing diagnoses and patient outcomes, use the following guide to help you distinguish among different patients' care needs. Category C patients usually need the most intense care.

Physical needs
Category A
• Patient with rheumatoid arthritis (RA) in remission (admitted for another disorder)
• Patient with chronic RA who is capable of independent activities of daily living (ADLs) admitted for another disorder or minor surgery
Category B
• Patient with subacute or chronic RA who can perform ADLs and exercise with some assistance
Category C
• Patient with acute RA or with a major complication of RA
• Patient with crippling joint deformities or with recent joint-replacement surgery

Timesaving measures
Set priorities for your nursing care according to urgency and the patient's need. Delegate and supervise activities when appropriate, and consult with specialists, such as physical and occupational therapists, for help with related care. Also, encourage patient independence whenever possible.

Teaching needs
Category A
• Patient who has adequate knowledge of RA and its management and complies with treatment

Category B
• Patient who requires reeducation in some areas of management
• Patient who has adequate knowledge of RA, but has new teaching needs, such as for planned surgery
Category C
• Patient newly diagnosed with RA
• Patient with significant learning problems
• Patient with a history of RA, but insufficient knowledge

Timesaving measures
To teach effectively in a timely manner, consider group teaching, video tapes, and printed information. Also consider consulting with a home health care nurse to complete the teaching, referring the patient to arthritis organizations, and consulting with the hospital's patient education department.

Emotional needs
Category A
• Patient who accepts the diagnosis and demonstrates adequate coping mechanisms
Category B
• Patient who experiences moderate emotional flare-ups after successful adjustment to illness
Category C
• Patient who experiences severe emotional reaction
• Patient who demonstrates inadequate coping mechanisms

(continued)

Determining the patient's care needs *(continued)*

• Patient with a history of noncompliance based on emotional reactions
• Patient with few or no support systems

Timesaving measures
Build in time for talking with the patient. Consult with a mental health specialist and, if the patient approves, seek other emotional support, such as clergy, self-help groups, and visits from persons who have successfully adjusted to RA.

occupational therapist for other ways to adapt equipment.
• Provide emotional support. Remember that the patient can easily become depressed, discouraged, and irritable. Encourage discussion of her fears about role loss, dependency, disability, sexuality, body image, and self-esteem. Help her to identify positive coping mechanisms and sources of support. Reinforce her strengths and encourage her participation in self-help groups. Refer her for appropriate counseling as needed.
• If the patient is scheduled for joint replacement surgery, provide comprehensive preoperative and postoperative care.
• Begin planning early for discharge. Consult with the social service department to arrange any needed home care services, equipment, and home adaptations, such as installation of ramps.

Patient teaching
• Explain that RA is a chronic disease that may require major changes in lifestyle.

Timesaving tip: Involve all team members in teaching the patient and her family so that you won't need to teach all topics yourself. For example, if the physical therapist explains the exercise program, you can concentrate on encouraging the patient's performance. For consistency, however, you should always be familiar with the topics taught and exercises ordered.
• Explain all diagnostic tests and procedures.
• If the patient requires total knee or hip arthroplasty, she'll need special teaching. (See *Teaching about joint replacement,* pages 116 and 117.)
• Provide information about all prescribed medications, including adverse reactions and precautions.
• Recommend hot showers or baths at bedtime or in the morning to reduce the need for pain medication. Explain the purpose and procedure for using paraffin foot and hand baths.
• Teach the patient how to use splints or other immobilization devices, if needed.
• Emphasize the need for a balanced diet and weight control, since obesity further stresses the joints.
• Teach the patient to maintain erect posture when standing, walking, and sitting. Recommend a raised toilet seat and chairs with high seats and armrests to keep the patient's knees lower than her hips and make rising easier. Describe how to adapt any

Treatments

Medical care of the patient with rheumatoid arthritis

Treatment for a patient with rheumatoid arthritis (RA) consists generally of drug therapy, supportive measures, and surgery.

Drug therapy
Drug therapy is the main treatment for RA. Choice of drugs is contingent upon the disease's progression and severity, how well the patient responds, and, when possible, the patient's preference. Some doctors now advocate aggressive second-line therapy before erosive articular changes occur.

First-line drugs
- Aspirin
- Nonsteroidal anti-inflammatory drugs, including ibuprofen, fenoprofen, naproxen, and indomethacin

Second-line drugs
- Gold salts (oral or parenteral)
- Penicillamine
- Antimalarials, such as hydroxychloroquine
- Corticosteroids (oral, parenteral, or intra-articular injection)
- Immunosuppressants, such as methotrexate sodium, azathioprine, and cyclophosphamide

Methotrexate sodium, commonly replacing highly toxic penicillamine, can result in rapid improvement of symptoms. Azathioprine, an antimetabolite, may be used if the patient doesn't respond to other second-line agents.

Supportive measures
When providing support, consider the following measures:

- increased sleep (8 to 10 hours every night)
- frequent rest periods between daily activities
- splinting to rest inflamed joints (although immobilization may stimulate osteoporosis)
- physical therapy (including individualized range-of-motion exercises and muscle and endurance strengthening) to forestall the loss of joint function
- application of moist heat (such as hot soaks, paraffin baths, and whirlpool baths) to relax muscles and relieve pain in chronic disease
- ice packs for acute episodes.

Surgery
Possible surgery for patients with RA includes:

- metatarsal head and distal ulnar resectional arthroplasty, with insertion of a silastic prosthesis between the metacarpophalangeal and proximal interphalangeal joints
- arthrodesis (joint fusion) to stabilize a joint and relieve pain
- synovectomy (removal of destructive, proliferating synovium), usually in the wrists, fingers, and knees, to halt or delay disease progression
- osteotomy (cutting of bone or excision of a bone wedge) to realign joint surfaces and redistribute stresses
- tendon transfers to prevent deformities and relieve contractures, and surgical repair of tendons that rupture spontaneously
- joint reconstruction or total joint arthroplasty in advanced disease.

Teaching about joint replacement

Your patient may have a joint totally or partially replaced with a synthetic prosthesis to restore stability and relieve pain. Joint replacement may also provide an increased sense of independence and self-worth. The illustrations below depict common joint replacement sites, with the hip and knee the most common.

Hip

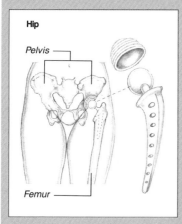

Pelvis

Femur

Knee

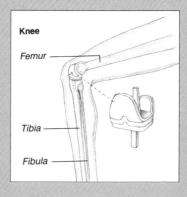

Femur

Tibia

Fibula

Elbow

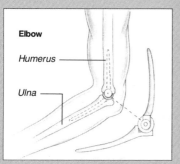

Humerus

Ulna

Shoulder

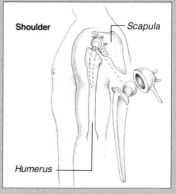

Scapula

Humerus

Preparing the patient for recovery

Explain to the patient that she'll begin an exercise program to maintain joint mobility, even though she's required to remain in bed for up to 6 days. Show her range-of-motion exercises, or demonstrate the continuous-passive-motion device that she'll be using.

If appropriate, teach the patient how to use crutches or a walker. When a patient requires total hip replacement, stress the importance of keeping the affected leg abducted and of avoiding hip flexion. Caution the patient that she may continue to experience pain immediately after surgery, and possibly even an increased level of pain for several weeks. Reassure her that analgesics will be prescribed as needed and that the pain will diminish dramatically after edema subsides.

Preparing the patient for home care
Reinforce the importance of the exercise regimen prescribed by the doctor and physical therapists. Remind the patient to adhere closely to her schedule and not to rush rehabilitation, no matter how well she feels.

Review with the patient her required limitations of activity. Depending on the surgery's location and extent, the doctor may order the patient to avoid bending, lifting, extensive stair climbing, and sitting for prolonged periods. He'll also caution against overusing the joint, especially if it's weight-bearing.

Caution the patient to promptly report signs and symptoms of a possible infection, such as persistent fever and increased pain, tenderness, and stiffness in the joint and surrounding area. Remind her that infection may develop several months after surgery. Also urge her to report a sudden increase in pain, which may indicate dislodgment of the prosthesis.

chair by putting blocks of wood under the legs.
• Caution the patient to pace her daily activities by resting 5 to 10 minutes each hour and alternating sitting and standing tasks. Stress the importance of adequate sleep and correct sleeping posture to avoid flexion deformity, including sleeping on her back on a firm mattress with no pillow under the knees.

Timesaving tip: Ask the occupational therapist to teach the patient how to simplify activities and protect involved joints. The patient should use the largest joint available for a task (for example, closing a door with a hip instead of hands), support weak or painful joints, use extension and avoid flexion, hold objects parallel to the knuckles as briefly as possible, use her hands at the center of her body, and slide — not lift — objects whenever possible.

Timesaving tip: If gripping tools or utensils is a problem, suggest buying foam pipe insulation in various diameters, cutting it to the desired length, and gluing it to handles.
• Reinforce exercises taught by the physical therapist. Provide a handout showing ROM exercises.
• Stress the importance of wearing shoes with proper support.

Timesaving tip: You can save valuable nursing time and promote independence by encouraging the patient to dress herself. Suggest buying dressing aids (a shelf-reacher, a long-handled shoehorn, elastic shoelaces, a zipper pull, and a buttonhook), installing helpful household items (easy-to-open drawers, a hand-held shower nozzle, handrails, and grab bars), and using mittens instead of gloves. Explain to the patient that she can dress more easily while sitting because of better balance.

Discharge TimeSaver

Ensuring continued care for the patient with rheumatoid arthritis

Review the following teaching topics, referrals, and follow-up appointments to make sure that your patient is adequately prepared for discharge.

Teaching topics

Make sure that the following topics have been covered and that your patient's learning has been evaluated:

☐ the nature of the disease, including its remissions, exacerbations, and complications

☐ drug information, including dosages, adverse reactions, and precautions

☐ explanation of apheresis, if ordered

☐ surgical options, when appropriate, and related preoperative, postoperative, and rehabilitation measures

☐ performing activities of daily living independently within limitations, including use of assistive devices if warranted

☐ rest and activity guidelines

☐ exercise program, including use of good body mechanics

☐ pain-relief measures, including application of heat or cold

☐ reduction in physical and emotional stress

☐ sources of information and support

☐ need for follow-up.

Referrals

Make sure that the patient has been provided with necessary referrals to:

☐ social service agencies

☐ physical therapist

☐ occupational therapist

☐ mental health specialist

☐ sex therapist if necessary.

Follow-up appointments

Make sure that the necessary follow-up appointments have been scheduled and that the patient has been notified:

☐ rheumatologist

☐ surgeon

☐ physical therapist

☐ occupational therapist

☐ diagnostic tests for reevaluation.

• Discuss the patient's sexual concerns. If pain interferes with intercourse, suggest alternative positions or using analgesics or moist heat beforehand to increase mobility. If fatigue interferes, suggest that the patient attempt intercourse after she is well rested.

Timesaving tip: You can save teaching time and encourage independence by directing the patient to sources of information and support, such as the College of Rheumatology and the Arthritis Foundation. Also, many cities have local Arthritis Foundation chapters, which sponsor self-help classes. (See *Ensuring continued care for the patient with rheumatoid arthritis*.)

EVALUATION

When evaluating the patient's response to your nursing care, gather reassessment data and compare it with the patient outcomes specified in your plan of care.

Teaching and counseling

Begin by determining the effectiveness of your teaching and counseling. Consider the following questions:

• Do the patient and her family understand the nature of the disorder, its possible complications, and its treatment?

• Do they know the signs and symptoms they should report to the doctor?

• Does the patient show reduced anxiety and sufficient ability to cope?

• Can she perform ADLs independently within limitations, using assistive devices as needed?

Physical condition

If treatment has been successful, you should note the following outcomes:

• The patient makes decisions about the treatment and management of her illness.

• She functions in her usual role within recognized limitations.

• She maintains maximum muscle strength and ROM.

• She remains free of complications, such as contractures, skin breakdown, or venous stasis.

• She identifies pain-relief measures, including appropriate application of heat and cold, and informs you of pain reduction or relief.

• She exercises to relieve stiffness and pain and avoids activities that cause or increase joint pain.

• She identifies symptoms of activity intolerance and shows a willingness to balance rest with activity.

Systemic lupus erythematosus

An inflammatory autoimmune disorder, systemic lupus erythematosus (SLE) affects connective tissues and organs throughout the body, including the skin. Discoid lupus erythematosus, a milder form, usually affects only the skin. SLE is characterized by recurrent seasonal remissions and exacerbations. Lack of a characteristic clinical pattern complicates the diagnosis. (See *Diagnosing systemic lupus erythematosus,* page 120.)

Although the survival rate has improved dramatically in the last decade, SLE can be fatal. Causes of death include renal failure, cardiac disease, and central nervous system (CNS) involvement. Other complications may include hemolytic anemia and pulmonary hemorrhage. (See *Key points about systemic lupus erythematosus,* page 121.)

Causes

SLE's cause remains unknown, but evidence points to interrelated immune, environmental, hormonal, and genetic factors. The primary cause appears to be autoimmunity, in which the patient's immune system produces antibodies directed against his own body. Although these autoantibodies usually affect nucleic acids, they may also target erythrocytes, platelets, phospholipids, lymphocytes, neuronal cells, coagulation proteins, and other factors.

Predisposing factors

SLE may be associated with certain predisposing factors, such as stress, streptococcal or viral infection, exposure to sunlight or ultraviolet light, immunization, pregnancy, and abnormal estrogen metabolism. The use of certain drugs may also provoke a lupus-like syndrome. (See *Drug-induced lupus-like syndrome,* page 122). A higher incidence of SLE occurs in identical twins and certain families, pointing to a genetic predisposition.

Diagnosing systemic lupus erythematosus

Diagnosing systemic lupus erythematosus (SLE) is far from easy because the disease often mimics other disorders. Signs may be vague and may vary from patient to patient. For these reasons, the American Rheumatism Association has devised criteria for identifying SLE. Usually, four or more of the following signs must appear at some time for a diagnosis of SLE:
• discoid rash
• facial erythema (butterfly rash)
• hematologic abnormality, such as hemolytic anemia, leukopenia, lymphopenia, or thrombocytopenia
• immune dysfunction, which may be identified by the following test results: positive lupus erythematosus cell test or anti-deoxyribonucleic acid antibody test, or false-positive tests for syphilis for more than 6 months
• neurologic disorder
• nonerosive arthritis
• oral or nasopharyngeal ulcers
• photosensitivity
• positive antinuclear antibody test results in the absence of drugs known to cause lupus-like syndrome
• renal disorder, such as persistent proteinuria of more than 0.5 g per day
• serositis.

ASSESSMENT

Your assessment should include a careful consideration of the patient's health history, physical examination findings, and diagnostic test results.

Health history

Onset of SLE may be acute or insidious. The patient may complain of nonspecific signs and symptoms, such as a low-grade fever (99° to 100.4° F [37.2° to 38° C]), anorexia, weight loss, malaise, and fatigue. Or she may report specific signs and symptoms related to the involved site, such as swollen joints, pain on movement, morning stiffness, myalgia, the symptoms of Raynaud's phenomenon (blanching, cyanosis, and erythema of the fingers and toes), rash, alopecia, hematuria, oliguria, abdominal pain, chest pain, and dyspnea.

Ask the patient about irregular menstruation or amenorrhea, particularly during flare-ups of SLE. Watch for neuropsychiatric symptoms, such as anxiety, depression, emotional instability, and confusion.

Also ask if sunlight and fluorescent and ultraviolet light provoke or aggravate skin eruptions. Additionally, inquire about any recent physical and emotional stress factors, including surgery, infection, injury, possible pregnancy, and emotional upset, that may have precipitated the disease.

Ask the patient's family members whether she has exhibited any of the typical neurologic signs, such as seizures, psychoses, emotional instability, or irritability.

Watch for medications that may cause a lupus-like syndrome, and be sure to note any sign of infection, especially in the patient receiving immunosuppressive drugs. Check the family history for a predisposition to SLE.

Assess what coping strategies and sources of support are available to your patient and what psychological, social, and financial effects SLE

FactFinder

Key points about systemic lupus erythematosus

- More than 95% of patients with systemic lupus erythematosus (SLE) survive at least 5 years after diagnosis.
- SLE can occur as a fulminant disease, but more commonly occurs as a chronic disorder with remissions and exacerbations.
- SLE does not follow a set course. Patients experience varying signs and symptoms and different rates of disease progression.
- Evidence indicates that SLE occurs nine times more often in women than in men and 30 times more often in women of child-bearing age than in other women.
- SLE occurs more commonly in blacks.

---

might have on the patient and her family.

Physical examination

Observe the patient for skin lesions that appear as an erythematous rash when exposed to light. The rash may vary in severity from malar erythema to discoid lesions (plaque); the classic sign of lupus erythematosus — a butterfly rash over the nose and cheeks — appears in less than 50% of patients. You may see ulcers on the mucous membranes that the patient reports as painless. Peripheral vascular involvement may produce skin redness, ulcers, lesions, or gangrene. Pallor accompanies anemia, and bruises and abnormal bleeding may indicate thrombocytopenia. Patchy alopecia is common.

Joint involvement may produce hand and foot deformities and impaired mobility. Pulmonary involvement alters breathing patterns and induces dyspnea. Peripheral and periorbital edema indicate kidney involvement.

Palpation reveals lymph node enlargement that's either diffuse or local and nontender. You may detect hepatomegaly and splenomegaly. Auscultation may reveal cardiopulmonary abnormalities, such as pericardial friction rub, tachycardia, myocarditis, endocarditis, hypertension, and pleural friction rub.

Diagnostic test results

The following tests may reveal factors that indicate SLE:

- A complete blood count with differential may show anemia and reduced white blood cell (WBC) and platelet counts during active disease.
- The erythrocyte sedimentation rate usually signals inflammation.
- Serum electrophoresis may detect hypergammaglobulinemia.
- Autoantibody tests may reveal various antibodies, including antinuclear, anti–double-stranded deoxyribonucleic acid (ds DNA), anti–single-stranded DNA (ss DNA), and anti-ribonucleoprotein (RNP).
- Serum complement tests may show reduced $C1$, $C2$, and $C4$ levels and increased $C5$ to $C9$ levels during active disease.

Drug-induced lupus-like syndrome

Nearly 25 drugs can cause a reaction similar to systemic lupus erythematosus.

Commonly implicated drugs
The most commonly implicated drugs include procainamide, hydralazine, isoniazid, phenytoin, and other anticonvulsants. Less commonly implicated drugs include penicillins, sulfa drugs, oral contraceptives, chlorpromazine, primidone, quinidine, reserpine, streptomycin, and tetracycline.

Clinical features
Keep in mind that drug-induced lupus-like syndrome usually has mild clinical features, such as skin rash, fever, and arthralgia, but not kidney or central nervous system involvement. Symptoms usually resolve when the medication in question is discontinued and the patient receives a brief course of corticosteroid therapy.

• Urine studies may reveal red blood cells (RBCs), WBCs, urine casts, sediment, and significant protein loss (more than 3.5 g in 24 hours).
• Chest X-rays can disclose cardiomegaly, pleurisy, platelike atelectasis, or lupus pneumonitis.
• Electrocardiogram can show a conduction defect with cardiac involvement or pericarditis.
• Renal biopsy can show the extent of renal involvement, which occurs in 50% of patients with SLE. Biopsy

also can reveal the progression of SLE.
• Skin biopsy commonly shows disposition of immunoglobulins (IgG and IgM) and complement.

NURSING DIAGNOSIS
Common nursing diagnoses for a patient with SLE include:
• Body image disturbance related to chronic skin eruption and altered body functioning
• Impaired physical mobility related to chronic inflammation of connective tissue
• Pain related to chronic inflammation of connective tissue
• Activity intolerance related to chronic anemia, pain, and multiorgan involvement
• Altered protection related to autoimmune disease and associated drug therapy.

PLANNING
Based on the nursing diagnosis *body image disturbance,* develop appropriate patient outcomes. For example, your patient will:
• acknowledge a change in body image
• express positive feelings about herself.
Based on the nursing diagnosis *impaired physical mobility,* develop appropriate patient outcomes. For example, your patient will:
• perform activities of daily living (ADLs) independently within limitations
• show no evidence of complications, such as contractures, thrombus formation, or pressure ulcer formation.
Based on the nursing diagnosis *pain,* develop appropriate patient outcomes. For example, your patient will:

• inform you of reduced pain.

Based on the nursing diagnosis *activity intolerance,* develop appropriate patient outcomes. For example, your patient will:

• identify symptoms of activity intolerance

• discuss plans to balance rest periods with activity in daily routine

• express need for bed rest during an acute flare-up

• perform ADLs without undue fatigue, dyspnea, or pain.

Based on the nursing diagnosis *altered protection,* develop appropriate patient outcomes. For example, your patient will:

• express intent to comply with the treatment regimen to control as much tissue damage as possible

• discuss plans to reduce or avoid factors known to precipitate flare-ups

• acknowledge the need to notify the doctor promptly of recurring symptoms of SLE or infection.

IMPLEMENTATION

Focus your nursing care on monitoring drug therapy and helping the patient adjust to body changes, reduced mobility and activity levels, and pain. (See *Medical care of the patient with systemic lupus erythematosus,* page 124.)

Nursing interventions

When caring for the SLE patient, institute the following measures:

• Continually assess for signs and symptoms of organ involvement.

• Encourage the patient to discuss feelings about body image and to participate in social activities and self-help groups.

• Monitor for decreased urine output, hypertension, weight gain, and other signs of renal involvement.

• Assess for possible neurologic damage signaled by personality changes, paranoid or psychotic behavior, depression, ptosis, and diplopia. Consult with a psychiatric or neurologic specialist as needed.

• Check urine, stools, and GI secretions for blood. Check the scalp for hair loss. Check skin and mucous membranes for petechiae, bleeding, ulceration, pallor, and bruising.

• Encourage the patient to perform good oral hygiene, including rinsing with 0.9% sodium chloride solution or a water–hydrogen peroxide mixture.

• Consult with a dietary specialist to provide a balanced diet. Protein, vitamins, and iron help prevent anemia. Renal involvement may mandate a low-sodium, low-protein diet. Bland, cool foods are best if the patient has a sore mouth.

• Urge the patient to get plenty of rest, and schedule diagnostic tests and procedures accordingly.

• Explain all tests and procedures, including the need for periodic blood samples to monitor progress.

• Apply heat packs to relieve joint pain and stiffness. Administer analgesics as prescribed.

• Encourage regular exercise to maintain full range of motion and to prevent contractures. When SLE isn't fulminant, encourage ambulation three to four times a day. If the patient is bedridden, reposition her every 2 hours.

• Administer medications and monitor for adverse effects, especially when giving high doses of corticosteroids or nonsteroidal anti-inflammatory drugs.

• Institute seizure precautions if you suspect CNS involvement.

Timesaving tip: Seek others' help in solving the problems caused by joint involvement. Ar-

Treatments

Medical care of the patient with systemic lupus erythematosus

Caring for the patient with systemic lupus erythematosus (SLE) involves drug therapy and other treatments.

Drug therapy

The mainstay of medical care for SLE is drug therapy. The patient with a mild case requires little or no medication, but the patient with severe, multisystem involvement may require corticosteroids or cytotoxic drugs.

• Aspirin is usually used to control arthritis and arthralgia symptoms when other organs are not involved.

• Nonsteroidal anti-inflammatory drugs, such as indomethacin, may also be used, but cautiously in the presence of renal involvement.

• Corticosteroids, especially prednisone, remain the treatment of choice for systemic symptoms, acute generalized exacerbations, and serious disease-related injury to vital organ systems from pleuritis, pericarditis, nephritis, vasculitis, and central nervous system involvement. Initial prednisone doses of 60 mg or more can markedly improve the patient's condition within 48 hours. With symptoms under control, the patient can slowly be weaned from prednisone. Remember, any amount of a corticosteroid administered in divided doses throughout the day has more adrenal-suppressing activity, and thus lupus-suppressing activity, than the same amount given in a single oral dose.

• Topical corticosteroid creams, such as triamcinolone and hydrocortisone, may be administered for skin lesions.

• Fluorinated steroids may control acute or discoid lesions. Refractory skin lesions may respond to intralesional or systemic corticosteroids or antimalarials, such as hydroxychloroquine and chloroquine. However, these drugs require that the patient have an ophthalmologic examination every 6 months to monitor for retinal damage. Antimalarials are also used for arthralgia.

• In some patients, chemotherapeutic immunosuppressants, such as azathioprine, cyclophosphamide, and methotrexate, may be used to suppress the immune response. They are typically used only when corticosteroids are ineffective because these immunosuppressants can cause serious adverse effects and complications.

• Intravenous cyclophosphamide is currently being used to treat lupus nephritis.

• Warfarin is indicated for antiphospholipid antibodies, which can cause clotting in vascular structures.

Other treatments

• Helpful dietary changes include a sodium-restricted diet if the patient is taking corticosteroids; high-protein, high-complex carbohydrates; and daily multivitamins with iron.

• If renal failure occurs despite treatment, dialysis, hemofiltration, or kidney transplantation may be needed.

• Physical therapy may relieve musculoskeletal discomfort. If chronic synovitis and pain remain a problem, joint replacement may be indicated.

• Bed rest is prescribed during an acute flare-up.

• Plasmapheresis may be performed to remove immune complexes from the blood.

range physical and occupational therapy consultations if musculoskeletal involvement compromises the patient's mobility and independent performance of ADLs.

• Support the patient's self-image. Suggest hypoallergenic cosmetics, hair care products, and shaving products. Refer to a hair stylist who specializes in scalp disorders if needed. Discourage use of hair dryers, which will further damage already thin, fragile hair.

Patient teaching

Include the following in your teaching program:

• Describe SLE, its treatment, and its complications.

• Instruct the patient about prescribed medications, including possible adverse reactions.

• Enlist the occupational therapist to discuss equipment adaptations that will allow the patient to remain independent.

• Teach the patient how to take her own temperature and to report any fever immediately because fever may indicate a flare-up or infection. Advise her to notify the doctor if fever, cough, oliguria, dysuria, or rash occurs or if fatigue or chest, abdominal, muscle, or joint pain worsens.

• Arrange for the physical therapist to teach an exercise program to the patient with joint involvement.

• Help the patient plan ways to balance rest periods with activity. Recommend about 10 hours of sleep nightly.

• Teach the patient about factors that may precipitate a flare-up, and help her identify ways to reduce or avoid them. Encourage her to maintain a stable, calm environment, and to practice relaxation exercises and other stress-reduction techniques.

• Teach the patient ways to avoid infection, including avoiding crowds and people with known infections.

• Tell the photosensitive patient to wear protective clothing and use a sunscreen when outdoors and to avoid undue exposure to the sun. Recommend using a sunscreen with a skin protection factor of at least 15. Tell the patient to avoid prolonged exposure even to fluorescent lighting.

• Instruct the patient with Raynaud's phenomenon to protect her feet and hands in cold weather and to use an oven mitt to remove items from a freezer.

• Teach the patient to perform meticulous mouth care to relieve discomfort and prevent infection.

• Provide birth control information as needed. Instruct the female patient to use a diaphragm and foam instead of oral contraceptives or intrauterine devices.

• Because pregnancy may exacerbate SLE and increase the risk of miscarriage and stillbirth, advise the female patient to discuss pregnancy plans with the doctor before trying to conceive.

• Teach the importance of keeping follow-up appointments.

• Refer the patient to the Lupus Foundation of America, the Arthritis Foundation, and local SLE support groups as necessary. (See *Ensuring continued care for the patient with systemic lupus erythematosus,* page 126.)

EVALUATION

When evaluating the patient's response to your nursing care, gather reassessment data and compare this information with the patient outcomes specified in your plan of care. (See *Assessing failure to respond to therapy in systemic lupus erythematosus,* page 127.)

Discharge TimeSaver

Ensuring continued care for the patient with systemic lupus erythematosus

Review the following teaching topics, referrals, and follow-up appointments to make sure that your patient is adequately prepared for discharge.

Teaching topics
Make sure that the following topics have been covered and that your patient's learning has been evaluated:
□ the nature of the disease, including remissions, exacerbations, and complications
□ medication information, including adverse reactions and necessary precautions
□ apheresis, if ordered
□ signs and symptoms that warrant an immediate call to the doctor
□ skin care
□ performing activities of daily living independently
□ rest and activity guidelines
□ infection prevention
□ pregnancy and family planning

□ avoidance of precipitating factors
□ sources of information and support.

Referrals
Make sure that the patient has been provided with necessary referrals to:
□ social service agencies
□ occupational therapist
□ physical therapist
□ mental health specialist.

Follow-up appointments
Make sure that the necessary follow-up appointments have been scheduled and that the patient has been notified:
□ doctor
□ diagnostic tests for reevaluation.

Teaching and counseling

Begin by determining the effectiveness of your teaching. Consider the following questions.
• Does the patient understand the need for complying with her treatment?
• Has she discussed plans to reduce factors known to precipitate SLE?
• Has she acknowledged the need to notify the doctor promptly if signs and symptoms of SLE or infection recur?
• Can she identify the signs and symptoms of infection and measures of prevention?
• How is she coping with changes in body image?

• Has she expressed positive feelings about herself?
• Does she report less pain?
• Can she identify symptoms of activity intolerance?
• Has she discussed plans to balance rest periods with activity in her daily routine?
• Is she aware of the need for bed rest during an acute flare-up?

Physical condition

Consider the following questions:
• Can your patient perform ADLs independently within limitations?
• Is she free of complications, such as contractures, thrombus formation, and pressure ulcer formation?

Evaluation TimeSaver

Assessing failure to respond to therapy in systemic lupus erythematosus

If your patient fails to respond to interventions, the following checklist can help you evaluate the reasons. When performing the evaluation, consult with the patient, doctor, and members of the health care team. The doctor can evaluate drug therapy if necessary. Remember, although optimum treatment and full compliance offer the best hope for successful disease management, flare-ups and complications are still possible.

Factors interfering with compliance
☐ Unclear instructions
☐ Failure to provide written instructions
☐ Inadequate patient teaching
☐ Neurologic symptoms due to systemic lupus erythematosus, such as loss of memory, disorientation, and impaired thinking
☐ Emotional instability
☐ Inability to afford medication
☐ Inability to tolerate adverse effects of medication
☐ Inconvenient medication administration schedule

Factors interfering with drug therapy
☐ Insufficient dosage
☐ Renal involvement interfering with drug elimination
☐ Predisposition to rapid drug metabolism
☐ Prescribed or over-the-counter drugs that cause lupus-like syndrome

Conditions interfering with treatment
☐ Infection
☐ Exhaustion
☐ Emotional stress
☐ Unprotected exposure to sunlight or excessive exposure to fluorescent light

Systemic sclerosis

Also called systemic scleroderma, systemic sclerosis is a chronic connective tissue disorder. It causes degeneration in the skin, blood vessels, synovial membranes, skeletal muscles, and various internal organs. Although similar to systemic lupus erythematosus, systemic sclerosis is unpredictable and gradually incapacitating and has a higher mortality. (See *Key points about systemic sclerosis,* page 128.)

Advanced systemic sclerosis can cause cardiac or pulmonary fibrosis, which can lead to respiratory or congestive heart failure. Renal involvement is common and usually results in malignant hypertension. Cardiomyopathy, bowel obstruction or perforation, and aspiration pneumonia are other possible complications.

Localized scleroderma, a more benign form, mainly affects the skin.

Causes
Although systemic sclerosis may result from autoimmunity, its exact cause is unknown.

FactFinder
Key points about systemic sclerosis

- Systemic sclerosis is twice as common in women as in men and usually affects persons from ages 30 to 50.
- It occurs in two distinct forms: limited subcutaneous scleroderma (CREST syndrome) and diffuse subcutaneous scleroderma.
- The acronym CREST stands for these symptoms: **C**alcinosis cutis, **R**aynaud's phenomenon, **e**sophageal dysfunction, **s**clerodactyly, and **t**elangiectasia.
- CREST syndrome accounts for 80% of cases.
- Diffuse systemic sclerosis, which accounts for 20% of cases, is marked by generalized skin thickening and invasion of internal organ systems. The prognosis is generally worse than with CREST syndrome.

ASSESSMENT

Your assessment should consider the patient's health history, physical examination findings, and diagnostic test results.

Health history
Months or even years before diagnosis, most patients complain of symptoms of Raynaud's phenomenon, such as blanching, cyanosis, and erythema of the fingers and toes. Later, the patient may complain of pain, stiffness, joint swelling, fatigue, and weakness.

Eventually, the patient may report frequent reflux, heartburn, dysphagia, and bloating after meals. Additional GI complaints include fibrosis, malabsorption, abdominal distention, diarrhea, constipation, and malodorous floating stools. Other findings include anorexia and weight loss, dyspnea on exertion and, with myocardial fibrosis, palpitations and dizziness.

Timesaving tip: First assess your patient's ability to perform daily activities to help you tailor your interventions and teaching efficiently. Next, assess the patient's coping mechanisms, sources of support, and any limitations imposed on her lifestyle.

Physical examination
Observe the patient's general appearance. Note early skin changes, such as edema that mainly affects the hands. (See *Early skin changes in systemic sclerosis*.)

Also note fibrosis that causes the skin to thicken, harden, and appear leathery. Facial skin may appear tight and inelastic, with a masklike appearance and a pinched mouth. You may also observe telangiectasis and areas of pigmentation and depigmentation.

Examine the patient's joints for contractures that can limit range of motion (ROM). Look for shortening of the patient's fingers (caused by progressive phalangeal resorption) and slow-healing ulcers on the fingertips or toes.

Expect to find dyspnea and decreased breath sounds or dependent crackles with pulmonary involvement. An irregular cardiac rhythm, a pericardial friction rub, and an atrial gallop may occur with cardiac involvement. Hypertension may signal renal involvement.

Diagnostic test results
The following tests are commonly used to detect systemic sclerosis:

• Blood studies can show mild anemia, a slightly elevated erythrocyte sedimentation rate, hypergammaglobulinemia, rheumatoid factor in 25% to 35% of patients, and a positive antinuclear antibody test in most patients. Elevated levels of blood urea nitrogen and serum creatinine may indicate renal involvement.

• Urinalysis may reveal proteinuria, microscopic hematuria, and casts.

• X-rays may show terminal phalangeal tuft resorption, subcutaneous calcification, and joint space erosion. Chest and GI X-rays can detect pulmonary and GI complications.

• Pulmonary function studies may reveal decreased diffusion, vital capacity, and lung compliance.

• Electrocardiogram may detect changes related to myocardial fibrosis.

• Skin biopsy may show marked thickening of the dermis and occlusive vessel changes.

NURSING DIAGNOSIS

Common diagnoses for a patient with systemic sclerosis include:

• Altered peripheral tissue perfusion related to exposure to cold and compromised circulation

• Altered protection related to adverse effects of immunosuppressive therapy

• Ineffective individual coping related to the effects of chronic, progressive disease

• Impaired skin integrity related to ulcerations and skin changes

• Altered nutrition: less than body requirements, related to anorexia and GI changes.

PLANNING

Based on the nursing diagnosis *altered peripheral tissue perfusion,* de-

Early skin changes in systemic sclerosis

Early in the course of systemic sclerosis, edematous changes occur as shown below. Later, the skin thickens and hardens, and contractures may occur. Accompanying ulcerations can lead to gangrene.

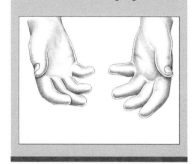

velop appropriate patient outcomes. For example, your patient will:

• show no severe tissue ischemia or gangrene

• identify and try to avoid factors that cause ischemia, such as cold and stress

• have pain-free extremities, especially fingers.

Based on the nursing diagnosis *altered protection,* develop appropriate patient outcomes. For example, your patient will:

• identify and promptly report signs and symptoms of complications

• remain free of secondary infection.

Based on the nursing diagnosis *ineffective individual coping,* develop appropriate patient outcomes. For example, your patient will:

• identify strategies to improve coping

• contact appropriate community support agencies.

Based on the nursing diagnosis *impaired skin integrity,* develop appropriate patient outcomes. For example, your patient will:
• demonstrate skill in caring for skin ulcerations
• regain skin integrity.

Based on the nursing diagnosis *altered nutrition: less than body requirements,* develop appropriate patient outcomes. For example, your patient will:
• consume a large amount of calories daily
• modify her diet to include soft or easily masticated foods to ease swallowing
• maintain normal body weight.

IMPLEMENTATION

Treatment consists primarily of supportive measures aimed at limiting the complications of the illness. (See *Medical care of the patient with systemic sclerosis.*)

Nursing interventions
• Regularly assess extremities, especially the fingers, for adequate peripheral perfusion.
• Provide gloves or mittens after warming therapy.
• Use plaster wraps or topical ointments to ease the pain of digital ulcerations.
• Assess ROM of all joints. Consult with the physical therapist and occupational therapist as needed.
• Monitor vital signs, daily weight, liquid intake and output, and urinary protein.
• Provide rest and pulmonary exercises if the patient has myocardial and pulmonary fibrosis. Coughing, deep breathing, and postural drainage and percussion will help clear the lungs.

• Consult with the dietitian to provide a nutritious, high-calorie diet that's smooth and palatable.
• Offer the patient small, frequent meals. Have her sit up after eating if she suffers from delayed gastric emptying.
• Treat GI disturbances with antacids and antidiarrheals as needed.
• Administer prescribed drugs, and monitor for effectiveness and adverse reactions.
• Let the patient participate in her own treatment. Allow her, for instance, to measure liquid intake and output and plan her diet.
• Help the patient and her family identify coping strategies and obtain support in the community.

Timesaving tip: You'll need to counsel the patient to help her adjust to living with a chronic, progressive disease. Before you do, consult with the psychiatric clinical nurse specialist to help you provide more effective and efficient nursing care.

Patient teaching
• Teach the patient and her family about the disease, its complications, and its treatment.

Timesaving tip: Assess your patient's knowledge of systemic sclerosis, and focus your teaching only on new or poorly understood areas. Involve other health care team members in patient teaching.
• Instruct her about all prescribed medications, including precautions and adverse reactions. Explain that drugs can relieve symptoms but can't cure the disorder.
• Reinforce the daily ROM exercise program taught by the physical therapist. (See *Performing facial exercises,* page 132.)
• Teach the patient to protect herself against cold. Warn her to avoid air

Treatments

Medical care of the patient with systemic sclerosis

Because no cure exists for systemic sclerosis, therapy is supportive. Your role is to treat symptoms and teach your patient to adjust to lifestyle changes.

Drug therapy

Administration of the following drugs may ease many of the symptoms of systemic sclerosis:

• Calcium channel blockers, such as nifedipine and diltiazem; direct vasodilators, such as hydralazine and topical nitrates; and sympatholytic agents, such as prazosin and methyldopa, may be prescribed to relieve severe symptoms of Raynaud's phenomenon.

• Nonsteroidal anti-inflammatory drugs (NSAIDs), such as ibuprofen and indomethacin, may be used for joint pain and swelling. However, NSAIDs should not be used in patients with renal disease.

• Corticosteroids in large doses are usually prescribed for pericarditis or inflammatory myopathy and for patients who don't respond to NSAIDs.

• Chemotherapeutic immunosuppressants, such as chlorambucil, azathioprine, cyclophosphamide, and methotrexate, are often used in large doses to help relieve symptoms of immune disorders generally.

• Antihypertensives, such as methyldopa, are prescribed for malignant hypertension. If hypertensive crisis develops, an angiotensin-converting enzyme inhibitor, such as enalapril maleate, may be prescribed.

• Antacids and histamine$_2$-receptor antagonists, such as omeprazole, cimetidine, and ranitidine, are used for heartburn and to protect the esophageal mucosa from acidic damage during reflux.

• GI stimulants, such as metoclopramide, are indicated to increase gastric emptying and to treat esophageal reflux.

Other therapies

The following therapies may be used to treat the effects of systemic sclerosis and to help the patient adjust to limitations imposed by the disease:

• Physical therapy can help preserve joint function and prevent contractures.

• Debridement is indicated for chronic finger ulcerations.

• Sympathectomy can relieve vascular symptoms.

• Resectioning the bowel or intestines can remove obstructions and repair perforations.

• Esophageal dilatation can treat esophagitis with stricture.

• Dialysis can provide life support in cases of malignant hypertension and renal failure.

• Plasmapheresis can remove the autoimmune component.

conditioning, cool showers and baths, and the use of cold running water to clean food or wash items. Stress the need to wear gloves outside, even in mild weather, and inside if needed.

Teaching TimeSaver

Performing facial exercises

By doing facial exercises, your patient can help keep facial muscles strong and toned at the same time. Instruct your patient to begin the daily facial exercise routine as directed below.

Exercising the mouth
Tell the patient to open his mouth wide, as if to say "ah." Then, have him round his lips as if to say "ooh." Finally, instruct him to close his mouth and smile as widely as possible.

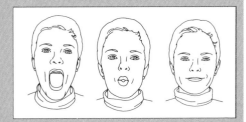

Exercising the cheeks
Have your patient begin by closing his lips and puffing up his cheeks. Tell him to hold this position, count to five, and then slowly blow out the air.

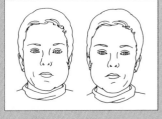

Next, he should suck in his cheeks. Instruct him to hold this position, count to five, and then relax.

To teach the next exercise, tell the patient to puff up one cheek with air, then swish the air to the other cheek without letting the air escape through the lips. He should alternate from one side to the other several times, then relax.

Exercising the lips
Instruct the patient to take a deep breath. With his lips just slightly apart, have him blow air out through his mouth, causing the lips to flap and make a vibrating sound.

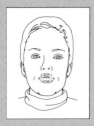

• Explain that smoking can trigger Raynaud's phenomenon. If the patient needs help quitting, refer her to her doctor, to effective group programs, or to the American Lung As-

Discharge TimeSaver

Ensuring continued care for the patient with systemic sclerosis

Review the following teaching topics, referrals, and follow-up appointments to make sure that your patient is adequately prepared for discharge.

Teaching topics
Make sure that the following topics have been covered and that your patient's learning has been evaluated:
☐ the nature of the disease, including its unpredictability and complications
☐ drug information, including adverse reactions and necessary precautions
☐ explanation of plasmapheresis, surgery, or dialysis if ordered
☐ explanation of signs and symptoms to report immediately to the doctor
☐ skin care measures
☐ performing activities of daily living independently within limitations
☐ rest and activity guidelines
☐ diet and measures for easing swallowing difficulties
☐ infection prevention

☐ avoidance of factors that precipitate Raynaud's phenomenon
☐ sources of information and support
☐ need for follow-up.

Referrals
Make sure the patient has been provided with necessary referrals to:
☐ social service agencies
☐ occupational therapist
☐ physical therapist
☐ mental health specialist
☐ dietitian.

Follow-up appointments
Make sure that the necessary follow-up appointments have been scheduled and that the patient has been notified:
☐ doctor
☐ surgeon if warranted
☐ diagnostic tests for reevaluation.

sociation or American Cancer Society.
• Teach stress management techniques. Help the patient pace activities and schedule periods of rest and exercise.
• Instruct the patient about daily skin care measures.
• Teach the patient to recognize and report signs of infection. Advise her to avoid people with active infections, especially upper respiratory tract infections.
• Help the patient plan a high-calorie diet if she's losing weight. Tell her to

avoid dietary supplements, which may cause diarrhea, and to monitor her weight weekly. (See *Ensuring continued care for the patient with systemic sclerosis.*)
• Advise the patient with GI involvement to avoid late-night meals and to sit up during and following meals. Tell her to cut her food into small pieces and to eat soft foods. Stress the importance of eating slowly. Explain that prescribed antacids and histamine$_2$-receptor antagonists will reduce the incidence of reflux.

• Teach the patient how to monitor her blood pressure, and tell her to report blood pressure elevations.
• Refer the patient to the National Kidney Foundation's local support group if she needs dialysis. Explain that she may have to permanently limit certain foods and liquids. Reassure her that dialysis can be done in the home or nearby.
• Have the patient contact the following organizations as needed: the Scleroderma Federation, the Scleroderma Research Foundation, or the United Scleroderma Foundation.

EVALUATION

When evaluating the patient's response to your nursing care, compare your reassessment data with the patient outcomes specified in your plan of care.

Teaching and counseling
To determine the effectiveness of your teaching, consider the following questions:
• Can the patient list ways to improve coping abilities?
• Can she explain her treatment, including precautions?
• Will she discuss her feelings about the disease and treatment?
• Has she contacted appropriate community support agencies?
• Has she learned to ingest a high level of calories daily to maintain normal body weight?
• Is her diet modified to ease swallowing?

Physical condition
Consider the following questions:
• Is the patient free of severe tissue ischemia and gangrene?
• Can she identify and avoid factors that cause ischemic tissue changes, such as cold and stress?

• Are her extremities, especially fingers, free of pain?
• Can she identify early signs and symptoms of complications?
• Is she free of secondary infection?
• Has she shown skill in caring for skin ulcerations and can she perform skin care measures?
• Has she regained general skin integrity?

Autoimmune thrombocytopenic purpura

Also known as idiopathic thrombocytopenic purpura, this form of thrombocytopenia results from platelet destruction. It's the most common cause of hemorrhagic disorders.

Initially, hemorrhage is a major complication. Although rare, cerebral hemorrhage may occur. Potentially fatal purpuric lesions can occur in vital organs, such as the brain and kidneys. Sensory and motor impairments and pain can occur from a hematoma that exerts pressure on nervous system structures. (See *Key points about autoimmune thrombocytopenic purpura.*)

Causes
Autoantibodies that reduce the life span of platelets appear in nearly all patients with autoimmune thrombocytopenic purpura. The disorder's acute form usually follows a viral infection, such as rubella or chicken pox, but can also follow immunization with a live vaccine. The chronic form is often linked with other immunologic disorders, such as systemic lupus erythematosus.

Autoimmune thrombocytopenic purpura commonly results from human immunodeficiency virus (HIV) infection. It can be the initial sign of

FactFinder
Key points about autoimmune thrombocytopenic purpura

• This disorder occurs in acute and chronic forms. The acute form usually affects children from ages 2 to 6, whereas the chronic form mainly affects adults, usually women, under age 50.

• The prognosis for the acute form is excellent. Nearly 4 out of 5 patients recover completely without specific treatment.

• The prognosis for the chronic form varies and can depend on the presence of other serious conditions. Transient remissions can last weeks or even years, especially among women. But sometimes the symptoms and abnormalities can last for years, except for occasional, brief remissions of purpura. A splenectomy usually results in a permanent remission of this disorder.

HIV infection or a complication of fully developed acquired immunodeficiency syndrome.

ASSESSMENT

Your assessment should consider the patient's health history, physical examination findings, and diagnostic test results.

Health history
The patient usually reports that she bruises easily. Epistaxis, oral bleeding, and menorrhagia may be present, as well as rectal bleeding, hematuria, and prolonged bleeding after minor abrasions. The patient may also complain of generalized weakness and fatigue.

Check for previous viral infection or recent immunization. Ask if the patient or her family has a history of autoimmune disorders. Note any risk factors for HIV infection.

Inquire about the recent use of medications that may decrease platelet aggregation, including aspirin, aspirin-containing products, and non-steroidal anti-inflammatory drugs

(NSAIDs). Also ask about the use of quinine, quinidine, sulfonamides, digitoxin, carbamazepine, heparin, indomethacin, rifampin, and methyldopa, which all may cause thrombocytopenia.

Ask how the disease has affected your patient's lifestyle. Note behavioral changes, such as abandonment of activities and exercise intolerance.

Physical examination
Observe the patient's general appearance. Note if she has mucous membrane bleeding or petechiae, ecchymoses, or hematomas on the arms, legs, or chest. Check for signs of elevated intracranial pressure (ICP), such as altered level of consciousness and pupillary changes. Watch for splenomegaly and hepatomegaly. Take vital signs, noting especially hypotension and tachycardia.

Diagnostic test results
The following tests and findings often help confirm diagnosis of autoimmune thrombocytopenic purpura:

• A platelet count that is less than 100,000/mm^3 and prolonged bleed-

ing time with normal coagulation time. Hemoglobin and hematocrit may be low if bleeding has occurred. Antiplatelet antibodies may be observed.
• Increased capillary fragility.
• Bone marrow studies with an increased number of megakaryocytes (platelet precursors).

NURSING DIAGNOSIS

Common diagnoses for a patient with autoimmune thrombocytopenic purpura include:
• Altered protection related to decreased platelet count
• High risk for infection related to immunosuppression from drug therapy or autoimmune disease
• Fear related to the risk of bleeding and the need for splenectomy.

PLANNING

Based on the nursing diagnosis *altered protection,* develop appropriate patient outcomes. For example, your patient will:
• remain free from injury
• comply with the treatment regimen prescribed to boost her platelet count
• take bleeding precautions routinely
• know the warning signs of increased bleeding.
  Based on the nursing diagnosis *high risk for infection,* develop appropriate patient outcomes. For example, your patient will:
• maintain a normal white blood cell (WBC) count
• list ways to minimize or prevent infection
• know the warning signs of infection.
  Based on the nursing diagnosis *fear,* develop appropriate patient outcomes. For example, your patient will:

• discuss fears with a person of choice
• identify strategies to reduce fear.

IMPLEMENTATION

Autoimmune thrombocytopenic purpura can cause severe complications and even fatalities. Direct your nursing care toward protecting the patient from injury and infection and allaying her fears. (See *Medical care of the patient with autoimmune thrombocytopenic purpura.*)

Nursing interventions
• Encourage your patient to discuss any concerns about the disease and its treatment.
• Protect all areas of petechiae and ecchymoses from further injury. Reassure the patient that they will heal as the disease resolves.
• Watch for bleeding, including surgical or GI bleeding and menorrhagia. Identify the amount of bleeding or the size of ecchymoses at least every 24 hours. Test stool, urine, and vomitus for blood.
• Provide rest periods between activities if the patient tires easily. During active bleeding, maintain the patient on strict bed rest. To avoid intracranial bleeding, elevate the head of the bed to prevent gravity-related pressure increases.
• Guard against bleeding by protecting the patient from trauma. Keep the bed's side rails raised, and pad them if possible. Promote the use of an electric razor and a soft toothbrush. Avoid invasive procedures, such as venipuncture or urinary catheterization if possible. When venipuncture is unavoidable, exert pressure on the puncture site until the bleeding stops.
• Monitor the patient's platelet count daily.

Treatments

Medical care of the patient with autoimmune thrombocytopenic purpura

The treatment regimen may vary, depending on whether the patient's condition is acute or chronic.

Treating chronic conditions

In chronic autoimmune thrombocytopenic purpura, corticosteroids are used to suppress phagocytic activity, promote capillary integrity, and enhance platelet production. More aggressive therapy uses low doses of chemotherapeutic agents, such as cyclophosphamide or vincristine. Using such toxic drugs requires careful consideration because of the risk of serious adverse reactions.

High-dose I.V. immune globulin administered to adults is 85% effective. Although this treatment can raise platelet counts rapidly, often in 1 to 5 days, its beneficial effect may last only about 1 to 2 weeks. Immune globulin is commonly prescribed to prepare severely thrombocytic patients for emergency surgery be-

cause it can reduce the destruction of antibody-coated platelets.

Adults with the chronic autoimmune thrombocytopenic purpura may undergo splenectomy. Permanent remission commonly results.

Treating acute conditions

The acute form of autoimmune thrombocytopenic purpura may be allowed to run its course without intervention, or it may be treated with corticosteroids or immune globulin.

Additional treatments

Analgesics, except for aspirin and aspirin-containing products and nonsteroidal anti-inflammatory drugs, can be given for pain control.

Platelet transfusions are required when the platelet count is less than 20,000/mm³ and the patient has life-threatening bleeding.

Plasmapheresis or thrombocytapheresis with transfusion has had only limited success.

• Provide a stool softener, if necessary, and encourage adequate fluid intake and a high-fiber diet.
• Administer prescribed medications, monitoring for effectiveness and adverse reactions.
• Before splenectomy, administer transfusions as ordered and according to hospital policy. Take the patient's vital signs immediately before the transfusion, and monitor them closely during the procedure. Watch for adverse reactions.
• After splenectomy, monitor the patient's vital signs and her liquid intake

and output. Administer analgesics, I.V. infusions, and transfusions as needed.

Patient teaching
• Teach the patient about her disorder, including its complications and treatment.
• Explain diagnostic tests and how platelet counts can help identify abnormal bleeding.
• Warn the patient that the lower her platelet count falls, the more precautions she'll need to take. Inform her that with severe thrombocytopenia,

Identifying purpuric lesions

Clarify for your patient the terms that the doctor may use for a rash or a bruise. Explain to the patient that the purpuric lesions, which are purplish discolorations caused by blood seeping into the skin, are related to spontaneous bleeding in thrombocytopenia and include petechiae, ecchymoses, and hematomas.

Petechiae
Painless, round, flat, and as tiny as pinpoints (1 to 3 mm in diameter), these red or brown lesions result from leakage of red blood cells into cutaneous tissue. Inform the patient that petechiae usually appear and fade in crops and sometimes group to form ecchymoses.

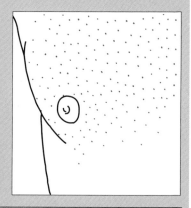

Ecchymoses
Another form of blood leakage, ecchymoses are purple or blue bruises that fade to yellow-green and, though larger than petechiae, can vary in size and shape. Tell your patient that although these can occur anywhere on the body, they usually appear on the arms and legs of patients with bleeding disorders.

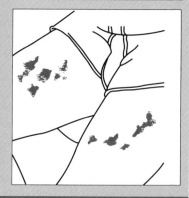

even minor bumps or scrapes can result in bleeding.
• Teach the patient to examine her skin for petechiae, ecchymoses, and hematomas. (See *Identifying purpuric lesions.*)

• Explain the medication regimen. If the patient takes any immunosuppressive drugs, teach her how to watch for adverse effects and signs of infection. Explain measures that reduce the risk of infection, such as

Identifying purpuric lesions *(continued)*

Hematomas
A palpable ecchymosis that's painful and swollen is a hematoma. Usually the result of traumatic injury, superficial hematomas are red, whereas deep hematomas are blue. Although their size can vary widely, hematomas typically exceed 1 cm in diameter.

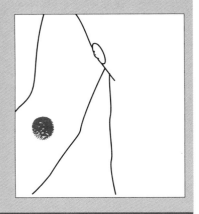

avoiding crowds during flu season. If the patient is taking prednisone, explain the importance of discontinuing therapy gradually.

• Caution the patient to avoid taking aspirin in any form or other drugs that impair coagulation. Teach her how to recognize aspirin compounds and NSAIDs on the labels of over-the-counter remedies.

• Explain to the patient how to make her home as safe as possible.

• Review your patient's daily routine and explain how to modify or avoid risky activities.

• Stress the need to report any signs of renewed bleeding, such as tarry stools, coffee-ground vomitus, epistaxis, menorrhagia, gingival bleeding, or urinary tract bleeding.

• If the patient experiences frequent nosebleeds, instruct her to use a humidifier at night.

• Advise the patient to avoid straining during defecation or coughing because both can lead to increased ICP, possibly causing cerebral hemorrhage.

• Teach the patient how to test her stools for occult blood.

• Teach her how to provide safe and effective oral and skin care.

• Advise her to carry medical identification stating that she has autoimmune thrombocytopenic purpura.

• Explain preoperative and postoperative care to the patient undergoing splenectomy. Make certain she knows to watch closely for signs of infection and to take preventive measures. (See *Ensuring continued care for the patient with autoimmune thrombocytopenic purpura,* page 140.)

EVALUATION

When evaluating the patient's response to your nursing care, compare your reassessment data with the pa-

Discharge TimeSaver

Ensuring continued care for the patient with autoimmune thrombocytopenic purpura

Review the following teaching topics, referrals, and follow-up appointments to make sure that your patient is adequately prepared for discharge.

Teaching topics
Make sure that the following topics have been covered and that your patient's learning has been evaluated:
☐ the nature of the disease and its complications
☐ drug information, including adverse reactions and necessary precautions
☐ measures to help prevent bleeding episodes
☐ signs and symptoms of increased bleeding, and the need to notify the doctor immediately
☐ infection prevention
☐ signs and symptoms of infection, and the need to report them immediately
☐ need for follow-up

☐ need for medical identification bracelet
☐ preoperative and postoperative care if necessary.

Referrals
Make sure that the patient has been provided with necessary referrals to:
☐ social service agencies
☐ mental health specialist if necessary.

Follow-up appointments
Make sure that the necessary follow-up appointments have been scheduled and that the patient has been notified:
☐ doctor
☐ surgeon if necessary
☐ diagnostic tests for reevaluation.

tient outcomes specified in your plan of care.

Teaching and counseling
Begin by determining the effectiveness of your teaching. Consider the following questions:
• Does your patient understand the disease, its complications, and its treatment?
• Does she know the warning signs of infection and increased bleeding and state what actions to take?
• Can she explain ways to minimize or prevent infection?
• Can she recognize aspirin compounds and NSAIDs?

• Can the patient discuss her fears with a person of choice?
• Can she identify strategies to reduce fear?

Physical condition
Consider the following questions:
• Is your patient free from injury?
• Is she complying with the treatment regimen prescribed to boost her platelet count?
• Does she routinely take precautions against potential causes of bleeding?
• Does she have a normal WBC count?

Hashimoto's disease

A chronic, progressive inflammatory disease, Hashimoto's disease is the most common form of thyroiditis. Untreated, it can destroy the thyroid gland or progressively alter its function. Initially, thyroid hormones released into circulation cause temporary hyperthyroidism. But as the disease progresses, destroying gland tissue, hypothyroidism results.

Problems related to hyperthyroidism or hypothyroidism can occur. For example, myxedema coma — which has a mortality of about 50% — may result from untreated hypothyroidism. A goiter often develops, compressing the surrounding tissues. Rarely, malignant lymphomas of the thyroid gland may occur. However, early diagnosis and monitoring, along with thyroid hormone replacement to treat or prevent hypothyroidism, offers the patient an excellent prognosis. (See *Key points about Hashimoto's disease.*)

Causes
Autoimmune factors are believed to play a prominent role in Hashimoto's disease, but the exact cause is unknown.

ASSESSMENT

Your assessment should consider the patient's health history, physical examination findings, and diagnostic test results.

Health history
The outstanding clinical feature of Hashimoto's disease (and usually the patient's chief complaint) is goiter, a painless enlargement of the thyroid.

FactFinder

Key points about Hashimoto's disease

- *Incidence:* Affects women more frequently than men; most common in people ages 30 to 50
- *Prognosis:* Excellent, with early diagnosis and treatment
- *Treatment:* Thyroid replacement hormone therapy
- *Leading complications:* Sporadic goiter in children; the most common cause of goitrous hypothyroidism in the United States
- *Other complications:* Dysphagia, hoarseness, slight dyspnea, asthenia, malaise, and local or referred pain

Early in the course of the disease, the patient may complain of symptoms of hyperthyroidism, such as heat intolerance, nervousness, and weight loss despite increased appetite. Later, the patient may also report symptoms of hypothyroidism, such as sensitivity to cold, fatigue, and weight gain.

The patient's medical history may reveal a recent viral or bacterial infection or traumatic thyroid injury. Because Hashimoto's disease is often related to other autoimmune disorders, check for systemic lupus erythematosus, Graves' disease, systemic sclerosis, rheumatoid arthritis, or pernicious anemia.

In assessing how the disease has affected your patient's lifestyle, consider behavioral changes, such as fatigue, abandonment of activities, and exercise intolerance.

Physical examination
On inspection, you'll probably notice reddened skin over an enlarged thy-

Thyroid enlargement in Hashimoto's disease

In Hashimoto's disease, the patient's thyroid gland is usually diffusely enlarged. The enlargement may be symmetrical. As fibrosis develops, nodules may be palpated.

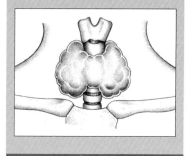

roid gland (goiter). Early in the disease, the thyroid will typically feel diffusely enlarged, firm, nontender, and smooth when palpated. Later, as fibrosis occurs, the gland may feel nodular. (See *Thyroid enlargement in Hashimoto's disease.*)

Vital signs and other findings may reflect hypothyroidism or hyperthyroidism. (See *Quick review: Hypothyroidism vs. hyperthyroidism.*)

Diagnostic test results

The following diagnostic tests and findings commonly aid diagnosis of Hashimoto's disease:

• Blood tests may show circulating autoantibodies present in varying levels.

• Needle biopsy may provide histologic confirmation.

• Serum thyroid hormone will be present in varying levels, depending on the progression of the disease. Thyroid failure shows a rise in thyroid-stimulating hormone (TSH) and a decrease in titers of triiodothyronine and thyroxine.

Timesaving tip: Monitor TSH levels because they're the most sensitive indicator of mild thyroid failure when hypothyroidism has an autoimmune cause.

NURSING DIAGNOSIS

Common diagnoses for a patient with Hashimoto's disease include:

• Decreased cardiac output related to hypothyroidism

• Impaired swallowing related to pressure of goiter on surrounding tissue

• Knowledge deficit related to unfamiliarity with the disease, its complications, and its management.

PLANNING

Based on the nursing diagnosis *decreased cardiac output,* develop appropriate patient outcomes. For example, your patient will:

• exhibit appropriate hemodynamic parameters and vital signs

• show appropriate skin color

• demonstrate a capillary refill time of less than 3 seconds

• have a urine output of more than 30 ml/hour

• demonstrate clear breath sounds upon auscultation.

Based on the nursing diagnosis *impaired swallowing,* develop appropriate patient outcomes. For example, your patient will:

• display improved swallowing

• show no signs of aspiration.

Based on the nursing diagnosis *knowledge deficit,* develop appropriate patient outcomes. For example, your patient will:

• demonstrate understanding of the disease

Assessment TimeSaver

Quick review: Hypothyroidism vs. hyperthyroidism

Monitor the patient with Hashimoto's disease for clinical indications of hypothyroidism or hyperthyroidism. Progressive glandular destruction associated with the disease characteristically leads to hypothyroidism and less commonly to hyperthyroidism. However, patients initially may be hyperthyroid because thyroid hormones escape into circulation. Also, shortly after thyroid hormone replacement therapy begins, the patient may show signs of hyperthyroidism.

Hypothyroidism	Hyperthyroidism
• Fatigue	• Restlessness, irritability
• Slowing of mental processes	• Tremor, nervousness
• Emotional instability	• Emotional lability
• Bradycardia	• Palpitations, tachycardia
• Arrhythmias	• Chest pain, arrhythmias
• Hypotension	• Increased systolic pressure
• Dyspnea	• Dyspnea, rapid respirations
• Anorexia	• Increased appetite
• Constipation	• Diarrhea
• Decreased libido	• Increased libido
• Infertility	• Amenorrhea
• Dry, coarse, flaky skin	• Smooth, moist skin
• Sensitivity to cold	• Heat intolerance, diaphoresis
• Unexplained weight gain	• Weight loss
• Facial puffiness	• Startled look

• recognize and report signs and symptoms and complications
• explain treatment and care measures.

IMPLEMENTATION

Direct your nursing care toward averting cardiac complications related to hypothyroidism, making sure your patient can swallow, and teaching her about the disease, its complications, and its management. (See *Medical care of the patient with Hashimoto's disease,* page 144.)

Nursing interventions
• Administer thyroid hormone replacement therapy as ordered. Expect to initiate therapy with low doses and progressively increase the dosage as needed. Monitor the patient's response carefully, especially if she has cardiovascular disease. Be sure to report arrhythmias, sudden dyspnea, and chest pain.
• Evaluate hormone replacement therapy by assessing the patient for relief of signs and symptoms and for a reduced goiter.
• Keep accurate records of vital signs, weight, fluid intake, and urine output.
• Watch for signs and symptoms of hyperthyroidism, such as restlessness and diaphoresis, after starting hormone replacement therapy.
• Help the patient with slight dyspnea find a position in bed (other than the

Medical care of the patient with Hashimoto's disease

A patient with Hashimoto's disease receives drug therapy and possibly surgery.

Drug therapy
Lifetime thyroid hormone replacement, such as synthetic levothyroxine sodium, is given to prevent symptoms of hypothyroidism, to suppress thyroid-stimulating hormone secretion, and to reduce the size of the gland.

Corticosteroids may be administered temporarily to treat thyroid inflammation.

Surgery
Though surgery is not preferred because it increases the risk of myxedema, a subtotal thyroidectomy may be performed if the goiter does not respond to medication or if it compresses other tissue or structures.

---

supine position) to facilitate breathing.
• If the patient has dysphagia, elevate the head of the bed 90 degrees during mealtimes and for 30 minutes afterward to decrease the risk of aspiration. Keep suction equipment available.
• Consult with the dietitian for nutritious, easy-to-swallow foods, and be sure the patient consumes adequate calories.
• Provide frequent mouth care, and lubricate the patient's lips to prevent cracks and blisters. Give meticulous skin care, and also lubricate dry skin.
• Provide a stool softener, if necessary, and encourage adequate fluid intake and a high-fiber diet.
• Measure the patient's neck circumference daily and record findings.
• Plan care so that the patient can have rest periods and sufficient time for activities.
• Give analgesics for pain as prescribed.
• Encourage the patient to discuss her feelings, and help her identify her strengths. Refer her to a mental health professional if necessary.
• Reassure the patient that treatment should relieve signs and symptoms of inadequate thyroid hormone, such as sluggishness, weight gain, and dry skin.

After thyroidectomy
• Monitor vital signs every 15 to 30 minutes until stable. Watch for signs of tetany, such as tingling in the toes and fingers and around the mouth, twitching, and apprehension. Keep 10% calcium gluconate available for I.V. use if needed.
• Check dressings frequently for excessive bleeding. Watch for signs of airway obstruction. Keep tracheotomy equipment handy.

Patient teaching
• Explain the nature of the illness, and teach the patient and her family to identify and report signs and symptoms of hypothyroidism or hyperthyroidism. Tell them to report chest pain immediately.

Discharge TimeSaver

Ensuring continued care for the patient with Hashimoto's disease

Review the following teaching topics, referrals, and follow-up appointments to make sure that your patient is adequately prepared for discharge.

Teaching topics

Make sure that the following topics have been covered and that your patient's learning has been evaluated:
☐ the nature of the disease and its complications
☐ drug information, including a method to ensure compliance, such as a pill container
☐ signs and symptoms to report immediately to the doctor
☐ preoperative and postoperative care if necessary
☐ need for follow-up
☐ symptom management
☐ need for medical identification bracelet.

Referrals

Make sure that the patient has been provided with necessary referrals to:
☐ social service agencies for financial considerations related to lifelong drug therapy
☐ mental health specialist if necessary.

Follow-up appointments

Make sure that the necessary follow-up appointments have been scheduled and that the patient has been notified:
☐ doctor
☐ surgeon if necessary
☐ diagnostic tests for reevaluation.

Timesaving tip: If hypothyroidism is evident, adjust your teaching program to allow full patient understanding. Explain all points slowly and clearly, in several short sessions. Be sure a family member is present in case the patient forgets information. Provide written handouts, and keep distractions to a minimum.

• Explain that the patient may also be susceptible to other autoimmune diseases, such as Addison's disease, pernicious anemia, and premature gonadal failure. Teach her to recognize and report the signs and symptoms of such diseases.

• Teach the patient about thyroid replacement therapy. Explain the medication's purpose, dosage, administration schedule, and adverse reactions. Stress the importance of continuing medications even when symptoms subside. Explain that failure to comply may result in myxedema coma.

• Encourage the patient to wear a medical identification bracelet and to always carry her medication with her.

• Explain preoperative, postoperative, and home care measures for thyroidectomy, if planned.

• Explain the importance of keeping follow-up appointments. (See *Ensuring continued care for the patient with Hashimoto's disease*.)

EVALUATION

When evaluating the patient's response to your nursing care, compare your reassessment data with the patient outcomes specified in your plan of care.

Teaching and counseling
To assess the effectiveness of your teaching, consider the following questions:
• Does the patient understand the disease?
• Can she recognize and report symptoms and complications?
• Can she explain treatment and care measures?

Physical condition
Consider the following questions:
• Does your patient exhibit appropriate hemodynamic parameters and vital signs?
• Does she show appropriate skin color?
• Is her capillary refill time less than 3 seconds?
• Does the patient's urine output exceed 30 ml/hour?
• Are her breath sounds clear upon auscultation?
• Has her swallowing improved?
• Has she avoided aspiration?

CHAPTER 6

Caring for patients with transplant complications

Transplant-related immunosuppression   *148*

Transplant rejection   *154*

Improved surgical techniques have lead to increasingly successful transplantation of a wide variety of organs and tissues, including the heart and its valves, the lungs, kidneys, liver, pancreas, corneas, bones, skin, small bowel, and saphenous veins. However, transplant rejection remains a major problem.

Rejection occurs when the patient's immune system recognizes donor cells as foreign and attacks and destroys them. Improvements in immunosuppressant drug therapy have resulted in fewer rejections. But immunosuppressant drugs may cause other serious problems, especially infection.

With the number of transplant patients increasing and their survival lengthening, chances are you'll encounter these patients in your practice. Even if the patient requires care for a problem unrelated to transplantation, you'll need to take special precautions. To provide care successfully, you must be familiar with the immunosuppressant therapy and the signs of infection or rejection.

Transplant-related immunosuppression

The body's normal immune response identifies and destroys foreign invaders, such as bacteria and viruses. During a solid organ transplant, histocompatibility differences between donor and recipient can trigger an unwanted immune response. For successful transplantation, the patient's immune response must be modified or suppressed by immunosuppressant drugs, which he must receive for the rest of his life. Immunosuppressants leave him vulnerable to bacterial, fungal, parasitic, and viral infections

and cancers, especially skin cancer and lymphomas. (See *Key points about transplant-related immunosuppression.*)

The first immunosuppressants, such as azathioprine, generally suppressed all immune response. More recently developed drugs, such as cyclosporine, act specifically on T lymphocytes, the major cause of damage to transplanted organs, reducing significantly the number and severity of acute transplant rejections. However, adverse effects remain serious, requiring the patient to adapt his lifestyle to daily drug therapy and to remain vigilant for the first signs of infection. (See *Monitoring posttransplantation infections,* page 150.)

ASSESSMENT

Your assessment should include a careful consideration of the patient's health history, physical examination findings, and diagnostic test results.

Health history
When taking the patient's health history, ask about the type of immunosuppressant drugs and their dosages and the duration of his therapy. Ask what type of transplant he had, when it occurred, and how many rejection episodes he's had. Determine the presence of associated diseases, invasive devices, or wounds. Also explore his dietary history.

Timesaving tip: If you're caring for a patient who has a history of tissue or organ transplants, be sure to call the original transplant center to coordinate care and avert later problems.

If infection is present, the patient will usually report fever. He may also complain of other signs and symptoms, such as nausea, vomiting, diarrhea, fatigue, anorexia, abdominal pain, sore throat, dyspnea, and productive cough.

Physical examination
Your examination of the immunosuppressed patient may reveal normal findings. Keep in mind that if infection is present, findings are often insidious or absent, making the investigation of even minor complaints imperative and your physical examination especially important.

Begin by assessing the skin. Check for signs of tinea and fungal infection of the nail beds, including toenails. Inspect for hematoma and petechiae, since easy bruising is a common adverse reaction to corticosteroids. Inspect surgical or traumatic wounds and any break in the skin very closely for signs of infection. Appraise the oral mucosa for ulcerations or signs of *Candida* infection, such as white patches or plaques on the buccal mucosa. Also check for jaundice.

Evaluate the lungs for any change in respiratory rate. Auscultate for breath sounds, noting any adventitious sounds that may indicate pulmonary infection, especially pneumonia. Auscultate for bowel sounds and palpate the abdomen, noting if it's soft. Look for any irregularities

that may be related to complications, especially cytomegalovirus infection. Check for hepatomegaly and assess for genitourinary lesions or discharge.

Inspect and palpate the lymph nodes; up to 4% of patients will experience posttransplant lymphoproliferative disease related to immunosuppression. This disease usually regresses if immunosuppressant drug therapy is reduced.

Check for signs of rejection. Take the patient's vital signs, noting especially any fever, tachycardia, or tachypnea.

Diagnostic test results
Cultures and other diagnostic tests will be ordered if fever or other signs of infection are present.
• A complete blood count can reveal leukopenia, thrombocytopenia, or anemia related to immunosuppressant therapy.
• Blood urea nitrogen and serum creatinine levels can evaluate kidney function related to drug-induced nephrotoxicity.
• Serum aspartate aminotransferase (AST, formerly SGOT), alanine aminotransferase (ALT, formerly SGPT), and lactate dehydrogenase levels can

Monitoring post-transplantation infections

Always ask the transplant patient the date of his operation, since different infections occur at specific intervals after a procedure. The following guidelines describe the most likely infections.

Up to 1 month after transplantation

Infections commonly relate to complications of the procedure, such as bacterial infections from I.V. devices, urinary catheters, and endotracheal tubes. Nosocomial infection, caused by such organisms as *Pseudomonas aeruginosa* and *Nocardia asteroides*, also pose a hazard; nocardiosis occurs most frequently in ambulatory care.

1 to 6 months after transplantation

Infection commonly results from viruses such as cytomegalovirus and hepatitis. Viral infection often precedes opportunistic infections caused by such organisms as *Pneumocystis carinii* or *Aspergillus*.

6 months or more after transplantation

The most frequent infections include community-acquired infections such as influenza, shingles, and opportunistic infections, which can be fatal, especially in patients frequently treated for rejection.

evaluate liver function related to drug-induced hepatotoxicity.
• Blood glucose and serum uric acid levels may be elevated in a patient who's taking cyclosporine, corticosteroids, or tacrolimus.

NURSING DIAGNOSIS

Common nursing diagnoses for a patient with transplant-related immunosuppression include:
• Altered protection related to immunosuppressant drugs
• Ineffective individual coping related to lifestyle changes caused by immunosuppressant drugs.

PLANNING

Based on the nursing diagnosis *altered protection,* develop appropriate patient outcomes. For example, your patient will:
• implement measures to reduce his risk of infection
• maintain normal body temperature, pulse rate, and blood pressure
• remain free of other signs and symptoms of infection, such as pain, shortness of breath, diarrhea, nausea, vomiting, increased fatigue, or increased drainage from or delayed healing of a wound
• report at scheduled times for blood tests to monitor infection and notify the transplant team immediately of any signs or symptoms of infection.

Based on the nursing diagnosis *ineffective individual coping,* develop appropriate patient outcomes. For example, your patient will:
• discuss his feelings about how therapy affects him
• explain why lifestyle changes are necessary
• identify and implement at least two coping mechanisms.

IMPLEMENTATION

When caring for the patient receiving immunosuppressant drug therapy, focus your nursing interventions on preventing complications. (See *Infection prophylaxis.*)

Nursing interventions

• Administer prescribed immunosuppressant drugs and carefully observe for adverse reactions. (See *Reviewing transplant-related immunosuppressant drugs*, pages 152 and 153.)
• Monitor the patient for signs and symptoms of infection.
• Minimize the risk of infection by implementing various supportive measures, such as washing your hands before touching the patient and between patients, and keeping the patient away from units undergoing construction to prevent aspergillosis. Isolation usually isn't required.
• Support the patient and his family emotionally.

Patient teaching

Timesaving tip: You can save time and provide additional support for transplant patients by teaching them in groups. Also, consider giving your patients written drug information, which will allow them review time before and after you teach.

• Explain how immunosuppressant therapy helps to control rejection and why it must be lifelong.
• Teach the patient about each prescribed drug's purpose, dosage, route, administration schedule, and possible adverse effects.
• Instruct the patient not to take any over-the-counter medications without his doctor's approval. Also, tell him to notify his transplant team or contact person before taking any medication prescribed by another

> ### Infection prophylaxis
>
> To prevent infection, you may give the following drugs, as prescribed, after transplantation:
> • trimethoprim-sulfamethoxazole to help prevent *Pneumocystis carinii* pneumonia and urinary tract infection
> • acyclovir and ganciclovir to help prevent viral infection, especially cytomegalovirus and herpes simplex
> • nystatin to help prevent fungal and yeast infection.

doctor because it may change the blood level of immunosuppressants or affect his white blood cell count.
• Teach the patient how to check for skin cancers and lymphomas, and stress to women the importance of having regular Papanicolaou tests as ordered.
• Teach the patient about signs and symptoms that should be reported, such as coughing, fever of 102° F (38.9° C) or higher, shortness of breath, diarrhea, nausea, vomiting, increased fatigue, or increased drainage from or delayed healing of a wound, even if the wound is not reddened or swollen.
• Explain the importance of keeping appointments for blood tests to check the level of immunosuppressants. Also emphasize the importance of keeping follow-up visits to the doctor.
• Advise the patient about the hazards of smoking. In addition to its known carcinogenic effects, the mucus accumulation caused by smoking can lead to pulmonary infection more

Reviewing transplant-related immunosuppressant drugs

Drug	Action	Adverse reactions
Preventing rejection		
Prednisone (Orasone)	Mainly decreases the inflammatory response but also acts on the monocyte-macrophage system to prevent release of interleukin-6 and interleukin-1, so that cell-mediated function is affected	Fluid and electrolyte disturbances (edema and sodium retention, metabolic alkalosis, hypocalcemia, or hypokalemia possibly leading to arrhythmias); weakness or myopathy and osteoporosis, leading to pathologic fractures of the long bones or vertebral compression. Also nausea, vomiting, and peptic ulcers; menstrual irregularities; growth suppression in children; cushingoid signs (moon face, buffalo hump, central obesity); decreased carbohydrate tolerance. Possibly acne, hirsutism, gynecomastia, impaired wound healing, cataract formation, emotional instability, and ophthalmic changes. Potentially fatal adrenal crisis following abrupt withdrawal from long-term, high-dose therapy.
Azathioprine (Imuran)	Nonselectively inhibits the synthesis of deoxyribonucleic acid, ribonucleic acid, or both, thus slowing proliferation of all dividing cells	Leukopenia, anemia, thrombocytopenia or pancytopenia; nausea, vomiting, diarrhea, mouth ulcerations, steatorrhea, esophagitis, hepatotoxicity, jaundice, rash, arthralgia, alopecia
Cyclosporine (Sandimmune)	Selectively inhibits proliferation of T lymphocytes	Tremor, nausea, vomiting, diarrhea, abdominal distention, cramps, paresthesia, nephrotoxicity, hepatotoxicity, hypertension, gingival hyperplasia, hirsutism, sinusitis, hearing loss, flushing, hyperglycemia

easily in an immunocompromised patient.

• Reinforce prescribed activity and rest guidelines.

• Teach the importance of eating a well-balanced diet with specific transplant-related modifications. Explain that good nutrition can help bolster the immune system. Tell the patient who is taking prednisone or tacrolimus to limit his sugar intake because these drugs increase blood glucose levels. If he is initially anorexic or feels full easily, suggest frequent small meals and snacks.

• Encourage the patient to wear a medical identification bracelet.

• Make certain that the patient has the names and the telephone numbers of key transplant team members and medical centers. (See *Ensuring continued care for the patient with transplant-related immunosuppression,* page 154.)

Drug	Action	Adverse reactions
Tacrolimus (Prograf)	Selectively inhibits proliferation of T lymphocytes (more potent than cyclosporine)	After I.V. administration: neurotoxicity, including headache, paresthesia, photophobia, tinnitus, sleep disturbances, and mood changes; nephrotoxicity; GI irritation. Better tolerated when administered orally.

Treating rejection

Drug	Action	Adverse reactions
Muromonab-CD3 (Orthoclone OKT-3)	Monoclonal antibody that acts specifically in the T-lymphocyte membrane to block the CD3 receptor site needed for antigen recognition, thus rendering T lymphocytes inactive	Fever, chills, tremor, dyspnea, nausea, vomiting, diarrhea, chest pain, fatigue, joint pain, severe pulmonary edema
Lymphocyte immune globulin (antithymocyte globulin [equine], ATG) (Atgam)	Exerts a greater action on cell-mediated immunity to graft tissue than humoral immunity by coating lymphocytes with antibody, which causes opsonization and macrophage destruction of lymphocytes, thus decreasing the number of circulating lymphocytes	Malaise, headache, seizures, febrile reactions, serum sickness, nausea, vomiting, hypotension, anaphylaxis

EVALUATION

When evaluating the patient's response to your nursing care, gather reassessment data and compare this information with the patient outcomes specified in your plan of care.

Teaching and counseling

Begin by determining the effectiveness of your teaching and counseling. Consider the following questions:

• Can your patient discuss his feelings about how his therapy affects him?
• Can he explain why his lifestyle changes are necessary?
• Is he able to identify and use effectively at least two coping mechanisms?

Physical condition

A physical examination and diagnostic tests will provide additional information. If treatment has been suc-

cessful, you should note the following outcomes:
• Your patient has initiated measures to reduce the risk of infection.
• He has maintained normal body temperature, pulse rate, and blood pressure.
• He has remained free of other signs and symptoms of infection, such as pain, shortness of breath, diarrhea, nausea, vomiting, increased fatigue, or increased drainage from or delayed healing of a wound.
• He reports at scheduled times for blood tests to monitor infection.

Transplant rejection

Transplant rejection occurs when the patient's immune system recognizes

transplanted tissue as foreign and attacks it. This recognition largely reflects histocompatibility differences between donor and recipient.

Several types of transplants exist. Those with identical or similar cell-surface antigens are less likely to be rejected. (See *Types of grafts.*) The two antigen systems most important for a successful transplant are the ABO blood group and the major histocompatibility complex (MHC). ABO antigens are present on erythrocytes and in most body tissues. In humans, MHC antigens are called human leukocyte antigens (HLA). To reduce the chances of transplant rejection, donors are sought with identical or similar immune characteristics, especially ABO antigens and HLA. (See *Preventing transplant rejection,* page 156.)

Even with improved tissue typing and immunosuppressant drugs, rejection remains the most common transplant complication and can occur at any time while the graft is in place. Rejection can be classified as hyperacute, acute, or chronic, depending on the mechanism of rejection and the amount of time between transplantation and the appearance of signs of rejection. (See *Three types of transplant rejection*, page 157.)

Graft-versus-host disease (GVHD), a potentially fatal variation of transplant rejection, can follow infusion of immunocompetent donor cells into an immunosuppressed patient. GVHD may be acute or chronic and mainly affects the skin, liver, and GI tract. Treatment and prevention resemble that prescribed for standard transplant rejection.

Causes

In standard transplant rejection, the recipient cells mount an immune response against the transplanted donor tissue or organ. In GVHD, the reverse occurs: The successfully transplanted donor cells attack immunosuppressed recipient (host) cells.

ASSESSMENT

Your assessment should include a careful consideration of the patient's health history, physical examination findings, and diagnostic test results. Because of the complex nature of the disorder, detecting transplant rejection requires careful assessment. For example, your patient may be asymptomatic or display only vague, nonspecific symptoms. Rejection may occur moments after transplantation, or it may occur months or even years later.

FactFinder

Types of grafts

Tissues and organs used for transplantation are classified according to the genetic relationship between the donor and the recipient.

• Autograft is a transplant of the patient's own tissue from one part of his body to another, such as skin grafts for burns and autologous bone marrow infusion for leukemia, lymphoma, or other malignant diseases.

• Isograft (also called syngeneic graft) refers to a transplant between a genetically identical donor and patient, such as between identical twins.

• Allograft (formerly called homograft) is a transplant between a genetically different donor and patient of the same species.

• Xenograft (formerly called heterograft) is a transplant involving different species, such as the transplant of hearts and kidneys from animals into humans.

Transplant rejection is less likely with autografts or isografts, since the antigens of the donor and patient are identical or very similar.

Health history

Commonly, the patient's main complaints are malaise and fatigue, although he may also report anorexia, nausea, restlessness, or anxiety. Decreasing blood pressure and dyspnea may also indicate rejection. (See *Signs and symptoms of solid organ transplant rejection*, page 158.)

Because the patient and his family often fear the consequences of rejection and worry about paying for the

Preventing transplant rejection

Measures to help prevent rejection include histocompatibility testing and immunosuppressant therapy that begins before the transplant procedure.

ABO blood typing
This measure helps ensure compatibility by identifying and comparing the antigens on donor and patient erythrocytes. If a donor's erythrocytes carry foreign ABO antigens, a patient's isohemagglutins may react against those antigens, resulting in injury to the vascular epithelium of the graft and subsequent rejection.

Tissue typing
Tissue typing identifies and compares a wide range of human leukocyte antigens in the patient and potential donors. The more genetically similar the donor and patient tissues, the less possibility of rejection.

Crossmatching
This technique determines the presence of preformed cytotoxic antibodies in the patient's serum against donor antigens. If the patient's serum contains preformed antibodies, he has a high risk of hyperacute transplant rejection.

Immunosuppressant drug therapy
Drug therapy prevents rejection by suppressing the immune response to the donor graft. Drug therapy starts prior to the transplant and continues afterward. Usually therapy involves a combination of drugs rather than a single agent. Regimens vary among transplant centers and among patients. Commonly used drugs include a combination of corticosteroids, cyclosporine, and azathioprine.

Radiation therapy
Radiation therapy may be performed before a bone marrow transplant to provide immunosuppression and to eradicate tumor cells.

necessary care, be sure to assess their coping mechanisms and sources of support.

Timesaving tip: If you're caring for a patient who has had a previous tissue or organ transplant, be sure to call the original transplant center about the date and place of surgery, the medical diagnosis, which doctor he visits for follow-up, which medications he's taking, and any history of rejection or other complications. This will give you immediate access to necessary information in case of transplant-related complications such as rejection.

Physical examination
Inspection typically reveals swelling, tenderness, and enlargement of the involved organ or site, especially in a patient who has undergone a kidney, liver, or pancreas transplant. Low-grade fever may be evident.

Diagnostic test results
No single test or combination of tests is definitive. Diagnosis often becomes a matter of exclusion, depend-

Three types of transplant rejection

Rejection may be classified as hyperacute, acute, or chronic.

Hyperacute rejection
This type of rejection occurs quickly, often within minutes to hours following transplantation. Preformed cytotoxic antibodies in the recipient's serum (usually from previous blood transfusions, pregnancy, or an earlier transplant) recognize, bind with, and quickly destroy donor cells. Standard immunosuppressant therapy is ineffective, although improved tissue typing and crossmatching have reduced the incidence of hyperacute rejection.

Acute rejection
The most common type of rejection, acute rejection usually occurs about 1 to 3 weeks after a transplant, but may occur months later. Sensitized recipient helper T cells begin the attack against donor cells, which are recognized as foreign. (Antibodies and complement aren't involved.) The helper T cells release cytokines that activate macrophages and recruit cytotoxic T cells. Both macrophages and cytotoxic T cells damage grafted tissue, compromising graft vascularity and rendering the graft necrotic. Immediate treatment with increased doses of immunosuppressant drugs may reverse the process.

Chronic rejection
Chronic rejection occurs months to years following transplantation. Both T and B cells participate in this type of rejection. Gradual occlusion of vessel walls with fibrin, platelets, and complement slowly interrupts blood supply to the graft. High-dose immunosuppressant therapy is ineffective, and the graft usually doesn't survive.

ing on careful evaluation of signs and symptoms, results of specific organ function tests, and standard laboratory studies. The following laboratory studies can reveal clues to rejection:
• Elevated levels of serum creatinine and blood urea nitrogen followed by a renal flow study can reveal renal transplant rejection by showing decreased perfusion.
• Elevated levels of serum bilirubin, serum transaminase, and alkaline phosphatase can indicate liver transplant rejection.
• Reduced urine amylase levels and low urine pH followed by elevated blood glucose levels can reveal pancreas transplant rejection.
• A low platelet and neutrophil count can indicate bone marrow rejection.

Tissue biopsy provides the most reliable diagnostic information for heart, liver, lung, and kidney transplants. Repeat biopsies help monitor histologic changes common to rejection, differences from previous biopsies, and the course and success of treatment. Biopsies of pancreatic transplants are not often performed because of their location. Instead, a technetium scan for evaluating blood flow is usually performed.

Signs and symptoms of solid organ transplant rejection

Heart rejection
Signs of rejection include right axis shift, atrial arrhythmias, conduction defects, S_3 gallop, and jugular vein distention. Additional signs and symptoms include malaise, lethargy, fever, weight gain, right ventricular failure, hypotension, hepatomegaly, and pedal edema.

Lung rejection
Signs of rejection include fever, crackles or wheezes, and shortness of breath. Respiratory function declines as evidenced by such serial spirometry results as reduced forced expiratory volume in 1 second or forced vital capacity.

Liver rejection
Rejection of this organ alters the color of urine or stool. It also causes jaundice, hepatomegaly, fever, and pain in the center of back, right flank, or right upper quadrant.

Kidney rejection
Besides fever, signs and symptoms of kidney rejection include decreased urine output, hypertension, weight gain, edema, and malaise. The patient may have kidney pain and swelling.

Pancreas rejection
In pancreas rejection, the patient may experience signs of diabetes mellitus. These include increased blood glucose levels, polyuria, polydipsia, polyphagia, and weight loss.

NURSING DIAGNOSIS

Common nursing diagnoses for a patient with transplant rejection include:
• High risk for altered body temperature related to transplant rejection
• High risk for infection related to effects of immunosuppressant therapy
• Knowledge deficit related to transplantation, signs and symptoms of rejection, and importance of follow-up care
• Ineffective management of therapeutic regimen related to lack of support systems and inadequate finances
• Fear related to potential loss of graft function due to transplant rejection.

PLANNING

Based on the nursing diagnosis *high risk for altered body temperature,* develop appropriate patient outcomes. For example, your patient will:
• maintain a normal temperature
• exhibit cool, dry skin.

Based on the nursing diagnosis *high risk for infection,* develop appropriate patient outcomes. For example, your patient will:
• remain free of infection throughout his therapy.

Based on the nursing diagnosis *knowledge deficit,* develop appropriate patient outcomes. For example, your patient will:

• identify signs and symptoms of rejection
• explain the importance of follow-up care in detecting rejection
• state that he will seek follow-up care.

Based on the nursing diagnosis *ineffective management of therapeutic regimen,* develop appropriate patient outcomes. For example, your patient will:
• acknowledge the importance of following his treatment regimen
• discuss potential reasons for not following his treatment regimen
• identify positive strategies that can help him follow the treatment regimen.

Based on the nursing diagnosis *fear,* develop appropriate patient outcomes. For example, your patient will:
• discuss his fear
• show reduced signs of fear
• identify three strategies for reducing fear.

IMPLEMENTATION

Start your nursing care before the transplant takes place by focusing on preventive measures. If transplant rejection develops despite preventive measures, you'll treat the reaction.

Nursing interventions
• Monitor the patient's temperature, and assess for other signs of improving or worsening graft function.
• Administer prescribed medications to treat acute rejection; then monitor the patient very closely for adverse reactions.
• Check for signs of infection related to immunosuppressant therapy, which commonly leaves the patient at increased risk for potentially fatal infection from opportunistic organisms,

such as cytomegalovirus, fungi, mycobacteria, and protozoa.
• Keep the patient informed of his progress.
• Encourage the patient to discuss his feelings about his disorder. Support the patient and his family by helping identify positive coping mechanisms, especially if the rejection is irreversible. Suggest psychological counseling if warranted. Consult with the social services department early to plan the patient's discharge.

Patient teaching
Timesaving tip: Furnishing written information on all prescribed drugs will save you teaching time by providing the patient with a ready source of review.
• Explain transplant rejection to the patient.
• Teach him the signs and symptoms indicating either improvement or worsening of the rejection.
• Review his drug therapy, including possible adverse effects and related precautions.
• Explain measures to help prevent infection, such as observing good hygiene and avoiding individuals with infections.
• Stress the importance of immediately reporting to the doctor any signs or symptoms of infection or further rejection.
• Stress the importance of follow-up therapy and compliance with the medication regimen. (See *Ensuring continued care for the patient with transplant rejection,* page 160.)

EVALUATION

When evaluating the patient's response to your nursing care, gather reassessment data and compare this information with the patient outcomes specified in your plan of care.

Discharge TimeSaver

Ensuring continued care for the patient with transplant rejection

Review the following teaching topics, referrals, and follow-up appointments to make sure that your patient is adequately prepared for discharge.

Teaching topics
Make sure that the following topics have been covered and that your patient's learning has been evaluated:
☐ signs and symptoms of rejection or infection
☐ need to report the first sign of rejection or infection to the doctor
☐ medications and adverse effects
☐ need for follow-up care and life-long compliance with the treatment regimen.

Referrals
Make sure that the patient has been provided with necessary referrals to:
☐ social service agencies for financial consultation
☐ mental health counseling if necessary.

Follow-up appointments
Make sure that the necessary follow-up appointments have been scheduled and that the patient has been notified:
☐ doctor
☐ surgeon
☐ diagnostic testing.

Teaching and counseling

Begin by determining the effectiveness of your teaching and counseling. Consider the following questions:
• Can your patient identify the signs and symptoms of transplant rejection?
• Can he explain the importance of preventing infection?
• Will he follow the prescribed treatment regimen?
• Will he discuss potential reasons for not following the treatment regimen?
• Can he identify positive strategies that can help him follow the treatment regimen?
• Does he discuss his fears related to transplant rejection? Will he seek counseling if it's recommended?
• Does he show physical signs of fear?

• Can he describe three strategies for reducing fear?
• Can he explain the importance of follow-up care in detecting rejection?
• Has he stated that he will seek follow-up care?

Physical condition

A physical examination and diagnostic tests will provide additional information. If treatment has been successful, you should note the following outcomes:
• The patient has remained free of infection.
• He has maintained a normal body temperature and demonstrated signs of adequate graft function.
• He has maintained cool, dry skin.

CHAPTER 7

Applying the nursing process to infectious disorders

Assessment   162

Nursing diagnosis 171

Planning   174

Implementation   178

Evaluation   180

Infectious disorders represent a major cause of death worldwide and a primary cause of illness in North America. They continue to challenge health care workers because of the following factors:

• The incidence of many infectious diseases once thought to be under control has increased.

• Efforts to prevent and control some infectious disorders — most notably gonorrhea, pneumococcal disease, salmonellosis, shigellosis, tuberculosis, and staphylococcal infections — have been hampered by drug-resistant strains.

• New pathogens and syndromes — such as hepatitis C virus, human immunodeficiency virus (HIV), Legionnaire's disease, Lyme disease, and toxic shock syndrome — have been discovered.

• The number of immunocompromised patients has risen dramatically.

• Rapid technological advances have increased the number of surgical and other invasive procedures performed each year, with a corresponding increase in the risk of infection. (See *Overview of infectious disorders.*)

Because of these factors, nurses in all health care settings can expect to care for growing numbers of patients with infectious disorders. Using the nursing process to guide this care will help ensure prompt and effective treatment. You'll use the nursing process to:

• identify patient problems you can treat

• identify patient problems you can help to prevent

• select goals for the patient and determine whether they've been achieved

• develop a plan of care that addresses the patient's actual and potential problems

• determine what kind of assistance the patient needs and who can best provide it

• accurately document your contributions to achieving patient outcomes.

The five steps of the nursing process — assessment, nursing diagnosis, planning, implementation, and evaluation — help you address specific patient needs in an orderly and timely way. Keep in mind, however, that these steps are dynamic and flexible and often overlap.

Assessment

The first step in the nursing process, assessment is crucial to the early detection and treatment of infection. The quality of data gathered during assessment will determine the success of all subsequent steps in the nursing process.

Assessment may focus on a known or suspected site of infection. For example, an assessment of a patient complaining of cough, shortness of breath, fever, and chest pain will include a detailed assessment of his respiratory system. However, assessing for the cause of generalized complaints, such as fever and fatigue, can be more difficult. (See *Risk factors for infectious disorders,* page 164.)

Assessment usually includes taking a health history, performing a physical examination, and reviewing the results of diagnostic tests.

Health history
The health history allows you to explore the patient's chief complaint and its relationship to other symptoms, assess the impact of illness on the patient and his family, and begin to develop and implement a plan of

Overview of infectious disorders

Microorganism	Examples	Related disorders
Bacteria	*Brucella* species, *Escherichia coli, Mycobacterium tuberculosis, Neisseria gonorrhoeae, N. meningitidis, Pseudomonas aeruginosa, Salmonella* species, *Staphylococcus aureus* (coagulase-positive), *Streptococcus* (beta-hemolytic group A), *Streptococcus pneumoniae* (pneumococcus)	Brucellosis, cellulitis, conjunctivitis, food poisoning, gastroenteritis, gonorrhea, impetigo, meningitis, meningococcal disease, otitis media, pharyngitis, pelvic inflammatory disease (PID), pneumonia, rheumatic fever, sepsis, septic arthritis, skin infection, tuberculosis, urinary tract infection, wound infection
Chlamydiae	*Chlamydia trachomatis*	Inclusion conjunctivitis, lymphogranuloma venereum, pneumonia, trachoma, urethritis
Fungi	*Aspergillus* species, *Blastomyces dermatitidis, Candida albicans, Coccidioides immitis, Cryptococcus neoformans, Histoplasma capsulatum*	Brain abscess, disseminated coccidioidomycosis, disseminated histoplasmosis, disseminated pulmonary blastomycosis, endocarditis, meningitis, pneumonia, pneumonitis, sinusitis, thrush, vaginitis
Helminths	*Ancylostoma duodenale* (hookworm), *Ascaris lumbricoides* (roundworm), *Enterobius vermicularis* (pinworm, threadworm), *Schistosoma* species, *Taenia solium* (tapeworm), *Trichinella spiralis*	Anemia, fistula, headache, hemorrhage, intestinal obstruction, intestinal stricture, perianal pruritus, pneumonitis, portal hypertension, renal failure, seizures, trichinosis, uncontrolled diarrhea
Mycoplasma	*Mycoplasma hominis, M. pneumoniae*	PID, pneumonia, pyelonephritis
Protozoa	*Entamoeba histolytica, Giardia lamblia, Plasmodium* species, *Pneumocystis carinii, Toxoplasma gondii*	Chorioretinitis, colitis, diarrhea, dysentery, encephalitis, liver abscess, malabsorption, malaria, pneumonia
Rickettsiae	*Rickettsia prowazekii, R. rickettsii*	Rocky mountain spotted fever, typhus
Virus	Epstein-Barr virus, hepatitis B virus, herpes simplex II virus, human immunodeficiency virus, influenza A virus, rhinovirus	Acquired immunodeficiency syndrome, common cold, genital herpes infection, hepatitis, infectious mononucleosis, influenza, neonatal vesicular disease

FactFinder

Risk factors for infectious disorders

Review the following list of risk factors to quickly determine if your patient is at high risk for infection:
- known exposure to an infectious agent
- recent invasive procedure or surgery
- tracheotomy
- malnourishment
- history of smoking or excessive consumption of alcohol
- exposure to toxic chemicals
- disrupted skin integrity
- impaired cough reflex
- altered gastric secretions
- immobility
- chemotherapy, immunosuppressive therapies (such as corticosteroids)
- very young or elderly
- autoimmune disease or immunodeficiency
- antibiotic therapy (interference with normal intestinal flora)
- diabetes mellitus, other endocrine disease, cancer.

care. It also provides information to guide medical diagnosis and treatment.

When taking the health history, use a systematic approach to avoid overlooking important clues. Be sensitive to the patient's concerns and feelings, and encourage him to formulate his own responses. Begin by recording the patient's sex, age, address, occupation, and work location.

Be alert for nonverbal signs that seem to contradict verbal responses. For example, the patient may deny shortness of breath yet exhibit signs of breathing difficulties. Explore these apparent contradictions.

Chief complaint
Begin by asking about the patient's reason for seeking treatment. Common complaints for infectious disorders include lymphadenopathy, pain, fever, purulent discharge, rash, and fatigue. Localized complaints may include cough, diarrhea, and urinary frequency and urgency.

If the patient has trouble identifying a single complaint ask, "What made you seek medical care today?" Then let him describe his problem in his own words. Record his response verbatim whenever possible. Ask him to describe the onset, location, frequency, and duration of the chief complaint. Consider asking the following questions:
- When did the symptom first occur?
- Did it appear suddenly or gradually?
- How often does it occur?
- How long does it last?
- Has it become more or less severe, or does it remain constant?

Next, ask the patient if he's aware of any precipitating, aggravating, or alleviating factors, such as exercise, changes in position, environmental conditions, or medications.

Past illnesses and treatments
Find out if the patient has any disorder or is receiving a treatment that can precipitate his condition or influence his recovery. Include a thorough medication and immunization history. Consider asking the following questions:
- Have you recently had contact with a person with a known or suspected infection?
- Have you been injured recently?
- Have you recently undergone an invasive procedure?

• Have you recently been bitten by an animal or insect?

• Have you been diagnosed as having a chronic illness or cancer?

• Are you currently taking any prescribed drugs?

• Have you recently received a blood transfusion?

Lifestyle factors

When exploring the patient's lifestyle, look for factors that can influence his disorder and his method of dealing with it. Ask about the patient's daily activities, personal habits, diet, interpersonal relationships, mental status, occupational history, and work, community, and home environments. Consider asking the following questions:

• Do you smoke cigarettes? Have you smoked in the past?

• Do you drink alcohol? If so, how often and how much?

• Do you use any recreational drugs, especially I.V. drugs?

• Can you describe your social life and sexual practices? Do you practice safe sex?

• Do you live in a house, apartment, or shelter? Are your living conditions unsanitary or overly crowded?

• Did you go on a vacation recently? Were you camping or traveling overseas? (This may suggest possible exposure to contaminated food or liquids.)

Coping patterns

Assess the patient's stress management techniques and his ability to cope with an infectious disorder. Consider asking the following questions:

• Has your illness caused drastic changes in your lifestyle?

• How have you coped with crises in the past?

• Do you feel that your current coping strategies are helping or hindering your progress?

• Are you having trouble coming to terms with your illness?

Use your assessment of the patient's coping patterns to determine his teaching needs. Does he understand his diagnosis? How willing is he to accept changes in his lifestyle? How important is good health to him? Is he willing to work to improve his health? If the patient isn't ready or willing to accept change, he's unlikely to respond to your teaching.

Physical examination

Your next step is to perform a physical examination. Using a systematic sequence of assessment techniques will help ensure that you don't miss an important finding, even if you're rushed. However, if your patient is acutely ill and requires emergency intervention, you'll need to remain flexible in your approach.

Generally, physical examination of a patient with an infectious disorder includes observing the patient's general appearance, recording vital signs, and assessing the patient's lymph nodes. If signs and symptoms suggest a specific infection or route of infection, further assessment of specific structures and systems is warranted. (See *Physical examination checklist,* pages 166 and 167.)

Before you begin, make sure that you have all the necessary equipment, including a stethoscope, sphygmomanometer, thermometer, pair of gloves, tongue blade, penlight, speculum, and otoscope. In case cultures are ordered, make sure that you also have the appropriate containers and labels.

Perform the physical examination in a quiet, well-lit room that ensures privacy. If necessary, adjust the

Assessment TimeSaver

Physical examination checklist

After measuring vital signs, use the information below to help you gather additional assessment data. Focus more closely on specific areas alluded to in the health history. If the health history reveals generalized complaints, a thorough examination of all body systems is in order. Be especially alert for any of the following signs or symptoms of infection.

Central nervous system
□ Altered level of consciousness
□ Nuchal rigidity
□ Brudzinski's sign
□ Kernig's sign

Skin
□ Swelling
□ Rash
□ Erythema
□ Wounds or lesions
□ Characteristics of any exudate
□ Jaundice
□ Lesion warmth, tenderness, presence or absence of fluid
□ Dryness or moisture
□ Poor skin turgor

Eyes
□ Periorbital edema
□ Eyelid lesions
□ Crusting
□ Tearing
□ Pain
□ Conjunctival redness

Ears
□ Auricular pain or lesions
□ Swelling, redness, drainage, or crusting in external auditory canal
□ Bright pink to red tympanic membrane

□ Yellow to white tympanic membrane (serum or pus accumulation)
□ Convex bulging of tympanic membrane (fluid accumulation)

Nose and sinuses
□ Nasal discharge
□ Swelling over sinuses

Oropharynx
□ Edema
□ Redness
□ Tenderness
□ Lesions
□ Characteristics of any exudate

Lungs and chest
□ Tachypnea
□ Shortness of breath
□ Abnormal breathing pattern
□ Diminished chest excursion
□ Increased tactile fremitus
□ Dullness on percussion
□ Crackles
□ Wheezing
□ Rhonchi
□ Sputum characteristics

Heart
□ Tachycardia
□ Murmur
□ Pericardial friction rub

Abdomen

☐ Hyperactive bowel sounds (may suggest gastroenteritis)
☐ Hypoactive bowel sounds (may suggest peritonitis)
☐ Rebound tenderness
☐ Guarding
☐ Abdominal rigidity
☐ Enlarged liver or spleen
☐ Suprapubic tenderness

Kidneys and genitalia

☐ Flank tenderness
☐ External edema, redness, lesions, characteristics of any discharge
☐ Presence of lice or nits
☐ Oliguria (ominous sign)
☐ Cervical lesion or discharge

Rectum

☐ Perianal redness, swelling, tenderness, or lesion
☐ Discharge or bleeding

Extremities

☐ Edema
☐ Delayed capillary refill time
☐ Diminished peripheral pulses
☐ Red, swollen, tender joints
☐ Limited range of motion
☐ Impaired mobility

thermostat; cool temperatures may alter the patient's skin temperature and color, heart rate, and blood pressure.

General appearance

Observe the patient. Note his body type, overall appearance, and muscle composition. Does he seem well nourished and alert? Does his appearance coincide with his given age? Also note his posture, gait, movements, and hygiene. Look for signs of fatigue, weakness, or overt distress, such as acute pain, coughing, or shortness of breath. Also look for obvious signs of infection, such as a draining skin lesion.

Measure and record the patient's height and weight. These measurements will help guide treatment, determine medication dosages, and direct nutritional counseling.

Timesaving tip: Save time by making general observations about the patient's appearance as you take the health history. Confirm your observations quickly at the beginning of the physical examination.

Observe the patient's breathing pattern. Is he experiencing any difficulty? If so, how many words can he say with each breath? As you speak to him, observe his posture. Many patients experiencing breathing difficulty adopt a tripod position (resting the elbows or arms on the knees, a table, or the arms of a chair) to ease breathing.

Vital signs

The patient's vital signs — temperature, blood pressure, pulse rate, and respirations — provide baseline data for your assessment.

Temperature

Take the patient's temperature and watch for fever (an oral temperature greater than 101° F [38.3° C]), the hallmark of infection. Keep in mind that fever also accompanies many noninfectious disorders and that infection may be present without fever, especially in debilitated older patients and infants and preschool children.

Make sure that you obtain an accurate reading. When using an oral thermometer, be aware that you may obtain a false-low reading if the patient has trouble keeping his lips closed (or typically breathes through his mouth), is receiving humidified oxygen, is tachypneic (respirations more than 20 breaths/minute), or recently smoked a cigarette or consumed a cold beverage. In these circumstances, use a rectal thermometer or a thermometer placed in the ear (tympanic thermometer) to ensure an accurate reading.

Look for signs that typically accompany fever, such as chills, flushing, malaise, myalgia, and irritability. In some infections, especially those that are associated with acquired immunodeficiency syndrome (AIDS) or tuberculosis, fever is often accompanied by night sweats. If the patient's temperature is greater than 104° F (40° C), watch for seizures (febrile seizures are common, especially in children).

Timesaving tip: Place an airway, oxygen equipment, and suction equipment in the room as soon as you identify the risk for seizures. When a patient begins seizure activity, you won't have time to gather equipment.

Blood pressure

Measure the patient's blood pressure. Although infection rarely affects blood pressure, hypotension may indicate advanced sepsis.

Pulse rate and respirations

Check the patient's pulse and respiratory rates. Infection commonly increases the pulse rate (usually 10 beats/minute for each 1° F [0.6° C] rise in temperature). The patient's respiratory rate usually rises as well.

Timesaving tip: Consider using a portable pulse oximetry device on your patient. It can supply you with data on the patient's respiratory status within 30 seconds. Use it on all initial assessments and on any patient you suspect is having respiratory distress. Document results and report any abnormal readings or significant changes to the doctor.

Lymph nodes

Inspect and palpate the patient's lymph nodes for evidence of systemic infection. Focus more intently on nodes where you suspect infection. Note any swelling, erythema, enlargement, warmth, or tenderness.

Diagnostic test results

The results of diagnostic tests complete the objective data base. Together with the health history and physical examination findings, they form a profile of your patient's condition. Common tests for diagnosing infection focus on the body's immune and inflammatory responses to the infection and on determining the infectious organisms.

White blood cell count with differential

In a patient with infection, leukocytosis and neutrophilia are normal and desirable findings. Leukocytosis (a total white blood cell [WBC] count greater than 10,000 cells/mm³) represents a normal initial response to acute infection. The WBC differential shows neutrophilia, with a dramatic rise in the percentage of segmented neutrophils (up to 99%).

If the infection persists for several days, microorganism growth may outpace the immune system's ability to produce leukocytes. Total WBC count drops to normal or below normal. The WBC differential reflects a shift in the population of circulating neutrophils. The percentage of mature segmented neutrophils (segs) decreases while the percentage of less mature forms (bands) increases. This shift signals overwhelming infection.

Direct microscopic examination
Direct examination of a specimen often provides important clues about the microorganism, such as its size, shape, and staining characteristics, and may permit positive identification. Often, staining provides valuable diagnostic leads, which may support a presumptive diagnosis and prompt antimicrobial therapy.

Staining techniques
Common staining techniques include Gram stain and acid-fast stain.
• The Gram stain technique rapidly distinguishes between gram-negative and gram-positive organisms. It also helps identify some anaerobes that fail to grow in culture and the type of inflammatory cells present.
• The acid-fast stain technique helps identify organisms of the genus *Mycobacterium* (including the pathogens that cause tuberculosis and leprosy) and often facilitates a prompt presumptive diagnosis.
• Other staining procedures, such as the periodic acid-Schiff (PAS) stain and the methenamine silver stain, may reveal characteristic reactions useful in diagnosing fungal infection

and infection due to *Pneumocystis carinii.*

Cytologic examination
Microscopic cytologic examination can confirm the presence of a viral or a fungal infection, although it doesn't identify the specific microorganism.

Cultures
Cultures may be performed on almost any body tissue or fluid to isolate and identify a microorganism. Bacterial cultures are commonly ordered when an infection is suspected. Accurate results depend on proper techniques for collecting, handling, and processing specimens. Major considerations include:
• using aseptic technique when obtaining specimens (except stool specimens)
• obtaining fresh specimens
• obtaining an amount sufficient for the culture ordered
• placing the specimen in an appropriate sterile container
• presuming that all specimens are potentially infectious and implementing appropriate precautions before, during, and after obtaining the specimens
• sending the specimen to the laboratory promptly to ensure accurate results. (See *Collecting specimens for bacterial culture,* page 170.)

If you're taking a specimen for a specific viral culture, check with the laboratory for exact directions on collection and handling.

How quickly the pathogen can be identified depends on it's growth rate and nutritional requirements. For example, results of cultures of common bacterial pathogens (such as streptococci and staphylococci) are usually available within 48 hours. Slower growing bacteria (for example, *My-*

Collecting specimens for bacterial culture

Specimen	Nursing considerations
Blood	• Clean skin over venipuncture site with hospital-approved antiseptic solution (usually povidine-iodine solution). • Clean caps on blood culture tubes. • With a syringe, draw 10 ml of blood; then inject 5 ml into an unvented blood culture bottle and 5 ml into a vented blood culture bottle. • If the patient is taking antibiotics, indicate which ones on the laboratory slip.
Cervical	• Wipe the cervix clean of mucus. • Insert a dry, sterile cotton swab into the external os for 10 seconds.
Gonorrheal	• Take specimen from urethra on males and from cervix on females. • *Males* — Instruct the patient to refrain from voiding during the hour before specimen collection. Clean the meatus with sterile gauze. Insert a sterile urogenital swab or a small bacteriologic loop into the urethra and rotate the implement. • *Females* — Wipe the cervix clean of mucus. Insert a dry, sterile cotton swab into the external os for 10 seconds. • Inoculate "chocolate" agar plate or special culture medium provided in gonorrhea test kit.
Pharyngeal	• Swab tonsillar areas and any visible pustular material. • Don't allow swab to touch tongue, mouth, teeth, cheeks, or lips. • On the laboratory slip, indicate which antibiotics the patient is taking or has taken during the previous week and indicate the suspected microorganism.
Rectal	• Insert culture swab about 1″ (2.5 cm) into the rectum and rotate gently.
Skin	• *Do not* clean skin areas before obtaining specimen. Cultures are more accurate if specimens are taken from drainage or a wound area. • Lift crusts off wounds or pustules, and swab the area immediately beneath the crust. • Aspirate fluid from blisters.
Sputum	• Collect the specimen soon after the patient has awakened from a night's sleep and before he eats. • Ask the patient to inhale deeply, cough forcefully, and expectorate into the appropriate container. • If obtaining the specimen by suction, use a sterile mucus trap collection tube. • Lubricate the outside of the catheter with sterile 0.9% sodium chloride solution, but don't aspirate the solution through the catheter before or after obtaining the specimen.
Stool	• Stool collection does not have to be sterile. • Send as much of the stool specimen as possible (including blood and mucus) to the laboratory. • Send the specimen to the laboratory immediately.
Urine	• Clean meatus with an antiseptic solution. • Obtain a clean-catch specimen. • Immediately take the specimen to the laboratory or refrigerate it. • If the patient is taking antibiotics, indicate which ones on the laboratory slip.

cobacterium tuberculosis) take 3 to 6 weeks to identify.

Sensitivity testing
After identification of a microorganism, sensitivity testing is often performed to determine its susceptibility to specific antimicrobials.

Immunodiagnostic testing
If the microorganism can't be isolated and identified, diagnosis relies on demonstrating an increasing titer of antibodies (the measure of antigen-antibody reaction) to a specific pathogen or its product, or detecting antigens unique to a specific pathogen. To demonstrate a rise in antibody titer, serum obtained early in the course of illness is compared with serum obtained 2 to 3 weeks later. Generally, a fourfold or greater increase confirms infection with a specific pathogen.

Other immunodiagnostic tests also detect various antigens or antibodies to them in clinical specimens. Some common test methods include:
• immunodiffusion and counter immunoelectrophoresis
• agglutination
• complement fixation
• direct and indirect immunofluorescence
• radioimmunoassay (RIA)
• enzyme-linked immunoabsorbent assay (ELISA).

RIA and ELISA prove extremely sensitive for detecting antigens or antibodies. In fact, they're probably the most widely used assays for antibodies. For instance, ELISA is used to screen for HIV antibodies; RIA helps confirm hepatitis B.

Technical advances in immunodiagnostic techniques have resulted in test kits that can quickly identify certain infectious pathogens. Examples include the rapid plasma reagin test (a serologic test for syphilis) and a test kit that takes only 7 minutes to identify group A streptococci from a throat-culture swab.

Polymerase chain reaction
This extremely sensitive test amplifies nucleic acid sequences of target pathogens in a specimen, thus expediting diagnosis of certain infectious diseases, especially those caused by viruses, such as HIV. It may also be used to type genital human papillomavirus.

Radiographic testing
Radiographic tests often support a diagnosis of infection but rarely establish the cause. For example, chest X-ray may reveal the interstitial infiltrates typical with *Pneumocystis carinii* pneumonia. Computed tomography may help diagnose an abscess.

Nursing diagnosis

The next step in the nursing process — nursing diagnosis — describes the patient's actual or potential response to a health problem. As you formulate a nursing diagnosis, review your assessment data for patterns that indicate specific problems. Consider asking yourself the following questions:
• What are the patient's signs and symptoms?
• Which assessment findings are abnormal for this patient?
• Did assessment reveal a cluster of findings that suggests a specific infectious disorder?
• How do the patient's behavior patterns and environment affect his risk for infection?
• Is the patient at risk for complications related to infection?

• Does the patient understand his health status?

• How has the patient's condition affected his ability to perform activities of daily living? How has it affected his social relationships?

• What is the patient's response to his infectious disorder? Is he willing and motivated to change his health status?

When formulating nursing diagnoses, use a diagnosis approved by the North American Nursing Diagnosis Association (NANDA) that fits your patient or, if necessary, create your own. To foster greater accuracy, you should also write an etiology, or "related to" statement, for each nursing diagnosis. The etiology should include conditions or circumstances that contribute to the development or continuation of the diagnosis, such as environmental, physiologic, psychological, cultural, or spiritual influences identified during assessment. For example, if you suspect that the patient's diarrhea is associated with a GI infection, your diagnostic statement might be "diarrhea related to infectious process."

Chapters 9 through 11 contain common nursing diagnoses for specific infectious disorders. Keep in mind, however, that diagnostic statements must be tailored to your patient's individual circumstances and needs. Each patient responds differently, and your nursing diagnoses should never become so standardized that they fail to reflect the individual needs of each patient under your care.

Developing diagnoses for each patient with an infectious disorder can be difficult. You can make this task easier and save time by becoming familiar with the more common nursing diagnoses encountered in infectious disorders. (See *Common nursing diagnoses in infectious disorders.*)

Activity intolerance

This nursing diagnosis refers to the state in which a patient has insufficient physiologic or psychological energy to endure or complete required or desired daily activities.

Characteristics of activity intolerance include:

• increased or decreased heart rate, blood pressure, or respiratory rate

• poor nutrition

• high metabolic needs

• changes in baseline electrocardiogram during activity

• discomfort or dyspnea during activity

• redness, cyanosis, or pallor of the skin during activity

• impaired ability to change position, stand, or walk without assistance

• weakness that necessitates frequent rest periods.

Common related factors include:

• generalized weakness

• fatigue

• immobility

• loss of muscle tone due to inactivity

• hypovolemia

• electrolyte imbalance

• imbalance between oxygen supply and demand

• discomfort

Activity intolerance commonly occurs in infectious mononucleosis, hepatitis, influenza, and AIDS.

Pain

This nursing diagnosis describes a state in which the patient experiences and reports severe discomfort or an uncomfortable sensation.

Defining characteristics for this diagnosis include:

• communication (verbal or nonverbal) of pain

Common nursing diagnoses in infectious disorders

Certain nursing diagnoses can be used frequently to describe the response patterns of patients with infectious disorders. This list identifies and defines these diagnoses.

Activity intolerance • Insufficient physiologic or psychological energy to endure or complete required or desired daily activities

Altered oral mucous membrane • Disrupted mouth integrity

Altered sexuality patterns • State in which an individual expresses concern about engaging in sexual activity

Altered urinary elimination pattern • Impairment of urinary function

Decreased cardiac output • Cardiovascular or respiratory symptoms resulting from insufficient blood being pumped by the heart

Diarrhea • A change in normal bowel elimination habits characterized by frequent passage of fluid and loose or unformed stools

High risk for fluid volume deficit • Presence of risk factors that can lead to excessive fluid and electrolyte loss

High risk for impaired skin integrity • Presence of risk factors for interruption or destruction of skin surface

Impaired tissue integrity • Damage to mucous membranes or to corneal, integumentary, or subcutaneous tissue

Hyperthermia • Elevation of body temperature above normal range

Ineffective airway clearance • Inability to clear secretions or obstructions from the respiratory tract

Ineffective breathing pattern • Inspiratory or expiratory pattern that fails to provide adequate lung inflation or deflation

Knowledge deficit • Inadequate understanding of information or an inability to perform skills needed to practice health-related behaviors

Noncompliance • Unwillingness to practice prescribed health-related behaviors

Pain • Subjective sensation of discomfort derived from multiple sensory nerve interactions generated by physical, chemical, biological, or psychological stimuli

Social isolation • State in which a patient experiences aloneness that he perceives as negative or threatening and caused by others

• distracting behavior (for example, moaning, crying, seeking out people or activities, restlessness)
• guarding behavior
• alterations in muscle tone ranging from rigidity to listlessness
• facial mask of pain
• increased blood pressure, pulse rate, and respiratory rate.

In infectious disorders, pain is most often related to a biological, chemical, physical, or psychological injuring agent.

Hyperthermia

This nursing diagnosis describes a state in which the patient's body temperature rises above the normal range.

Hyperthermia is characterized by:
- fever
- flushed skin
- increased respiratory rate
- seizures
- shivering
- skin that's warm to the touch
- tachycardia
- weakness
- perspiration
- verbal reports of feeling "hot."

Hyperthermia in a patient with an infectious disorder may be related to illness or trauma, dehydration, increased metabolic rate, or an inability (or reduced ability) to perspire.

High risk for fluid volume deficit

This nursing diagnosis describes a state in which the patient is at risk for experiencing vascular, cellular, or intracellular dehydration.

This diagnosis is more common in very young patients, older patients, or patients who are extremely overweight or underweight. High risk for fluid volume deficit may be related to the following factors:
- loss of fluids through abnormal routes (for example, an indwelling catheter)
- an excessive loss of fluid through normal routes (for example, diarrhea)
- a hypermetabolic state
- a knowledge deficit
- the effects of medications
- conditions (or deviations) that limit the patient's access to, intake of, or absorption of fluids (for example, physical immobility).

Ineffective breathing pattern

This nursing diagnosis describes a state in which the patient's inhalation or exhalation pattern, or both, fails to provide adequate lung inflation or deflation.

Ineffective breathing pattern is characterized by:
- dyspnea
- nasal flaring
- cough
- fremitus
- cyanosis
- bradypnea, orthopnea, or tachypnea
- use of accessory muscles, pursed-lip breathing, and splinting or guarding during respirations
- reluctance to breathe deeply because of pain.

In infectious disorders, the most common related factors include decreased lung expansion, effects of medications, fatigue, pulmonary infection, pain, immobility, and inactivity.

Planning

The next step of the nursing process involves creating a plan of action that will direct your patient care toward achieving specific goals. This step includes writing a plan of care to serve as a record of your nursing diagnoses, expected patient outcomes, nursing interventions, and evaluation data. In most hospitals, the plan of care forms a permanent part of the patient's health record to help ensure the quality and effectiveness of health care delivery.

Early in the planning process, you'll need to determine priorities for nursing care. Using your nursing diagnoses, you'll need to decide which problems require immediate attention and which can wait. Always give the highest priority to problems that pose immediate safety risks, and then address health-threatening and psychosocial concerns. For example, when managing the care of a patient with pneumonia, your first priority will be correcting altered breathing patterns; after that, you'll be able to deal with issues related to impaired individual coping. (See *Setting priorities for nursing diagnoses in infectious disorders,* pages 176 and 177.)

To save time and create a plan of care that is meaningful and attainable, enlist the help of staff members who are familiar with the patient. Be sure to involve your patient and members of his family in the planning process. Ask what problems are most important to him because these may differ from the problems you perceive as priorities. A patient with an infectious disorder is more likely to comply with treatment if you take time to learn his priorities.

Effective communication is essential when you're working with the patient and his family. To enhance communication with them, create a quiet, private, and relaxed environment, and encourage them to ask questions about the infectious disorder and its treatment. Be sure to translate medical terms into simple, clear language.

Establishing patient outcomes
After evaluating the patient's priorities, you'll need to establish patient outcomes — measurable goals derived from the patient's nursing diagnoses. A patient outcome should describe a behavior or result that's to be achieved within a specific time frame. (Target dates help motivate the patient and help you keep the patient on schedule for discharge.)

Patient outcomes are used to evaluate the effectiveness of nursing care; therefore, they should be realistic. For a patient with a urinary tract infection with the nursing diagnosis *pain related to bladder spasms and dysuria secondary to the infectious process,* an expected outcome might be *Patient will report an absence of pain and discomfort.* However, for this goal to be realistic, the patient must first achieve several preliminary outcomes; for example:
• Patient will comply with prescribed therapeutic drug regimen.
• Patient will describe how to use a topical antiseptic for pain relief.
• Patient will identify factors that aggravate and alleviate pain.

The success of your plan of care depends on accurate documentation of patient outcomes. Outcome statements that are vague, hard to measure, or unrealistic may invalidate a plan that is otherwise accurate and useful. When choosing patient outcomes, consider asking yourself the following questions:
• What type of behavior will show that the patient has reached the specific goal you've set?
• Which criteria will be used to measure the behavior (how much, how long, how far)?
• Under what conditions should the behavior occur?
• What is a realistic time frame for the behavior to be achieved?

For example, if your patient's nursing diagnosis is *hyperthermia related to dehydration,* appropriate outcome statements might include the following:
• Patient's oral temperature will be within a normal range (97.7° to 99.5° F [36.5° to 37.5° C]) within 24 hours.

(Text continues on page 178.)

Setting priorities for nursing diagnoses in infectious disorders

As you plan care for your patient with an infectious disorder, you'll need to establish priorities. Consider the significant assessment findings underlying your nursing diagnoses and address life-threatening problems first.

Consider this example.

Subjective data

Suppose that you're caring for 68-year-old Mr. Butler, who was transferred to your unit after evaluation for upper GI bleeding. Earlier endoscopic examination identified a small duodenal ulcer. Your initial assessment reveals that Mr. Butler is dyspneic with a nonproductive cough. He complains of chills and mild right-sided chest discomfort aggravated by the coughing spells.

Mr. Butler reports a pack-a-week history of cigarette smoking but is unaware of any allergies or contact with anyone having a respiratory infection. He does not have a history of significant occupational or environmental exposure to pulmonary irritants. He has never before been hospitalized, does not regularly see a doctor or nurse practitioner, and takes no medications except aspirin twice daily for joint pain. Occasionally, he has had blood pressure checks at a shopping mall and admits that the readings have been high.

When Mr. Butler was admitted to your unit, you learned that he had a nasogastric (NG) tube for several hours that was removed before endoscopy. He also received a short-acting sedative (I.V. midazolam) before the procedure. Before transfer, clear liquids were started by mouth. His bleeding is now under control and an I.V. of 1,000 ml of 0.9% sodium chloride solution is infusing at a keep-vein-open rate.

Objective data

Your examination of Mr. Butler reveals the following:

- general appearance — sitting slightly forward, with head of bed elevated, supported by two pillows; patient alert and oriented to person, place, and time
- height 5'8" (173 cm); weight 212 lb (96.2 kg)
- oral temperature, 101° F (38.3° C); blood pressure, 118/84 mm Hg; pulse rate, 94 beats/minute and regular with diminished volume
- respirations, 28 breaths/minute and slightly labored
- heart sounds normal; no neck vein distention or peripheral edema
- tubular (bronchial) breath sounds over right lower lobe, posteriorly
- abdomen soft and nontender, with hypoactive bowel sounds
- skin warm, dry, and flushed
- mucous membranes and axillae dry
- intake and output record showing a negative balance. Last recorded voiding was 150 ml, 6 hours ago.

Diagnostic test results

- Arterial blood gas (ABG) analysis indicates a pH of 7.33, partial pressure of arterial carbon dioxide of 49 mm Hg, partial pressure of arterial oxygen of 68 mm Hg, and bicar-

bonate level of 24 mEq/liter.
• Chest X-ray shows a right lower lobe infiltrate.
• Sputum and blood cultures are pending.
• White blood cell count with differential shows leukocytosis with an increased number of immature neutrophils (bands), indicating infection.
• Hematocrit is 37% and hemoglobin is 10 g/dl.

Findings

The findings suggest that Mr. Butler may have developed a nosocomial pneumonia. There are several reasons why this may have occurred:
• The use of the NG tube altered the normal protective glottic reflex and mucociliary clearance of the upper respiratory tract.
• During the endoscopy, the patient may have regurgitated and aspirated gastric or pharyngeal contents, which promotes bacterial growth.
• Because the patient was sedated for the endoscopy, his depressed level of consciousness may have contributed to ineffective airway clearance.
• His history of cigarette smoking places him at increased risk, because it's associated with increased mucus production and decreased ciliary motion.

Setting priorities

Your first concern is Mr. Butler's respiratory status. His ABG levels reflect respiratory acidosis and hypoxemia. You realize he'll need aggressive management so that his respiratory status does not deteriorate. You select *impaired gas exchange related*

to infectious pulmonary process as your first priority nursing diagnosis.

Your next priority is to improve the patient's airway clearance. His mucus production has increased and he isn't coughing effectively. You know that smoking paralyzes the cilia and impairs mucociliary clearance. Therefore, you choose *ineffective airway clearance related to increased mucus production* as your second priority nursing diagnosis.

Your next priority is to take steps to improve his fluid status. Your assessment findings suggest mild dehydration. You'll need to administer I.V. fluids to ensure adequate organ perfusion. As your third priority nursing diagnosis, you select *fluid volume deficit related to inadequate volume replacement, poor oral intake, and fever*.

After addressing your immediate concerns, you examine the health-related aspects of Mr. Butler's lifestyle. You realize that he may need to become better informed about risks to his health. You are concerned about his excessive aspirin ingestion, cigarette smoking, hypertension, as well as failure to obtain regular checkups. Therefore, to help reduce risks, you select *knowledge deficit related to health maintenance* as your final nursing diagnosis.

Having set priorities for Mr. Butler's problem, you can now proceed to establish patient outcomes and implement care.

• He will achieve and maintain fluid balance within 24 hours.
• He will verbalize increased comfort within 8 hours.
• He will identify risk factors for hyperthermia within 48 hours.

Developing nursing interventions

After establishing patient outcomes, you'll develop nursing interventions — specific strategies that will help the patient achieve those outcomes. Information obtained during your assessment of such factors as your patient's age, emotional status, any physical or mental impairments, developmental and educational levels, environment, and cultural values is helpful. Talk with the patient and members of his family. The more you know about the patient, the easier it will be to formulate appropriate interventions.

Write each intervention in precise detail. Include how and when to perform the intervention (including supplies or equipment) as well as any special instructions. Clearly state the necessary actions so they can be continued or modified by other nurses in your absence. Examples of clearly stated interventions include the following:

• Provide cool, humidified air, changing the water daily to prevent *Pseudomonas* superinfection. Clean the humidifier thoroughly and change the filter according to established procedures at your hospital.
• Assess the patient's emotional reaction to his condition, especially if the condition is chronic and produces skin lesions. Provide a nonthreatening, nonjudgmental atmosphere that encourages the patient to verbalize feelings about perceived changes in sexual attractiveness, behavior, and body image. Contact a psychiatric clinical nurse specialist or other mental health specialist if the patient requires services you can't provide.
• Take the patient's temperature at least every 4 hours. Administer antipyretics as ordered. If the patient's fever is very high, assess his level of consciousness. If necessary, provide a hypothermia blanket.

To ensure cooperation, make sure that the patient and his family members understand each intervention and the reason behind it.

Implementation

During the fourth step of the nursing process, you put your plan of care into action. During this phase, you'll have direct and prolonged contact with the patient. You'll also coordinate and direct the activities of other health care team members.

It's important to use your time effectively when implementing patient care. Use your plan of care to help you organize your day and manage your time wisely. As you document your interventions, note changes in the patient's condition, new problems, the status or resolution of old problems, the patient's responses to treatments or medications, and the responses of the patient's family members to your interventions. The following is a brief review of nursing interventions you may need to implement during your care of a patient with an infectious disorder.

Therapeutic interventions

These interventions focus on alleviating the effects of illness and restoring optimal function. Common therapeutic interventions for infectious disorders include:

• administering prescribed medications, such as antimicrobials
• performing and teaching pulmonary hygiene measures, such as postural drainage and percussion, coughing and deep breathing, and incentive spirometry, as needed
• providing hydration
• administering supplemental oxygen
• positioning the patient carefully, turning him often, and assisting with range-of-motion exercises
• consulting with the dietitian to ensure that the patient receives a nutritious diet.

Emergency care

Infection can necessitate emergency interventions. For example, if your patient has worsening sepsis, you must be prepared to recognize and respond to signs and symptoms of septic shock. Untreated septic shock can cause multiple organ failure and death. In this case, emergency interventions may include:
• establishing or safeguarding the airway
• promptly notifying the doctor
• immediately establishing a vascular access site
• administering oxygen and prescribed emergency medications
• administering prescribed antimicrobials
• initiating hemodynamic monitoring
• transferring the patient to the intensive care unit, if necessary
• providing him and his family with emotional support.

Monitoring

Periodic or continuous evaluation of your patient's status and response to therapy is just as important as the initial assessment. In many cases, you'll monitor the following:
• temperature
• complete blood count

• arterial blood gas (ABG) levels
• pulse oximetry values
• blood levels of drugs and any adverse reactions
• culture and sensitivity results.

Patient teaching

Teaching can help the patient with an infectious disorder maintain his health and avoid future problems. Many of your lessons will focus on providing the patient and his family with information about the specific infection and the infectious process, including:
• symptoms to report to the doctor
• possible complications
• factors that may precipitate complications
• the prescribed medication regimen, including the need to complete the entire regimen even if the patient feels well
• proper hand-washing technique
• proper methods of disposing of used tissues
• importance of covering the mouth when coughing or sneezing.

Emotional support

You may plan and implement interventions to enhance your patient's emotional well-being. This would include taking into account physiologic, emotional, social, sexual, or financial concerns. For example, if your patient has gonorrhea, encourage him to express his feelings and fears about his condition. Also provide information that helps him understand his disorder better. These interventions may help reduce the patient's anxiety.

Schedule a specific time to talk with the patient and establish a trusting, supportive relationship. This will promote patient compliance with therapeutic interventions and help him resume his usual role more easily upon discharge.

For patients who are coping poorly, you may need to provide a referral for psychological counseling. Family members may also need help in coping with the patient's disorder and any associated increase in demands it places on them.

Preparation for discharge

For some patients with infectious disorders, the thought of going home and having to care for themselves is overwhelming. At discharge, the patient may still be weak and feel unprepared to leave the security and care of the hospital.

By preparing the patient for discharge, you can help make the transition from the hospital to the patient's home safe and smooth and ensure continued quality of care. Preparation for discharge may include:

• reinforcing the teaching plan
• reviewing the infectious disorder, including possible complications
• reviewing signs and symptoms to report to the doctor
• reviewing prescribed medications (especially the need to continue taking antimicrobial medications even after the patient feels better) and possible adverse effects
• reviewing any nutritional or activity guidelines
• reminding the patient when to return for follow-up appointments and diagnostic tests
• providing necessary referrals (for example, to a home health care service or medical equipment supplier).

The implementation phase concludes when the nurse's actions are completed and the results of actions and the patient's response to them have been recorded.

Evaluation

During evaluation, the last step in the nursing process, you judge the effectiveness of nursing care and gauge your patient's progress in achieving expected outcomes. The evaluation process begins as soon as you implement a plan of care and continues until the patient is discharged or all of the goals are met. Evaluating the patient gives you a chance to:

• determine if original assessment findings still apply
• identify complications
• validate the appropriateness of nursing diagnoses, expected patient outcomes, and interventions
• analyze patterns or trends in your patient's care and his responses to care
• assess his response to all aspects of care, including medications, changes in diet and activity, procedures, unusual incidents or problems, and patient teaching
• determine how closely care conforms with established standards
• measure the effectiveness of your care
• assess the performance of other health care team members
• discover opportunities to improve the quality and effectiveness of your nursing care.

Evaluation is an ongoing activity that overlaps other phases of the nursing process; therefore, your evaluation findings may trigger a new cycle of assessment, nursing diagnosis, planning, implementation, and further evaluation.

To ensure a successful evaluation, keep an open mind. Never hesitate to consider new patient data or to revise previous judgments. Remember, no plan of care is perfect. In fact, you should anticipate revising the plan of care during the course of treatment.

Reassessment

Reassessing the patient's condition is the basis for evaluation. You'll reassess the patient at regular intervals, depending on his status and your hospital's policy. You may not need to complete a multisystem physical assessment again; just focus on areas identified in the nursing diagnoses. You'll also reassess the patient any time his status changes unexpectedly.

Next, compare reassessment data with criteria established in the patient outcomes documented in your plan of care. As you analyze reassessment data, consider asking yourself the following questions:

• Do the reassessment data support the expected outcomes?

• Has the patient's condition improved, deteriorated, or stayed the same?

• Have new complications developed?

• Which outcomes were achieved? Which were partially achieved? Which were not achieved?

If you find that your expected outcomes have not been met by the projected dates, you must assess what factors might be interfering with the patient's progress. Consider all possible reasons that the patient may not be able to achieve a desired outcome. Below are some examples:

• The purpose and goals of the plan of care aren't clear.

• The expected outcomes aren't realistic in light of the patient's condition.

• The plan of care is based on incomplete or inaccurate assessment data.

• Nursing diagnoses are inaccurate.

• The nursing staff experienced conflicts with the patient or medical staff.

• Staff members didn't follow the plan of care.

• Interventions weren't documented in detail, resulting in confusion or inconsistency.

• The patient failed to carry out activities outlined in the plan of care.

• The patient's condition changed or complications developed.

Writing evaluation statements

Evaluation statements provide a method for documenting the patient's response to care. These statements indicate whether expected outcomes were achieved and list the evidence supporting your conclusions.

The importance of clearly written evaluation statements can't be overemphasized. Documentation of patient outcomes is necessary to substantiate the rationales for nursing care and to justify the use of nursing resources. You'll record your evaluation statements in your progress notes or on the revised plan of care, according to your hospital's documentation policy.

Writing clear, concise evaluation statements is easy if you wrote precise patient outcome statements during the planning phase of care. The patient outcome statements provide a model for evaluation statements. When writing an evaluation statement, you should describe the patient's progress using active verbs, such as "discusses," "demonstrates," and "maintains." Include criteria used to measure the patient's response to care and describe the conditions under which the response occurred (or failed to occur).

Write a separate evaluation statement for each patient response or behavior that you wish to describe. Remember to date the evaluation statement.

For example, possible evaluation statements for the nursing diagnosis

ineffective breathing pattern related to decreased energy or fatigue include:
• Patient's respiratory rate remains within 5 breaths/minute of baseline.
• Patient's ABG levels returned to and remain within established limits.
• Patient indicates, either verbally or through behavior, feeling comfortable when breathing.
• Each day, patient reports that he feels rested.
• Patient performs diaphragmatic pursed-lip breathing.
• Patient demonstrates skill in conserving energy while carrying out activities of daily living.

Modifying the plan of care

During evaluation, you may discover that the plan of care needs to be modified. If patient outcomes have been achieved, make sure that you record the date the outcome was achieved and whether any nursing diagnosis has been resolved. Revise other outcome statements as necessary, and determine which nursing interventions need to be revised or discontinued. If outcomes are not met or a change in the patient's condition has occurred, you may need to assign new priorities to existing nursing diagnoses or add new diagnoses. The same is true for interventions.

Like all steps in the nursing process, evaluation is ongoing. Continue to assess, diagnose, plan, implement, and evaluate for as long as you care for the patient.

CHAPTER 8

Exploring chief complaints in infectious disorders

Pain   *184*

Purulent discharge   *187*

Several important signs and symptoms commonly occur in patients with infections. These include pain, purulent discharge, lymphadenopathy, fever, fatigue, and skin lesions. This chapter focuses on the first two chief complaints, pain and purulent discharge. For information about the other four chief complaints, see Chapter 2, Exploring chief complaints in immune disorders.

In addition to general chief complaints, the patient may have a chief complaint specific to the infection site. Common infection sites and associated signs and symptoms are as follows.

• *Central nervous system:* behavioral changes, confusion, drowsiness, headache, motor deficit, paresthesia, seizure, stiff neck

• *Eyes, ears, nose, and throat:* disturbed vision, dizziness, vertigo, hearing loss, pain (eye, ear, sinus, throat, jaw), photophobia, pruritus, purulent discharge, redness, swelling, sneezing, tearing, tinnitus

• *Respiratory system:* chest pain, congestion, cough, dyspnea

• *GI system:* abdominal pain or cramps, diarrhea, jaundice, nausea and vomiting

• *Urinary system:* dysuria, flank pain, frequency, hematuria, pyuria, urgency

• *Reproductive system:* abnormal bleeding, genital pain, lesions, pelvic pain or cramps, purulent discharge, vaginal pruritus

• *Musculoskeletal system:* joint, muscle, or bone pain; joint deformity; impaired mobility; stiffness; swelling; redness

• *Skin:* rash, redness, swelling, lesions, purulent drainage, petechiae and purpura, pain, pruritus.

Pain

Although pain is the most common complaint when disease is present, it may be difficult to assess. A patient's perception of pain is influenced by numerous cultural, economic, psychological, social, and physiologic factors.

In infectious disorders, pain occurs as a reaction to inflammation. It may result from the pressure of the exudate on nerve endings in surrounding tissue. It also may result from the inflammatory process — release of substances such as serotonin, histamine, and prostaglandins from damaged tissue, and bradykinin from the circulation or from local nerve endings themselves. These substances increase the irritability of pain receptors and initiate pain impulses. (See *Causes of pain.*)

History of the symptom
To further understand the patient's pain, consider asking the questions listed below.

• When did the pain begin?

• Is the pain continuous, or does it sometimes go away? If it's intermittent, how long does each episode last?

• How would you describe the pain?

• Did the pain start suddenly or build gradually?

• Where do you feel pain? (Ask the patient to point to the site.)

• Does the pain radiate to other areas? If so, what areas are involved? (See *Common referred pain sites,* page 186.)

• Can you rate your pain on a scale of 1 to 10, with 1 representing no pain and 10 the worst pain you've ever felt? (Rating scales vary, but should be used consistently within the facility.)

• What measures alleviate the pain?
• What factors aggravate the pain?
• Are you taking any medication, including over-the-counter drugs, to relieve pain? If so, what drugs are you taking, what dosage, and how often? How effectively does the medication relieve the pain?
• Has the pain interfered with your eating or sleeping?

If the patient has chronic pain, consider also asking these questions:
• How has the pain affected your life?
• Has the pain affected your relationship with others? If so, in what way?
• Do you work? How has the pain affected your ability to work?
• Has the pain interfered with your ability to care for yourself?
• How do you think we can help you?

If the patient is currently in severe pain, don't obtain a detailed history. Instead, limit your questions to those most pertinent to his pain. When the patient is more comfortable, you can complete the assessment.

Associated findings

Note whether the patient has experienced any of the following signs or symptoms that may accompany pain:
• anorexia
• diaphoresis
• fatigue
• nausea and vomiting
• rapid breathing
• reduced attention span
• restlessness.

Previous conditions and treatments

Consult with the patient, his family members, or his companion about the patient's medical history. Note any conditions or treatments that may be related to pain, such as:
• acute or chronic infection
• arthritis or bursitis

Causes of pain

Infectious disorders that commonly cause pain include:
• genital warts
• herpes simplex
• herpes zoster
• pneumonia
• hepatitis
• gastroenteritis
• meningitis
• pyelonephritis
• otitis media.

• calculi
• cancer
• dental work
• diverticulitis
• gallbladder disease
• heart disease
• herniated disk
• inflammatory bowel disease
• injury
• pancreatitis
• peptic ulcer
• peripheral vascular disease
• pleurisy
• pneumonia
• psychiatric illness
• radiation therapy
• sickle cell anemia
• surgery.

Drug history

Obtain a drug history. Note if the patient is taking drugs that may cause pain, such as:
• podofilox
• carboplatin injection
• sargramostim, by I.V. infusion
• etretinate capsules.

Common referred pain sites

Visceral pain — deep pain from structures within the body — is often poorly localized and may be referred to an area supplied by the same spinal root. These anterior and posterior views show the locations of pain referred from various visceral organs.

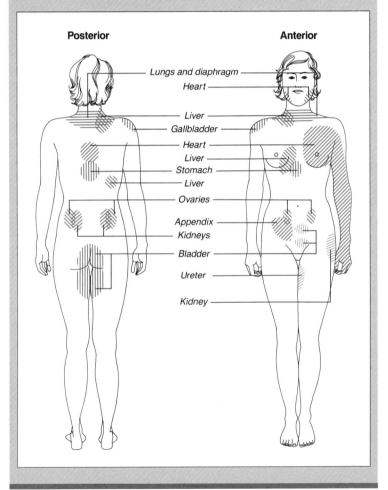

Posterior   Anterior

Lungs and diaphragm
Heart
Liver
Gallbladder
Heart
Liver
Stomach
Liver
Ovaries
Appendix
Kidneys
Bladder
Ureter
Kidney

Physical examination

Focus this examination on observation of the patient's nonverbal behavior, posture, and movements and on his physiologic responses to pain. Observe for these nonverbal clues that may indicate the presence of pain:

• inability to concentrate
• grimacing, frowning, squinting
• moaning, crying, writhing
• tense facial muscles
• drawing arms or legs close to the body
• clutching or rubbing the painful area
• muscle guarding, unusual posture, rocking motion
• inactivity, lying still in bed
• restlessness
• splinting or holding painful part during movement
• withdrawal.

If the patient has a history of chronic pain, be alert for coping mechanisms that may be related to pain, such as dependency, manipulation, or overly demanding behavior.

Watch for autonomic nervous system changes (more common with acute than chronic pain):

• altered sleep or rest patterns
• diaphoresis
• hypertension
• pupil dilation
• skin color changes (pallor, flushing)
• tachycardia
• tachypnea.

Purulent discharge

The result of inflammation, purulent exudate consists of live and dead leukocytes and microorganisms, serous exudate, and liquefied products of necrotic tissue. After forming at the infection site, the exudate may be absorbed, spread to other areas, or expelled from the body in any of several ways: in the sputum or urine; from the eye, ear, nose, or genitourinary tract; or from a break in the skin. (See *Causes of purulent discharge*, page 188.)

History of the sign

To further understand your patient's complaint, consider asking these questions:

• When did you first notice the discharge?
• What do you think caused it?
• Where is the discharge occurring?
• What does it look and smell like (frothy, foul smelling, etc.)?
• Has its appearance changed since you first noticed it?
• How much discharge is occurring daily?
• Have any factors aggravated or increased the amount of discharge, such as movement or body position?
• Have any factors reduced the amount of discharge?
• Are you currently taking medication for this problem? If so, what is its name and what dosage are you taking? Have you taken the medication exactly as prescribed? If not, why not? Has the medication helped? Has it caused any adverse reactions?
• Have you ever had a similar problem with discharge in the past? If so, what was the cause?
• Has anyone with whom you are in close contact experienced a similar problem? If so, provide details.

Timesaving tip: Consider the patient's answers to these questions and the site of the drainage. Then use your remaining questions to focus in on potential problems quickly and effectively. For example, if the patient recently had a similar vaginal discharge and was diagnosed with chlamydia, obtain a detailed sexual history, assess her level of knowledge about sexually transmitted diseases,

Causes of purulent discharge

Several common infectious microorganisms that cause purulent discharge are listed below, along with their distinguishing characteristics.

• Anaerobes (*Bacteroides* species, *Clostridium* species, *Staphylococcus aureus*) produce a strong odor.
• *Candida albicans* produces a thick, curdlike drainage.
• *Clostridium difficile* causes a liquid or semi-solid yellow-brown-orange bowel movement.
• *Clostridium perfringens* causes foamy, foul-smelling stools.
• *Klebsiella pneumoniae* produces brick red or currant jelly sputum.
• *Pseudomonas aeruginosa* discharge has a slight green tint and characteristic grapelike odor.
• *Trichomonas vaginalis* produces copious amounts of frothy yellow or yellow-green discharge.

Associated disorders

Disorders that may produce visible purulent discharge include pneumonia, tonsillitis, sexually transmitted diseases, infected wounds, external otitis, and bacterial conjunctivitis.

and assess her compliance with treatment.

Associated findings

Note whether the patient has experienced any of the following signs or symptoms:
• abnormal bleeding
• fever
• fatigue
• pain
• redness, swelling, warmth at site
• skin rash or lesion
• swollen glands.

Previous conditions and treatments

Ask the patient about any of the following in his health history:
• traumatic injury causing a break in the skin
• surgery
• sexually transmitted disease
• any other recent or continuing infection, including human immunodeficiency virus
• primary immunodeficiency disease
• cancer, chemotherapy, or radiation therapy
• immunosuppressive drug therapy
• intravascular access device
• any other invasive procedure.

Physical examination

Observe the patient's general appearance and physical and emotional state. Note if he appears clean and well nourished. Look for nonverbal behavior indicating pain or discomfort.

Inspect the infection site. Note the location, color, consistency, and amount of drainage and any associated odor. Inspect the area for a lesion and for signs of inflammation, including redness, edema, tenderness, and warmth. Also inspect the surrounding skin or mucous membrane for signs of excoriation.

You may need to obtain additional assessment data based on the involved site. For example, if purulent discharge runs from the eye, you'll need to assess its effect on vision.

Obtain the patient's vital signs and note the presence of fever, tachycardia, or tachypnea. If hypotension is present, report it immediately; this sign suggests a more serious progression of the infection.

CHAPTER 9

Caring for patients with viral infections

Viral hepatitis   190

Influenza   197

Herpes simplex   202

Herpes zoster   207

Genital warts   211

Infectious mononucleosis   214

Viral encephalitis   218

Viruses lack independent metabolism and can replicate only within the cells of a living host. These microorganisms spread in various ways, such as by inhalation, ingestion, or sexual contact.

Viral hepatitis

This common systemic disease is characterized by hepatic cell destruction, necrosis, and autolysis, which lead to anorexia, fatigue, and hepatomegaly. In most patients, hepatic cells eventually regenerate with little or no residual damage, allowing relatively quick recovery in 2 to 3 months. However, in elderly patients and in those with severe underlying disorders, complications are more likely. They may include edema and hepatic encephalopathy, fulminant hepatitis, and chronic liver disease. Rarely, hepatitis may lead to pancreatitis, myocarditis, atypical pneumonia, aplastic anemia, transverse myelitis, or peripheral neuropathy.

Causes
Hepatitis results from infection by one of five categories of virus: hepatitis A virus, hepatitis B virus, hepatitis C virus, hepatitis D virus, and hepatitis E virus. (See *Comparing types of viral hepatitis.*)

ASSESSMENT

Your assessment should include consideration of the patient's health history, physical examination findings, and diagnostic test results.

Health history
Signs and symptoms of hepatitis vary little among strains but occur in stages. In the prodromal stage, the patient generally complains of fatigue and anorexia, possibly with moderate weight loss. He also may report generalized malaise, headache, weakness, arthralgia, myalgia, photophobia, a cough, and nausea with vomiting. Frequently, he describes changes in his sense of taste and smell.

With the onset of jaundice, the earlier symptoms diminish, but some patients may complain of continued weight loss (moderate) and of right upper quadrant pain (due to an enlarged liver), pruritus, and indigestion. Hepatitis may also occur without jaundice.

During the recovery stage, most symptoms have subsided. (See *Determining the source of viral hepatitis,* page 192.)

Physical examination
Assessment of vital signs may reveal a fever of 100° to 104° F (37.8° to 40° C) — most often in hepatitis A. As the prodromal stage concludes, usually within 5 days of the onset of jaundice, specimens may reveal dark-colored urine and light or clay-colored stools.

Jaundice, which can last for 1 to 2 weeks, may be evident in the sclerae, mucous membranes, and skin. Rashes, erythematous patches, or hives may accompany jaundice, especially if the patient has hepatitis B or C. Palpation may disclose an enlarged and tender liver and, in some cases, splenomegaly and cervical adenopathy.

During the recovery stage, assessment may reveal a decrease in liver enlargement on palpation. The recovery phase generally lasts from 2 to 12 weeks — sometimes longer in patients with hepatitis B, C, or E.

Comparing types of viral hepatitis

TYPE A	TYPE B	TYPE C	TYPE D	TYPE E
Age of incidence				
Children, young adults	Any age	Any age	Any age	Any age
Major mode of transmission				
Fecal-oral route Feces, saliva, and contaminated water, food, and shellfish	*Parenteral, sexual, and maternal-fetal routes* Blood and blood products, body fluids, perinatal contact, and unknown causes	*Parenteral route* Blood and blood products (via transfusion, needle stick, or I.V. drug use) and unknown causes	*Same as hepatitis B* Appears as a coinfection with hepatitis B	*Fecal-oral route* feces-contaminated water
Incubation and infectivity period				
15 to 50 days incubation; infectivity lasts from later half of incubation period until 1 to 2 weeks after symptoms start	40 to 180 days incubation; infectivity begins before symptoms develop and may continue for life if patient becomes a carrier	15 to 160 days incubation; infectivity begins before symptoms develop and may continue for life if patient becomes a carrier	15 to 64 days incubation; infectivity extends throughout disease	15 to 64 days incubation; unknown duration of infectivity
Serum markers				
Anti-HAV IgM	HBsAg, HBeAg, anti-HBs, HBcAb, HBsAb, anti-HBc, and anti-HBc IgM	Anti-HCV	Anti-HDV	No test available
Prognosis				
Good, rarely fatal, no carrier state or chronicity	Worsens with age; 5% to 10% of patients become chronic carriers, rest become immune; chronic hepatitis B associated with liver cancer	50% of patients progress to chronic hepatitis; 20% progress to cirrhosis	Patient may become chronic carrier; chronic, active hepatitis may lead to death	Doesn't progress to chronic hepatits but has a 10% mortality during pregnancy

Assessment TimeSaver

Determining the source of viral hepatitis

A complete patient history can help to determine the source of infection. Be sure to:
• ask the patient about recent blood transfusions, known exposure to patients with hepatitis A or B, or hemodialysis
• question him about his personal activities, including sexual practices, I.V. drug use, travel to foreign countries where hepatitis is endemic, or living in overcrowded conditions
• look for evidence of recent ear piercing or tattooing because contaminated instruments can transmit hepatitis
• ask about the possibility of contaminated water or shellfish as the source of hepatitis A
• check the patient's employment history for potential occupational exposure. For example, a hospital or laboratory worker's risk of viral exposure from contaminated instruments or waste could be high.

Diagnostic test results

A hepatitis profile identifies serum antigens and antibodies (serum markers) specific to the causative virus, establishing the type of hepatitis. Liver function studies, which may help support the diagnosis, reveal the following findings:
• Serum aspartate aminotransferase (AST), formerly SGOT, and serum alanine aminotransferase (ALT), formerly SGPT, levels increase in the prodromal stage of acute viral hepatitis (preceding the rise in bilirubin levels).

• Serum alkaline phosphatase levels are slightly increased.
• Serum bilirubin levels are elevated by jaundice and may remain high late in the disease, especially if the patient's infection is severe. Urine bilirubin levels are also elevated.
• Prothrombin time (PT) may be prolonged. A PT more than 3 seconds longer than normal may indicate severe liver damage.

In addition, white blood cell counts commonly reveal transient neutropenia and lymphopenia followed by lymphocytosis. Liver biopsy may be performed if chronic hepatitis is suspected. Liver biopsy is performed for acute hepatitis only if the diagnosis is questionable.

NURSING DIAGNOSIS

Common nursing diagnoses for a patient with viral hepatitis include:
• Altered nutrition: Less than body requirements, related to anorexia, nausea, and vomiting
• Fatigue related to effects of the disease
• High risk for impaired skin integrity related to rashes and itching brought on by jaundice
• Fear related to potential for permanent liver damage.

PLANNING

Based on the nursing diagnosis *altered nutrition: less than body requirements,* develop appropriate patient outcomes. For example, your patient will:
• eat a balanced, high-carbohydrate, low-fat diet with frequent, small meals
• regain lost weight
• maintain weight within his normal range.

Based on the nursing diagnosis *fatigue,* develop appropriate patient outcomes. For example, your patient will:
• express understanding of how hepatitis causes fatigue and the need to restrict activities during acute episodes
• seek assistance, when needed, to perform activities of daily living (ADLs)
• regain energy needed to perform ADLs as hepatitis subsides.

Based on the nursing diagnosis *high risk for impaired skin integrity,* develop appropriate patient outcomes. For example, your patient will:
• show no evidence of skin breakdown
• request medication for itching, when indicated
• demonstrate skin care measures to reduce rash and itching.

Based on the nursing diagnosis *fear,* develop appropriate patient outcomes. For example, your patient will:
• communicate his fears
• report decreased feelings of fear.

IMPLEMENTATION

Treatment of hepatitis usually focuses on maintaining adequate rest and nutrition. (See *Medical care of the patient with viral hepatitis,* page 194.)

Nursing interventions
• Always follow universal blood and body fluid precautions and adhere to your hospital's infection control policies. Make sure that visitors also observe these precautions.
• Although complete bed rest isn't necessary, schedule necessary treatments and tests at the same time of the day to allow the patient longer periods of uninterrupted rest. Gradually increase his daily activities as

his condition improves. Be sure to include the patient in planning activities to aid compliance. Because inactivity may increase the patient's anxiety, include diversions, such as television, video tapes, radio, and magazines, as part of his care. Encourage family members and friends to visit. Spend time with the patient and encourage him to express his feelings.
• Don't overload the patient's meal tray. Too much food may diminish his appetite. Offer small, frequent meals.
• Remove food covers outside the room to decrease nausea triggered by concentrated food odors.
• Include favorite foods in the patient's meal plan. Allow family members to bring food, especially high-carbohydrate, low-fat products. If the patient is nauseated late in the day, make breakfast his largest meal. Administer antiemetics as ordered.
• Administer supplemental vitamins and commercial formulas as ordered. If symptoms are severe and the patient can't tolerate oral intake, provide I.V. therapy and parenteral nutrition as ordered.
• Provide at least 2 quarts (liters) of fluid daily. Offer a choice of fruit juices, soft drinks, ice chips, or water.
• Apply water-based lotions to the patient's skin if jaundice has caused dryness and itching. If itching is severe, cholestyramine may be prescribed.
• Keep an accurate record of the patient's vital signs, especially his temperature. If his temperature is high, treat with tepid baths, acetaminophen if prescribed, or a hypothermia blanket.
• Report all cases of hepatitis to health officials. Ask the patient to name recent contacts. (See *Providing immunity against viral hepatitis,* page 195.)

Treatments

Medical care of the patient with viral hepatitis

Treatment of viral hepatitis aims to control symptoms through supportive measures and drug therapy. Rarely, a liver transplant may be performed.

Supportive measures
• Advise the patient to rest in the early stages of the illness and to combat anorexia by eating small, high-calorie, high-carbohydrate, low-fat meals. Large meals usually are better tolerated in the morning because of characteristic late-day nausea.
• Provide I.V. replacement of fluids and nutrients only if the patient can't maintain his dietary intake because of vomiting related to high fever.
• In acute viral hepatitis, hospitalization usually is required only for patients with severe symptoms or complications. Patients with persistent vomiting may need parenteral nutrition.

Drug therapy
• Antiemetics (trimethobenzamide or benzquinamide) may be given 30 minutes before meals to relieve nausea and prevent vomiting; phenothiazines have a cholestatic effect and should be avoided. For severe pruritus, cholestyramine may be given to sequester bile salts.
• Interferon alfa-2b helps to control symptoms of hepatitis B. It has achieved remission in 30% to 40% of patients who take it daily for about 4 months. Interferon alfa-2b, which may be used alone or after prednisone treatment, is the most promising drug for preventing the progression of chronic hepatitis.
• Prednisone and azathioprine (an immunosuppressant) have been effective in treating autoimmune chronic active hepatitis.

Liver transplantation
Transplantation is a last resort for patients with viral hepatitis and cirrhosis, localized tumor, or other signs of deteriorating liver function. Unfortunately, reinfection rates are high in patients with liver transplants.

• Monitor the patient for signs of improvement or deterioration, particularly daily weight changes (versus intake and output records), frequency of bowel movements, and color, consistency, and volume of stools.
• Watch for any signs of complications — for example, changes in level of consciousness, ascites, edema, dehydration, respiratory problems, myalgia, arthralgia, prolonged bleeding from puncture sites, easy bruising, and blood in urine or feces.

Patient teaching
• Teach the patient about the disease, including modes of transmission, recommended treatments, and the recovery process.
• Explain all diagnostic tests, reviewing any required special preparation.
Timesaving tip: Give the patient materials about hepatitis to read. Then check his understanding by questioning him and reinforcing missed points. As the patient's knowledge and independence im-

Providing immunity against viral hepatitis

Immune globulin may provide passive immunity against some types of viral hepatitis. Vaccination may provide active immunity against hepatitis B.

Immune globulin

No vaccine exists for hepatitis A, but immune globulin — or gamma globulin — effectively provides passive immunity. Immune globulin is generally recommended for anyone who has had contact with persons with hepatitis A and for travelers outside the United States. In confirmed exposure, the drug should be given as soon as possible after exposure or within 2 weeks after jaundice appears.

Although no vaccine exists for hepatitis C or E, immune globulin may contribute some passive immunity if given after exposure.

Most immune globulin made in the United States contains low titers of antibody against hepatitis B virus (HBV), providing some passive protection. Passive immunity may effectively prevent transmission from accidental needle sticks, open wound or lesion contamination, administration of HBV-contaminated blood, and sexual contact with a partner with acute hepatitis B (within 2 weeks of contact). It may also provide protection for infants living with a person with hepatitis B and for infants born to HBsAg-positive mothers.

For the best protection after exposure to hepatitis B, immune globulin should be given with HBV vaccine. Initial vaccination should be followed by two more doses of HBV vaccine.

HBV vaccine

Hepatitis B is the only form of hepatitis for which you can be actively immunized. Hospitals and other health care employers must provide this vaccine free of charge as a precaution for staff members whose jobs expose them to blood or body fluids. The vaccine provides protection for 5 years or longer. It's administered as a series of three I.M. injections, with the second and third injections given 1 month and 6 months after the first injection.

The vaccine is also recommended for residents of and workers in mental health facilities, hemophiliacs, homosexuals, heterosexuals with multiple sex partners, and long-term prison inmates.

prove, you can devote more time to other important nursing care functions.

• Explain prescribed medications, including possible adverse effects. Also warn of the potential dangers of over-the-counter drugs that are metabolized through the liver. Advise the pa-

tient to check with his doctor before taking over-the-counter medications.
• Stress that complete recovery takes time. Point out that the liver takes 3 weeks to regenerate and up to 4 months to return to a normal functioning level. Advise the patient to rest and to avoid contact sports. In-

Discharge TimeSaver
Ensuring continued care for the patient with viral hepatitis

Review the following teaching topics, referrals, and follow-up appointments to make sure that your patient is adequately prepared for discharge.

Teaching topics
Make sure that the following topics have been covered and that the patient's learning has been evaluated:
☐ disease and its course, including signs and symptoms of complications
☐ prevention of spread
☐ good nutrition.

Referrals
Make sure that the patient has been provided with necessary referrals to:

☐ social service agencies for financial and psychological counseling
☐ dietition for meal planning.

Follow-up appointments
Make sure that the necessary follow-up appointments have been scheduled and that the patient has been notified:
☐ doctor (for frequent follow-up visits).

struct him to check with his doctor before beginning strenuous activity.
• Review measures to prevent spread of the disease, stressing thorough, frequent hand washing. Tell the patient not to share food, eating utensils, toothbrushes, or razors.
• Remind the patient with hepatitis B, C, or D that he will never be able to donate blood.
• Instruct the patient to eat several small meals rather than three large meals and to drink 2 to 4 quarts (liters) of fluids daily.
• Tell the patient to weigh himself daily and report any weight loss greater than 5 lb (2.3 kg) to his doctor.
• Warn the patient to abstain from alcohol. Explain that alcohol puts undue stress on the liver.
• Explain to the patient and his family that anyone exposed to the disease through contact with him — for example, anyone who ate a meal prepared by him, had sexual contact

with him, came in contact with his blood, or shared a needle with him — should receive prophylactic treatment as soon as possible.
• Stress the need for continued medical care. Encourage a follow-up visit approximately 2 weeks after the diagnosis is made. Mention that monthly follow-up visits may be necessary for up to 6 months (or longer if he develops chronic viral hepatitis). (See *Ensuring continued care for the patient with viral hepatitis.*)

EVALUATION

When evaluating the patient's response to nursing care, gather reassessment data and compare this information with the patient outcomes specified in your plan of care.

Teaching and counseling
Begin by determining the effectiveness of your teaching and counseling. Consider the following questions:

• Does the patient understand viral hepatitis and how it's transmitted?
• Is he knowledgeable about his prescribed treatment?
• Does he adhere to his schedule of rest and activity, gradually increasing his level of activity as his condition and energy level improve?
• Does he know the measures that can help prevent the spread of the disease?

Physical condition

If interventions are successful, you should note the following in your patient:
• maintenance of adequate intake of both foods and liquids, as evidenced by absence of dehydration or malnutrition and by keeping weight within normal range
• minimal fatigue
• no evidence of skin breakdown
• diminished fear about the disease.

Influenza

Also called the grippe or the flu, influenza is an acute, highly contagious infection of the respiratory tract. The influenza virus commonly mutates, thereby overcoming the patient's immunologic barriers. Influenza is most severe in young children, elderly people, and those with chronic diseases.

Usually, influenza resolves in 1 to 2 weeks, leaving no permanent damage. However, it can lead to primary viral pneumonia and secondary bacterial pneumonia. Less common complications include myositis, Reye's syndrome and, rarely, myocarditis, pericarditis, transverse myelitis, and encephalopathy.

In children with reactive airways, influenza may provoke an asthmatic attack and may lead to febrile seizures.

Causes

Three types of myxoviruses cause influenza. Type A, the most prevalent, strikes every year, and its new serotypes cause epidemics every 3 years. Type B also strikes annually but causes epidemics at 4- to 6-year intervals. Type C is endemic and causes only sporadic cases. The infection is transmitted by inhaling a respiratory droplet from an infected person or by indirect contact with contaminated hands or surfaces.

ASSESSMENT

Signs and symptoms of influenza are easy to spot in the midst of an epidemic but, in other cases, may be confused with other respiratory disorders. Your assessment should include consideration of the patient's health history, physical examination findings, and diagnostic test results.

Health history

The patient's history usually reveals recent exposure to a person with influenza and no immunization with the influenza vaccine during the past season.

After an incubation period of 24 to 48 hours, the virus produces characteristic signs and symptoms. The patient may report a sudden onset of chills, fever (101° to 104° F [38.3° to 40° C]), headache, malaise, myalgia (particularly in the back and limbs), photophobia, sore throat, anorexia, a nonproductive cough and, occasionally, laryngitis, hoarseness, rhinitis, and rhinorrhea. These signs usually subside in 3 to 5 days, but a cough and weakness may persist. Some patients may feel tired and listless for several weeks.

Physical examination

Inspection initially may reveal red watery eyes, erythema of the nose and throat without exudate, and clear nasal discharge.

As the infection progresses, respiratory findings become more apparent. The patient frequently coughs and looks tired. If pulmonary complications occur, tachypnea, cyanosis, and shortness of breath may be noted. With bacterial pneumonia, you'll see purulent sputum.

Palpation may reveal cervical adenopathy and tenderness. Auscultation typically detects normal breath sounds. With pneumonia, however, breath sounds may be diminished in areas of consolidation.

Diagnostic test results

During epidemics, diagnosis typically requires only observation of clinical signs and symptoms. At times, the following tests may be needed to confirm the diagnosis:

• Nose and throat cultures may be ordered to help identify the virus.
• Blood tests may reveal a decreased white blood cell count and an increased lymphocyte count.
• Chest X-rays may show pneumonitis when a respiratory disorder is present.

NURSING DIAGNOSIS

Common nursing diagnoses for a patient with influenza include:

• Hyperthermia related to infection
• High risk for fluid volume deficit related to fever and decreased fluid intake
• Fatigue related to infection
• Pain (headache, myalgia) related to the effects of the disorder.

PLANNING

Based on the nursing diagnosis *hyperthermia,* develop appropriate patient outcomes. For example, the patient will:

• demonstrate decreased fever following antipyretic therapy
• regain and maintain a normal temperature
• avoid complications associated with hyperthermia, such as seizures or dehydration.

Based on the nursing diagnosis *high risk for fluid volume deficit,* develop appropriate patient outcomes. For example, the patient will:

• consume at least 3,000 ml of fluid, either orally or I.V.
• maintain a normal fluid volume, as evidenced by normal vital signs and an adequate urine output
• show no signs or symptoms of dehydration.

Based on the nursing diagnosis *fatigue,* develop appropriate patient outcomes. For example, the patient will:

• explain the relationship between influenza and fatigue, and express an understanding of how his level of activity can affect his level of fatigue
• employ measures to minimize fatigue
• regain his normal energy level after the influenza has resolved.

Based on the nursing diagnosis *pain,* develop appropriate patient outcomes. For example, the patient will:

• notify you immediately when pain occurs, indicating the intensity of his pain on a scale of 1 to 10
• inform you of reduced pain within 1 hour after receiving treatment.

IMPLEMENTATION

Treatment of influenza usually focuses on relieving discomfort and monitoring for complications. (See *Medical care of the patient with influenza*.)

Nursing interventions

• Administer analgesics, antipyretics, and decongestants, as ordered.
• Watch for signs and symptoms of developing pneumonia, such as crackles, diminished breath sounds, increased temperature, chest pain, dyspnea, and coughing accompanied by purulent sputum.
• Follow respiratory and universal precautions.
• Encourage a high-protein, high-calorie diet, especially if the patient has a fever.
• Provide cool, humidified air. Clean the humidifier thoroughly and change the filter. Change the water daily to prevent *Pseudomonas* superinfection.
• Encourage the patient to rest in bed and drink 3 to 4 liters of fluid daily. Monitor his fluid intake and output. Check for signs of dehydration, such as diminished skin turgor. Administer prescribed I.V. fluids if ordered.
• Regularly monitor the patient's vital signs, including his temperature.
• Administer oxygen therapy as ordered.
• Help the patient to gradually return to his normal activities as influenza resolves.

Patient teaching

• Influenza usually doesn't require hospitalization. Teach the home care patient about supportive care measures and signs and symptoms of serious complications.
• Advise the patient to use mouthwash or warm saline gargles to ease a sore throat.

Treatments

Medical care of the patient with influenza

Treatment of influenza may vary, depending on possible complications.

Uncomplicated influenza
The patient with uncomplicated influenza needs:
• bed rest
• adequate fluids
• guaifenesin or another expectorant to relieve nonproductive coughing
• acetaminophen or aspirin to relieve fever and muscle pain. (However, children should not take aspirin because of the threat of Reye's syndrome.)

Additional therapy
The antiviral agent amantadine has effectively reduced the duration of influenza A infection only when given within 48 hours of onset. Although not routinely used, this agent should be given to influenza patients who are at high risk for developing viral pneumonia, such as immunosuppressed patients. An experimental drug, rimantadine, has been found to cause fewer adverse reactions and may eventually be used to stop epidemics in non-vaccinated populations.

• Recommend that the patient take an analgesic or an antipyretic, such as acetaminophen, according to doctor's guidelines. A child or adolescent should not be given aspirin to prevent the possibility of Reye's syndrome.

Preventing influenza

Inactivated influenza virus vaccines are the most important means of preventing influenza. Other preventive measures include the antiviral drug amantadine, infection-control measures, and appropriate nursing interventions — especially thorough patient teaching.

Vaccines

Experts recommend that influenza virus vaccines be administered to the groups of patients described below (note that the virus should not be administered to infants under 6 months of age):

• patients at high risk for influenza morbidity or mortality, such those over age 65 and those with chronic cardiac, pulmonary, metabolic, or renal diseases

• military personnel and residents of nursing homes, to prevent outbreaks

• children and adolescents requiring long-term aspirin therapy (because of the increased risk for Reye's syndrome)

• health care workers and people living in the same household with a high risk individual

• patients with diabetes mellitus, cancer, or immunosuppression. (Patients with human immunodeficiency virus may receive the vaccine but often respond poorly and may require amantadine prophylaxis.)

Amantadine

This antiviral drug has been proven 70% effective against type A influenza. It may be used prophylactically for:

• adults at high risk for developing complications of influenza who haven't been vaccinated recently or shouldn't receive vaccination

• patients with immunodeficiencies, such as acquired immunodeficiency syndrome, who respond poorly to influenza vaccine

• home caregivers who have not been immunized, to reduce the spread of infection

• patients and staff in health care facilities (such as extended care facilities) that house persons at high risk. All such patients and staff, regardless of vaccination status, should receive amantadine for the duration of influenza's spread in the community.

Infection-control measures

These measures center on hygiene. To promote good hygiene, advise your patients to:

• wash their hands frequently

• disinfect surfaces touched by infectious persons

• properly dispose of used tissues and secretions

• avoid close contact with people in the infectious stage; otherwise, use a mask

• avoid crowds.

Nursing interventions

To help prevent unnecessary illness and deaths from influenza, you should:

• promote annual vaccination for those in high-risk groups. Explain that current vaccines are highly purified and therefore result in fewer adverse reactions, such as fever and local irritation. Clarify that only a few cases of Guillain-Barré syndrome have been reported since the 1976 cases associated with swine flu immunizations. Stress that annual vaccination is necessary because immunity usually lasts no longer than 1 year, and vaccines change to include the most prevalent types of influenza.

• recommend vaccination in the early fall to allow antibody buildup before the winter influenza season. Check for allergy to hen's eggs, which contraindicates use of the influenza vaccine.

• get your annual vaccination to help prevent contagion.

• Teach the patient the importance of increased fluids to prevent dehydration.

• Suggest a warm bath or a heating pad to relieve myalgia.

• Advise the patient to use a vaporizer to provide cool, moist air, but tell him to clean the reservoir and change the water every 8 hours.

• Teach the patient how to dispose of tissues properly, and demonstrate proper hand-washing technique to prevent the virus from spreading. Also teach the importance of cleaning surfaces, such as tables, chairs, and desks.

• Discuss influenza immunization and other preventive measures. (See *Preventing influenza.*)

EVALUATION

When evaluating the patient's response to nursing care, gather reassessment data and compare this information with the patient outcomes specified in your plan of care.

Teaching and counseling

Begin by evaluating the effectiveness of your teaching. Consider the outcome satisfactory if the patient:

• expresses an understanding of the relationship between activity and fatigue

• employs measures to minimize fatigue.

Physical condition

Continue your evaluation by reassessing the patient's physical condition. Consider the outcome satisfactory if the patient:

• maintains a normal temperature and avoids complications of hyperthermia

• demonstrates no signs of dehydration, such as diminished skin turgor

• maintains vital signs within the normal range
• regains normal energy levels after influenza has resolved
• verbalizes diminished or absent pain
• maintains a normal fluid volume and takes in at least 3,000 ml of fluid daily.

Herpes simplex

A common infection, herpes simplex occurs subclinically in about 85% of patients. In the rest, it causes localized lesions. After the initial infection, the patient becomes a carrier susceptible to recurrent attacks. The outbreaks may be provoked by fever, menses, stress, heat, cold, lack of sleep, sun exposure, and contact with reactivated disease (for example, by kissing or by sharing cosmetics). In recurrent infections, the patient usually has no systemic signs and symptoms. (See *Key points about herpes simplex*.)

Causes
This infection results from herpes simplex virus (HSV) types 1 and 2.

ASSESSMENT

Signs and symptoms may be more apparent if linked to behavior revealed in a thorough health history. Your assessment should also include consideration of physical examination findings and diagnostic test results.

Health history
In a patient with suspected primary herpes simplex, the health history may reveal oral, vaginal, or anal sexual contact with an infected person or other direct contact with lesions. With recurrent infection, the patient may identify various precipitating factors.

Physical examination
Signs of herpes simplex depend on the location of the virus and whether its primary or recurrent. Herpes simplex can be perioral, genital or, less commonly, ocular. (See *Detecting herpes simplex*, page 204.)

Diagnostic test results
Characteristic lesions often pinpoint the diagnosis. Confirmation of HSV infection requires isolation of the virus from local lesions and a histologic biopsy.
• In primary infection, a rise in antibodies and moderate leukocytosis may support the diagnosis.
• A Tzanck smear identifies giant cells characteristic of herpes; however, it will not distinguish between HSV and varicella-zoster virus.

NURSING DIAGNOSIS

Common nursing diagnoses for a patient with herpes simplex include:
• Altered oral mucous membrane related to the effects of the disease
• Impaired tissue integrity related to the effects of the disease
• High risk for infection related to the potential for recurrence
• Pain related to lesions.

PLANNING

Based on the nursing diagnosis *altered oral mucous membrane,* develop appropriate patient outcomes. For example, your patient will:
• explain prescribed treatments to alleviate oral lesions
• state intent to complete prescribed therapy

FactFinder

Key points about herpes simplex

• *Causes:* The infection results from herpes simplex virus (HSV) types 1 (HSV-1) and 2 (HSV-2).

• *Transmission:* Seen most commonly in children, HSV-1 is transmitted primarily by contact with oral secretions. It mainly affects oral, labial, ocular, or skin tissues. HSV-2, transmitted primarily by contact with genital secretions, mainly affects genital structures, typically in adolescents and young adults.

• *Occurrence:* HSV occurs equally in males and females worldwide. Lower socioeconomic groups are infected more often, probably because of crowded living conditions, lack of health education, and inadequate health care.

• *Incubation period:* The incubation period varies, depending on the infection site, but averages 2 to 12 days for generalized infection and 3 to 7 days for genital infection.

• *Complications:* HSV infection can cause perianal ulcers, colitis, esophagitis, pneumonitis, and various neurologic disorders in the immunocompromised patient. Primary HSV infection during pregnancy can lead to abortion, premature labor, microcephaly, and uterine growth retardation. Congenital herpes transmitted during vaginal birth may produce a subclinical neonatal infection or severe infection with seizures, chorioretinitis, skin vesicles, and hepatosplenomegaly. Ocular infection can cause infant blindness. Women may be at increased risk for cervical cancer and urethral stricture from recurrent genital herpes.

• exhibit healing of oral lesions.

Based on the nursing diagnosis *impaired tissue integrity*, develop appropriate patient outcomes. For example, your patient will:

• explain prescribed therapy to alleviate lesions

• state intent to complete prescribed therapy

• demonstrate improvement through healing of lesions.

Based on the nursing diagnosis *high risk for infection*, develop appropriate patient outcomes. For example, your patient will:

• express an understanding of how herpes simplex can recur

• take precautions to prevent recurrences.

Based on the diagnosis *pain*, develop appropriate patient outcomes. For example, your patient will:

• express pain relief with treatment

• become free of pain once lesions heal.

IMPLEMENTATION

Treatment of HSV consists of symptomatic and supportive therapy. (See *Medical care of the patient with herpes simplex*, page 205.)

Nursing interventions

• Answer the patient's questions and encourage him and his family to express their concern about the illness.

• Adhere to universal precautions.

Assessment TimeSaver
Detecting herpes simplex

Assessment findings will vary, depending on the infection site, the patient's sex, and the recurrence or nonrecurrence of lesions.

Primary perioral HSV
In primary perioral herpes simplex virus (HSV), the patient may have generalized or localized infection. Generalized infection usually causes sore throat, fever, increased salivation, halitosis, anorexia, and severe mouth pain. Signs of dehydration, such as poor skin turgor, may be present. After a brief prodromal tingling and itching, typical primary lesions erupt.

Examination of the pharyngeal and oral mucosa may disclose edema and small vesicles on an erythematous base. These vesicles eventually rupture, leaving a painful ulcer that's followed by yellow crusting. Vesicles most commonly occur on the tongue, gingiva, and cheeks, but any part of the oral mucosa may be involved. Palpation reveals cervical tenderness and adenopathy. A generalized infection usually runs its course within 10 days.

Primary genital HSV
With primary genital HSV, the patient usually complains first of malaise, dysuria, dyspareunia and, in females, leukorrhea. Then fluid-filled vesicles appear.

While examining a female patient, you may detect vesicles on the cervix (the primary infection site) and, possibly, on the labia, perianal skin, vulva, and vagina. In male patients, vesicles develop on the glans penis, foreskin, and penile shaft. Extragenital lesions may be seen on the mouth or anus. Ruptured vesicles appear as extensive, shallow, painful ulcers, with redness, marked edema, and characteristic oozing yellow centers. Lesions may persist for several weeks. Palpation may reveal inguinal tenderness and adenopathy.

Recurrent perioral or genital HSV
The patient with recurrent perioral or genital HSV may report prodromal symptoms (pain, tingling, or itching) at the site. Typically, the disease course is shorter than with primary infection. Recurrent perioral infection usually triggers no systemic symptoms, but the outer lip may be affected and painful. A male patient with recurrent genital herpes usually has fewer severe systemic symptoms and less local involvement than a female patient. Palpation may reveal cervical tenderness and adenopathy.

Primary ocular HSV
The patient with a primary ocular infection may report localized signs and symptoms, such as photophobia and excessive tearing. Follicular conjunctivitis or blepharitis with vesicles on the eyelid, eyelid edema, and chemosis also may occur. Systemic signs and symptoms include lethargy and fever. The infection usually is unilateral and heals within 3 weeks. Recurrent ocular infections may cause decreased visual acuity and even permanent vision loss. Palpation may reveal regional adenopathy.

Treatments

Medical care of the patient with herpes simplex

In herpes simplex, therapy involves treating the symptoms and providing support — there is no known cure.

Drug therapy

Acyclovir is a major agent for combating genital herpes, particularly primary infection. The drug may reduce symptoms, viral shedding, and healing time. Acyclovir therapy also may help treat primary perioral herpes infection. Although not usually effective in recurrent attacks, it may be prescribed to treat and suppress herpes simplex virus in immunocompromised patients and those with severe and frequent recurrences. The drug is available in topical, oral, and I.V. form (usually reserved for severe infection).

Generalized primary infection usually requires antipyretic and analgesic medications to reduce fever and pain.

Refer patients with eye infections to an ophthalmologist. Topical corticosteroids are contraindicated in active infection, but ophthalmic antiviral agents, such as idoxuridine, trifluridine, and vidarabine, may be effective.

Supportive therapy

Anesthetic mouthwashes, such as viscous lidocaine, may reduce the pain of gingivostomatitis, promoting eating and drinking and, thus, improved hydration. (Avoid offering alcohol-based mouthwashes, which can increase discomfort.) A bicarbonate-based mouth rinse may be used for oral care.

Drying agents, such as calamine lotion, may soothe labial and skin lesions. Avoid using petroleum jelly–based salves or dressings because they promote viral spread and slow healing.

- Instruct caregivers with active oral or cutaneous infections not to care for a patient in a high-risk group until the caregiver's lesions crust and dry. Also, insist that the caregiver wear protective coverings, including a mask and gloves.
- Administer pain medications and prescribed antiviral agents as ordered.
- Provide indicated supportive care, such as oral hygiene, nutritional supplements, and antipyretics for fever.
- As appropriate, refer the patient to a support group, such as the Herpes Resource Center.

Monitoring
- Observe the patient's response to treatment measures.
- Assess the patient for complications associated with herpes simplex.
- Monitor the patient with oral lesions for signs and symptoms of nutritional deficits and dehydration. Weigh the patient regularly.

Patient teaching
- Teach the patient about the disease, its signs and symptoms, and treatment.
- Instruct the patient with cold sores not to kiss anyone. Also, he shouldn't

engage in oral sex because oral herpes can be transmitted to the genitals.

• Tell the patient with genital herpes to wash his hands carefully after using the bathroom or touching his genitals, to avoid spreading the infection to infants or other susceptible people.

• Instruct the patient with oral lesions to use lip balm containing a sunscreen to avoid reactivating lesions.

• Encourage him to get adequate rest and nutrition and to keep lesions dry, except for applying prescribed drugs. Teach him to apply drugs using aseptic technique.

• Urge the patient with genital herpes to avoid sexual intercourse until his lesions heal completely and to inform any sexual partner of his condition. Advise patients and partners to be screened for other sexually transmitted diseases, including human immunodeficiency virus infection.

• If a female patient is pregnant, explain to her the potential risk to her infant during vaginal delivery. Answer her questions about cesarean delivery if she has an HSV outbreak when labor begins and her membranes haven't ruptured.

• Advise the female patient with genital herpes to have an annual Papanicolaou (Pap) test if previous results from this test have been normal. If Pap test results have been abnormal, suggest she be tested every 6 months or as her doctor recommends.

• Instruct the patient with herpetic whitlow not to share towels or eating utensils with uninfected people. Herpetic whitlow is a painful HSV infection of a terminal phalanx, usually the thumb or index finger. Educate hospital staff members and other susceptible people about the risk of contracting the disease. Nurses who have herpetic whitlow shouldn't work until the lesion heals.

• Accept the patient's feelings of powerlessness as normal. Help him identify and develop coping mechanisms, personal strengths, and support resources.

• Provide a nonthreatening, nonjudgmental atmosphere to encourage the patient to verbalize any feelings about perceived changes in sexuality and behavior. Provide patient and partner with current information about the disease and treatment options. Refer them for appropriate counseling as needed. (See *Ensuring continued care for the patient with herpes simplex.*)

EVALUATION

To evaluate the patient's response to your nursing care, gather reassessment data and compare this information with the patient outcomes specified in your plan of care.

Teaching and counseling

Begin by determining the effectiveness of your teaching. Consider the following questions:

• Does the patient understand the prescribed therapy and agree to complete it?

• Can he describe his plan to help prevent recurrences?

Physical condition

Conclude your evaluation by reassessing the patient's physical condition. Consider your nursing care effective if your patient:

• demonstrates the healing of lesions with no signs of infection

• expresses pain relief after analgesics have been administered or when lesions have healed.

Discharge TimeSaver
Ensuring continued care for the patient with herpes simplex

Review the following teaching topics, referrals, and follow-up appointments to make sure that your patient is adequately prepared for discharge.

Teaching topics
Make sure that the following topics have been covered and that the patient's learning has been evaluated:
☐ hygienic practices
☐ avoidance of sexual relations during flare-ups
☐ medication, including dosage and adverse effects
☐ counseling; if the patient feels socially isolated, ensure that he has a list of outreach organizations.

Referrals
Make sure that the patient has been provided with necessary referrals to:
☐ social service agencies as needed
☐ support groups.

Follow-up appointments
Make sure that the necessary follow-up appointments have been scheduled and that the patient has been notified:
☐ doctor or clinic.

Herpes zoster

Commonly known as shingles, herpes zoster is an acute unilateral and segmental inflammation of the dorsal root ganglia. It produces localized vesicular skin lesions confined to no more than two adjacent dermatomes. If more than two dermatomes are involved, the condition is said to be disseminated. The patient with herpes zoster may have severe neuralgic pain in the areas bordering the inflamed nerve root ganglia. (See *Key points about herpes zoster,* page 208.)

Causes
This disorder is caused by the varicella-zoster virus, a herpesvirus that causes two types of disease. The primary disease is varicella, or chicken pox. The second or recurrent disease is herpes zoster.

ASSESSMENT
Signs and symptoms of herpes zoster reveal a pattern of pain and lesion eruption. Your assessment should include careful consideration of the patient's health history, physical examination findings, and diagnostic test results.

Health history
Typically, the patient complains of pain or burning and itching affecting the area where lesions appear 2 to 3 days later. For example, if he reports eye pain, the trigeminal nerve is involved.

Physical examination
You'll typically observe small, red, nodular skin lesions spread unilaterally around the thorax or vertically along an arm or leg. The rash develops into vesicles that generally stop appearing by the fifth day in an otherwise healthy patient and eventually

Key points about herpes zoster

• *Incidence:* More than 300,000 cases of herpes zoster are reported each year in North America. The virus can affect people of any age but it most often strikes people over age 60. The recurrence rate in an otherwise healthy person is about 2%. Patients who are immuno-compromised have a considerably higher incidence of a second episode, with a more severe infection.

• *Prevalence:* Herpes zoster may be more prevalent in people who had chicken pox at a very young age, especially before age 1 — but this is still a hypothesis.

• *Dermatomes:* The most commonly involved dermatomes are those from T3 to L3.

• *Prognosis:* Most patients recover completely unless the infection spreads to the brain. The virus is more severe in immunocompromised patients but seldom is fatal.

• *Treatment:* Most treatment focuses on the relief of symptoms and prevention of complications.

• *Complications:* Depending on the involved dermatomes, complications may include vision loss, intractable neurologic pain, permanent scarring and, rarely, generalized central nervous system infection, muscle atrophy, motor paralysis (usually transient), acute transverse myelitis, or allergic granulomatous angiitis.

form scabs. The infection lasts 7 to 10 days, but the skin doesn't return to normal for several weeks. During palpation, you may detect enlarged regional lymph nodes.

If the facial nerves are involved, you may see lesion formation in the external auditory canal or tongue and ipsilateral facial palsy. Lesions will most likely occur unilaterally on the face and head if the cranial nerves are involved.

Diagnostic test results

Many cases of herpes zoster can be diagnosed by the characteristic lesions that appear unilaterally on the head, face, trunk, or extremities. The following tests may help confirm diagnosis:

• A Tzanck smear of the lesion base may confirm multinucleated giant cells, intranuclear inclusions, or both, indicating herpes. However, it can't distinguish between herpes zoster and herpes simplex.

• Culturing tissue cell lines is the most effective way to diagnose herpes zoster, but the lengthy process is infrequently used.

• Three commonly used antigen-antibody tests are immunofluorescent detection of antibodies to varicella-zoster virus membrane antigens, fluorescent antibody to membrane antigen, and enzyme-linked immunoabsorbent assay. Immune adherence hemagglutination may also be performed.

• With central nervous system involvement, results of a lumbar puncture indicate increased cerebrospinal (CSF) pressure, and CSF analysis demonstrates increased protein levels and, possibly, pleocytosis.

NURSING DIAGNOSIS

Common nursing diagnoses for a patient with herpes zoster include:
• Impaired skin integrity related to infection
• Pain and itching related to inflamed nerve root ganglia
• High risk for injury related to paresthesia and hyperesthesia secondary to the infection.

PLANNING

Based on the nursing diagnosis *impaired skin integrity,* develop appropriate patient outcomes. For example, your patient will:
• demonstrate skill in performing the prescribed skin care regimen
• avoid complications of skin lesions, such as infection and skin breakdown
• demonstrate healing of skin lesions and regain normal skin integrity.

Based on the nursing diagnosis *pain,* develop appropriate patient outcomes. For example, your patient will:
• express pain relief after analgesic administration
• comply with prescribed treatments to alleviate pain.

Based on the nursing diagnosis *high risk for injury,* develop appropriate patient outcomes. For example, your patient will:
• describe precautions to prevent injury to the affected areas
• avoid injury to affected areas
• regain normal sensory function once the infection heals.

IMPLEMENTATION

Much of the treatment of herpes zoster is aimed at relieving the symptoms of pain and itching and preventing complications. (See *Medical care*

of the patient with herpes zoster, page 210.)

Nursing interventions
• Maintain proper hygiene, including regular bathing and soaks. Administer topical drugs as directed. If the doctor prescribes calamine lotion, apply it liberally to the patient's lesions. Tepid baths and wet compresses relieve itching. Maintaining meticulous hygiene helps to prevent spreading the infection to other parts of the patient's body.
• Be prepared to administer drying therapies, such as oxygen, if the patient has severe disseminated lesions.
• Give analgesics exactly as scheduled to minimize severe neuralgic pain. For a patient with postherpetic neuralgia, consult with and follow a pain specialist's recommendations to maximize pain relief without risking tolerance to the analgesic.
• Take drainage and secretion precautions for the patient with shingles, using strict isolation in the case of disseminated shingles.
• Monitor the patient for signs of improved or worsening condition, including his response to treatment, signs of complications, and daily evidence of skin lesion healing or infection.

Patient teaching
• Teach your patient about the disease, modes of transmission, and prescribed treatment.
• Explain the course of medications, including adverse effects.
• Stress the need for adequate rest during the acute phase.
• Repeatedly reassure the patient that herpetic pain usually subsides eventually. Suggest diversions or relaxation activities to take his mind off the pain and pruritus. (See *Ensuring*

Medical care of the patient with herpes zoster

Primary therapeutic goals include relief of itching with antipruritics (such as calamine lotion) and relief of neuralgic pain with analgesics (such as aspirin, acetaminophen, or possibly codeine). In addition, you can prevent secondary infection by applying a demulcent and skin protectant (such as collodion or tincture of benzoin) to unbroken lesions.

Antiviral therapy
A dosage of 600 to 800 mg of acyclovir, five times a day, may be administered to patients at high risk for complications. I.V. acyclovir may be prescribed for immunocompromised patients and patients with an infected ophthalmic branch of the trigeminal nerve. This drug halts the rash progression, reduces the duration of viral shedding and acute pain, and prevents visceral complications. Vidarabine, though less effective than acyclovir, may also be used.

Herpes zoster affecting trigeminal and corneal structures requires instillation of idoxuridine ointment or another antiviral agent.

Antibacterial therapy
If bacteria infect ruptured vesicles, treatment includes an appropriate systemic antibiotic.

Pain relief
To help a patient cope with the intractable pain of postherpetic neuralgia, a systemic corticosteroid, such as cortisone or corticotropin, may be prescribed to reduce inflammation. The doctor also may prescribe tranquilizers, sedatives, or tricyclic antidepressants with phenothiazines.

As a last resort for pain relief, transcutaneous peripheral nerve stimulation, patient-controlled analgesia, or a small dose of radiotherapy may be considered.

continued care for the patient with herpes zoster.)

EVALUATION

To evaluate the patient's response to your nursing care, gather reassessment data and compare this information with the patient outcomes specified in your plan of care.

Teaching and counseling
Begin by determining the effectiveness of your teaching. Consider the following questions:

• Does the patient understand the disease, complications of skin lesions, and prescribed treatment?
• Does he know how to perform the prescribed skin care regimen?
• Can he describe precautions to prevent injury to the affected areas?

Physical condition
Conclude your evaluation by reassessing the patient's physical condition. Consider your nursing care effective if your patient:
• shows no signs of bacterial skin infection in lesions, demonstrates heal-

Ensuring continued care for the patient with herpes zoster

Review the following teaching topics, referrals, and follow-up appointments to make sure that your patient is adequately prepared for discharge.

Teaching topics
Make sure that the following topics have been covered and that your patient's learning has been evaluated:
☐ good hygiene and skin care
☐ any medications, including adverse effects
☐ the need to refrain from contact with anyone who has not had chicken pox.

Referrals
Make sure that the patient has been provided with necessary referrals to:
☐ pain specialist, if needed
☐ social service agencies for financial or psychological counseling.

Follow-up appointments
Make sure that the necessary follow-up appointments have been scheduled and that the patient has been notified:
☐ doctor.

---

ing of lesions, and regains normal skin integrity
• expresses a diminishing of pain with treatment and healing
• avoids injury to affected areas
• regains normal sensory function.

Genital warts

A common sexually transmitted disease, genital warts are papillomas that consist of fibrous tissue overgrowth from the dermis and thickened epithelial coverings. Also known as venereal warts and condylomata acuminata, these growths are rare before puberty or after menopause. (See *Key points about genital warts,* page 212.)

Causes
Genital warts result from infection with one of the more than 60 known strains of human papillomavirus (HPV).

ASSESSMENT

Clinical findings in genital warts are often confirmed by the patient's health history. Your assessment also should include consideration of the patient's physical examination findings and diagnostic test results.

Health history
Typically, the patient reports unprotected sexual contact (vaginal, anal, or oral) with a partner with a known infection, a new partner, or many partners. The history often reveals the presence of another sexually transmitted disease. Most patients report no symptoms; a few complain of itching or pain.

Physical examination
On examination, you'll observe warts growing on the moist genital surfaces, such as the subpreputial sac, the urethral meatus and, less commonly, on the penile shaft or scrotum in male patients and on the vulva and vaginal and cervical walls in female patients. (Colposcopy may be necessary to see cervical lesions.) In both sexes, papillomas may spread to the perineum and the perianal area. You may find warts that begin as tiny red or pink swellings. These warts may grow to as large as 4″ (10 cm) in diameter and frequently become pedunculated. Infected lesions become malodorous.

Diagnostic test results
Diagnosis usually hinges on clinical, cytologic, or histologic findings. To differentiate genital warts from other growths in the area, such as normal anatomic warts, tumors, and growths due to other infectious agents, the following tests may be ordered:
• Darkfield microscopy of wart cell scrapings will distinguish genital warts (condylomata acuminata) from warts associated with secondary syphilis (condylomata lata).
• Specific deoxyribonucleic acid probes may be used to identify the type of HPV, but these tests aren't yet available for screening.

NURSING DIAGNOSIS

Common nursing diagnoses for a patient with genital warts include:
• Altered sexuality patterns related to presence of genital warts
• Body image disturbance related to presence of skin lesions and odor
• Knowledge deficit regarding HPV as a sexually transmitted disease.

PLANNING

Based on the nursing diagnosis *altered sexuality patterns,* develop appropriate patient outcomes. For example, your patient will:

Treatments

Medical care of the patient with genital warts

Occasionally, genital warts resolve spontaneously. Usually, however, doctors recommend topical drug therapy to remove small warts and, in some cases, surgery.

Drug therapy
Medications may include 10% to 25% podophyllum resin in tincture of benzoin (contraindicated in pregnancy) and trichloroacetic acid. These drugs aim to remove exophytic warts and ameliorate signs and symptoms, not to eradicate the human papillomavirus (HPV).

Surgery
Warts larger than 1″ (2.5 cm) in diameter usually are removed by carbon dioxide laser (the treatment of choice), electrocautery and diathermy or, rarely, cryosurgery. Conventional surgery may be recommended to remove perianal warts.

Other treatments
Other treatments that have been used with some success include fluorouracil cream debridement, topical idoxuridine in patients with extensive genital warts, and systemic cytotaxic chemotherapy.

Treatments under investigation
Alpha interferon therapy is under evaluation and holds promise because it aims to eradicate the HPV reservoir, in addition to its antiproliferative effects. However, toxic effects and recurrences are possible with all of the interferons. Researchers are studying the benefits of combining interferon therapy with ablative therapy.

• express feelings about changes in sexuality patterns
• resume normal sexual activity when external lesions are healed
• follow safe sexual practices.

Based on the nursing diagnosis *body image disturbance,* develop appropriate patient outcomes. For example, your patient will:
• acknowledge his feelings about changes in body image
• express positive feelings about himself
• have genital warts removed, if indicated.

Based on the nursing diagnosis *knowledge deficit,* develop appropriate patient outcomes. For example, your patient will:

• identify HPV as a sexually transmitted disease
• describe the role of HPV in genital wart formation and list precautions to prevent infecting sexual partners.

IMPLEMENTATION

Treatment of genital warts usually focuses on relieving symptoms and teaching prevention. (See *Medical care of the patient with genital warts.*)

Nursing interventions
• Adhere to universal precautions when examining the patient, collecting a specimen, or performing associated procedures.

• Provide a nonthreatening, nonjudgmental atmosphere that encourages the patient to verbalize feelings about perceived changes in sexual identity, behavior, and body image.

• Regardless of the setting, take time to assess your patient's emotional reaction to his condition, especially if it is chronic and produces skin lesions. Don't hesitate to contact a psychiatric clinical nurse specialist or other mental health specialist if the patient requires services you can't provide.

Patient teaching

Timesaving tip: Have anatomic pictures and printed instructions ready before you begin teaching the patient about genital warts. It is a good idea to have printed information about safe sexual practices as well.

• Inform the patient about genital HPV infection. Explain the mode of transmission, treatment, and complications.

• Tell the patient who is being treated with podophyllum resin that tissues are first protected with an agent such as petroleum jelly and that the application remains for 1 to 4 hours. Tell the patient to then remove the podophyllum resin with soap and water. Explain that weekly treatments may be necessary. Systemic adverse reactions may occur. Inform the female patient that pregnancy is contraindicated during this therapy because podophyllum resin is teratogenic.

• Recommend sexual abstinence or condom use during intercourse until healing is complete. Review proper use of condoms.

• Advise the patient to inform his sexual partners about the risk of genital warts and the need for evaluation.

• Urge the patient and his sexual partners to be tested for other sexually transmitted diseases.

• Remind the patient to report for all scheduled treatments until all warts are removed. Then instruct him to schedule a checkup 3 months after all warts are gone. Emphasize that genital warts can recur and that the virus can mutate, causing infection with warts of a different strain. Repeated treatments may be necessary.

• Encourage female patients to have a Papanicolaou test every 6 months.

EVALUATION

When evaluating the patient's response to nursing care, gather reassessment data and compare this information with the patient outcomes specified in your plan of care.

Teaching and counseling

Establish realistic target times to evaluate outcomes. A successfully counseled patient will:

• verbalize his feelings about altered sexuality patterns

• resume normal and safe sexual practices when external lesions are cleared

• communicate positive feelings about himself

• explain the role of HPV in causing genital warts, measures to prevent transmission, treatment, and possible complications.

Infectious mononucleosis

This systemic disorder causes acute pharyngotonsillitis and typically affects the lymph nodes, spleen, liver, and peripheral blood. Rarely, it affects the kidneys, skin, myocardium, central nervous system, and lungs. (See *Key points about infectious mononucleosis.*)

FactFinder

Key points about infectious mononucleosis

- *Incidence:* Susceptible (seronegative) adolescents and young adults who come in contact with saliva infected by Epstein-Barr virus (EBV) are at high risk for infectious mononucleosis. Among college students, an estimated 30% to 50% are susceptible to EBV, and 10% to 15% of those are infected each year. Both sexes are affected equally.
- *Modes of transmission:* The virus is commonly transmitted by the oropharyngeal route and through blood transfusion.
- *Incubation period:* The virus incubates 30 to 50 days before symptoms appear.
- *Recovery period:* Fever and pharyngitis usually resolve in 1 to 3 weeks; lymphadenopathy and spleno-

megaly generally subside in 4 to 6 weeks.
- *Prognosis:* Excellent; serious illness rarely occurs.
- *Treatment:* Therapy is supportive, including bed rest and measures to alleviate symptoms.
- *Complications:* Although rare, complications can occur. These include splenic rupture, aseptic meningitis, encephalitis, hemolytic anemia, hepatitis, myocarditis, pericarditis, and Guillain-Barré syndrome.
- *Associated clinical findings:* Other findings include cervical lymphadenopathy, pharyngotonsillar exudation, splenomegaly, hepatomegaly, jaundice, palatal petechiae, and morbilliform rash.

Causes

Infectious mononucleosis is caused by primary infection with Epstein-Barr virus (EBV).

ASSESSMENT

Your assessment should include consideration of the patient's health history, physical examination findings, and diagnostic test results.

Health history

The patient's history may reveal contact with a person who has infectious mononucleosis. After an incubation period of about 30 to 50 days, the patient (typically an adolescent or young adult) usually experiences prodromal symptoms and reports headache, malaise, profound fatigue, an-

orexia, myalgia and, possibly, abdominal discomfort. After 3 to 5 days, he develops a sore throat, which he may describe as the worst he's ever had, and dysphagia related to adenopathy. Typically, the patient's late afternoon or evening fever will peak at 101° to 102° F (38.3° to 38.9° C).

Physical examination

Inspection commonly reveals exudative tonsillitis and pharyngitis and sometimes palatal petechiae, periorbital edema, and a maculopapular rash that resembles rubella. Rarely, jaundice is evident.

On palpation, you'll usually find mildly tender lymph nodes and cervical adenopathy with slight tenderness. The patient also may have inguinal and axillary adenopathy.

Timesaving tip: Anterior cervical adenopathy commonly occurs with a multitude of pharyngeal infections; however, posterior cervical adenopathy strongly suggests the illness is systemic. You may also detect splenomegaly and, less commonly, hepatomegaly.

Diagnostic test results
• White blood cell (WBC) count is elevated (10,000 to 20,000/mm³) during the second and third weeks of illness. Lymphocytes and monocytes account for 50% to 70% of the total WBC count; up to 20% of the lymphocytes may be atypical (a hallmark of the disorder).
• A fourfold rise in heterophil antibodies is shown in serum drawn during the acute phase and at 3- to 4-week intervals.
• Antibodies to EBV and cellular antigens appear on indirect immunofluorescence. Such testing usually is more definitive than heterophil antibodies but may not be necessary because most patients are heterophil-positive.
• Abnormal liver function studies may indicate EBV.

NURSING DIAGNOSIS

Common nursing diagnoses for a patient with infectious mononucleosis include:
• Fatigue related to infection
• Hyperthermia related to infection
• Pain related to throat inflammation and swelling.

PLANNING

Based on the nursing diagnosis *fatigue,* develop appropriate patient outcomes. For example, your patient will:
• avoid activities that increase fatigue
• obtain adequate rest to minimize fatigue
• regain his normal energy level when the infection is resolved.

Based on the nursing diagnosis *hyperthermia,* develop appropriate patient outcomes. For example, your patient will:
• demonstrate a decrease in fever following antipyretic therapy
• avoid complications associated with hyperthermia, such as seizures and shock
• regain and maintain a normal temperature.

Based on the nursing diagnosis *pain,* develop appropriate patient outcomes. For example, your patient will:
• express relief from discomfort after analgesic administration
• use diversionary activities to minimize pain
• verbalize absence of throat discomfort after infection is resolved.

IMPLEMENTATION

Most patients with infectious mononucleosis aren't hospitalized. Hospitalization may be warranted for complications, especially the possibility of airway compromise associated with severe pharyngitis. (See *Medical care of the patient with infectious mononucleosis.*)

Nursing interventions
• Administer medications, such as analgesics and antipyretics, to treat symptoms as needed.
• Provide warm saline gargles for relief of sore throat.

Medical care of the patient with infectious mononucleosis

Infectious mononucleosis is difficult to prevent and resistant to standard antimicrobial treatment. Thus, therapy is essentially supportive, including relief of symptoms, bed rest during the acute febrile period, and administration of aspirin (or another salicylate) for headache and saltwater gargles for sore throat. Acetaminophen is not generally recommended.

Treating complications
If severe throat inflammation causes airway obstruction, corticosteroids may relieve swelling and prevent a tracheotomy.

Splenic rupture, marked by sudden abdominal pain, requires splenectomy.

About 20% of patients with infectious mononucleosis also have streptococcal pharyngotonsillitis and should receive antibiotic therapy for at least 10 days.

A possible vaccine?
Epstein-Barr virus vaccine is currently unavailable; however, an experimental vaccine is expected to enter clinical trials within 1 or 2 years.

• Avoid vigorous splenic palpation because this may precipitate splenic rupture.
• Encourage fluid intake of about 3,000 ml daily.
• Plan care to provide rest periods.
• Monitor the patient's temperature and watch for signs and symptoms of complications.
• Monitor the patient's response to analgesics, antipyretics, and other supportive care measures.

Patient teaching
Timesaving tip: Supplement patient teaching with preprinted medication instructions, filling in the precise doctor-recommended time periods.
• Explain that convalescence may take several weeks, usually until the patient's WBC count returns to normal.

• Stress the need for bed rest during acute illness (usually for the first 3 to 5 days and during febrile episodes).
• If the patient is a student, tell him that he can continue less demanding school assignments and see his friends but that he should avoid long, difficult projects until after recovery.
• To minimize throat discomfort, encourage the patient to drink milk shakes, fruit juices, and broths and to eat cool, bland foods. Advise using warm saline gargles and prescribed analgesics and antipyretics as needed.
• Warn the patient to avoid activities that could lead to splenic rupture. These include heavy lifting, contact sports, rigorous exercise, and any other activities considered excessive exertion for the period defined by the doctor, usually 4 to 6 weeks.
• If liver enzymes are elevated, instruct the patient to refrain from alcohol use until test results are normal.

Discharge TimeSaver
Ensuring continued care for the patient with infectious mononucleosis

Review the following teaching topics, referrals, and follow-up appointments to make sure that your patient is adequately prepared for discharge.

Teaching topics
Make sure that the following topics have been covered and that your patient's learning has been evaluated:
□ nature of the disorder and possible complications
□ medications, including dosage and adverse effects
□ need for rest and fluids
□ need to avoid strenuous activities, such as heavy lifting, rigorous exercise, and contact sports for prescribed period
□ need to report abdominal pain
□ measures to relieve sore throat
□ need for follow-up evaluation.

Referrals
Make sure that the patient has been provided with necessary referrals to:
□ social service agencies as needed.

Follow-up appointments
Make sure that the necessary follow-up appointments have been scheduled and that the patient has been notified:
□ doctor
□ surgeon if needed
□ diagnostic tests for reevaluation.

• Tell the patient to immediately report abdominal pain, which could indicate a ruptured spleen. (See *Ensuring continued care for the patient with infectious mononucleosis.*)

EVALUATION

To evaluate the patient's response to your nursing care, gather reassessment data and compare this information with the patient outcomes specified in your plan of care.

Teaching and counseling
Begin by determining the effectiveness of your teaching. Consider the following questions:
• Does the patient know which activities to avoid to prevent fatigue and splenic rupture?

• Has he learned to use diversionary activities to minimize pain?

Physical condition
Conclude your evaluation by reassessing the patient's physical condition. Consider your nursing care effective if your patient:
• regains normal temperature and energy levels
• verbalizes absence of pain
• avoids complications of the disorder.

Viral encephalitis

A severe inflammation of the brain, viral encephalitis results when an invading virus destroys neuronal cells. The effects of viral encephalitis depend on the severity of infection and the brain area affected, but widespread cortical involvement results in decreased cognitive functioning. Most patients fail to return to their preexisting mental status. Focal neurologic deficits vary depending on localized brain involvement. (See *Key points about viral encephalitis.*)

Causes

Viral encephalitis is most often caused by arboviruses, enteroviruses, herpes simplex type 1 virus (HSV-1), and human immunodeficiency virus (HIV). Each associated virus can cause a variable disease course, ranging from an infection with no symptoms to fatal coma.

ASSESSMENT

Depending on the severity of the disease, most forms of viral encephalitis produce similar clinical features. HIV encephalitis (more commonly called HIV encephalopathy or HIV dementia) differs: The course is more insidious and subclinical and consists primarily of progressive cognitive or behavioral decline. Your assessment should include consideration of the patient's health history, physical examination findings, and diagnostic test results.

Health history

The patient may report systemic symptoms, such as headache, muscle stiffness, malaise, sore throat, and upper respiratory tract symptoms that existed for several days before the onset of neurologic symptoms.

After neurologic symptoms appear, the patient's history may reveal the sudden onset of altered levels of consciousness (LOC), from lethargy or drowsiness to stupor. The patient or a family member may also report

FactFinder
Key points about viral encephalitis

- *Causes:* Common causative viruses include the arboviruses, enteroviruses, herpes simplex type 1 virus (HSV-1), and human immunodeficiency virus.
- *Occurrence:* Mosquito-borne or, in some areas, tick-borne arboviruses (western equine, California, and St. Louis encephalitis) most commonly occur in rural areas. In urban areas, enteroviruses are more common causes. HSV-1 is the most common cause of nonepidemic encephalitis in North America.
- *Prognosis:* Most patients suffer neurologic effects. Viral encephalitis caused by HSV-1 causes death in up to 50% of patients.
- *Chief diagnostic tests:* Blood and serologic studies, lumbar puncture, EEG, computed tomography scan and, rarely, cerebrospinal fluid analysis help establish the diagnosis.
- *Treatment:* Therapy focuses on preventing complications in the acute phase.
- *Leading complications:* These include neurologic impairment, contractures, venous stasis, thrombus formation, and skin breakdown.

seizures, which may be the only evidence of viral encephalitis. Fever, nausea, and vomiting may also occur.

The patient may have a history of recent travel, recent exposure to infectious disease, ulcerations of the oral cavity or cold sores, or a recent tick or mosquito bite.

Timesaving tip: Because diagnosis can be difficult and prolonged, be sure to take a thorough history. Investigate all risk factors. Since the patient may be unaware of a recent insect bite, ask about outdoor recreation.

Physical examination

Typically, the patient with viral encephalitis looks acutely ill. Marked fever is a characteristic finding. Assessment usually reveals an altered LOC—for example, the patient may be confused, disoriented, comatose, or hallucinating. Use a standard tool, such as the Glasgow Coma Scale, to establish a baseline LOC.

Cranial nerve examination may reveal ocular palsies, facial weakness, and dysphagia. Assessment of the motor system may reveal paresis or paralysis of the extremities. You may detect exaggerated deep tendon reflexes, absent superficial reflexes, and a positive Babinski's sign.

Focal deficits (such as involuntary movements, poor memory retention, and ataxia) and sensory deficits (such as disturbances of taste and smell) may be present with cerebral hemisphere involvement. Meningeal irritation may be apparent, and the patient may demonstrate Kernig's or Brudzinski's sign and nuchal rigidity.

Diagnostic test results

During a viral encephalitis epidemic, a quick diagnosis is made from clinical findings and the patient history. However, sporadic cases are difficult to distinguish from other febrile illnesses, such as gastroenteritis or meningitis. The following tests help establish a diagnosis:

• Blood analysis or, rarely, cerebrospinal fluid (CSF) analysis may identify the virus and confirm the diagnosis.

• Serologic studies in some types of viral encephalitis may be diagnostic.

• Lumbar puncture discloses CSF pressure elevated in all forms of viral encephalitis. Despite inflammation, CSF analysis findings often reveal clear fluid. White blood cell count and protein levels in CSF are slightly elevated, but the glucose level remains normal. No bacteria are present.

• EEG reveals abnormalities such as generalized slowing of waveforms.

• Computed tomography scan may be ordered to check for temporal lobe lesions that indicate herpesvirus and to rule out cerebral hematoma. If localized lesions are found, a biopsy of the affected area can confirm HSV-1.

NURSING DIAGNOSIS

Common nursing diagnoses for a patient with viral encephalitis include:

• Hyperthermia related to infection

• Altered thought processes related to inflamed brain tissue

• Impaired physical mobility related to neurologic dysfunction

• Altered cerebral tissue perfusion related to increased intracranial pressure (ICP).

PLANNING

Based on the nursing diagnosis *hyperthermia,* develop appropriate patient outcomes. For example, your patient will:

• register an oral temperature not higher than 100° F (37.8° C) following the administration of antipyretics.

Based on the nursing diagnosis *altered thought processes,* develop appropriate patient outcomes. For example, your patient will:

• show orientation to person, place, and time

• communicate his needs

• participate in the decision-making process
• interact with others in a socially appropriate manner
• remain free of injury.

Based on the nursing diagnosis *impaired physical mobility,* develop appropriate patient outcomes. For example, your patient will:
• maintain maximum mobility within the limits of his neurologic impairment
• exhibit lack of complications due to immobility, such as contractures, venous stasis, thrombus formation, or skin breakdown, throughout course of illness.

Based on the nursing diagnosis *altered cerebral tissue perfusion,* develop appropriate patient outcomes. For example, your patient will:
• show ICP of 15 mm Hg or less
• record a Glasgow Coma Scale score of 11 to 15
• exhibit pupils that are equal and react to light
• demonstrate a normal respiratory pattern or a return to an acceptable baseline level
• record systolic blood pressure that is within 20 mm Hg of an acceptable baseline level
• have a pulse that is within the normal range for his age
• experience no vomiting or seizures
• demonstrate no increasing motor deficits.

IMPLEMENTATION

Treatment of viral encephalitis usually focuses on preventing complications in the acute phase. (See *Medical care of the patient with viral encephalitis,* page 222.)

Nursing interventions
• Monitor neurologic function, especially early indications of increased ICP. (See *Quick detection of worsening viral encephalitis,* page 223.) Later signs include widened pulse pressure, bradycardia, and irregular respirations; posturing; and fixed and dilated pupils.
• Maintain adequate fluid intake to prevent dehydration, but avoid fluid overload, which may increase cerebral edema. Monitor intake and output. Check for clinical signs of dehydration such as decreased skin turgor.
• If prescribed, give acyclovir I.V. for herpes encephalitis and monitor for adverse effects. Check infusion sites for infiltration and phlebitis. Alternatively, administer vidarabine as ordered.
• Administer antipyretics to control fever. Use a hypothermia blanket if necessary.
• Assess the patient's respiratory status frequently. Maintain a patent airway to prevent aspiration, atelectasis, and pneumonia. Assist with mechanical ventilation if the patient experiences respiratory failure.
• Assess the patient's mobility status. Carefully position the patient to prevent joint stiffness, contractures, and neck pain, and turn him often. Support affected extremities with pillows and adaptive devices. Assist with range-of-motion exercises. Consult with the physical therapist.
• Assess for signs of thrombophlebitis; apply antiembolism stockings or sequential compression devices as ordered. Provide skin care measures to prevent complications.
• If the patient has seizures, take precautions to prevent him from injuring himself. Pad the bed's side rails. Keep an artificial airway and suction equipment available.
• If the patient is delirious or confused, attempt to reorient him. For example, provide and mark a calen-

Treatments

Medical care of the patient with viral encephalitis

The antiviral agent acyclovir has replaced vidarabine as the treatment of choice for herpes encephalitis. The antiretroviral agent zidovudine (AZT) may benefit patients with human immunodeficiency virus type 1 encephalopathy.

Major supportive measures
Treatment of all other forms of viral encephalitis is purely supportive. Drug therapy includes I.V. mannitol to reduce intracranial pressure (ICP) and corticosteroids to reduce cerebral inflammation and resulting edema; phenytoin or another anticonvulsant, usually given I.V., to prevent seizures; sedatives to decrease restlessness; and acetaminophen to relieve headache and reduce fever.

Other measures
Isolation is unnecessary. Early rehabilitation is indicated to treat neurologic deficits and prevent complications. Other supportive measures include:
• fluid and electrolytes to prevent dehydration and control cerebral edema
• appropriate antibiotics for associated infections, such as pneumonia or sinusitis
• maintenance of a patent airway
• administration of oxygen to maintain normal arterial blood gas levels
• mechanical ventilation for a reduced level of consciousness or to treat increased ICP
• maintenance of adequate nutrition, especially during periods of coma.

dar, and keep a clock and familiar photographs at his bedside.
• Get the patient's attention before speaking. Speak slowly and calmly, and use short, simple sentences. Always explain what you're about to do. Repeat information or answer questions as often as necessary. Provide positive reinforcement about improving cognitive skills. When appropriate, consult with the occupational therapist about arranging meaningful activities. Divide tasks into multiple steps.

Timesaving tip: Clearly identify the patient with altered thought processes as a patient at high risk for injury. If your unit has no established system, suggest color coding the Kardex or the patient's identi-

fication band. This will alert the staff to maintain patient safety.
• Maintain adequate nutrition. Give the patient small, frequent meals, or provide nasogastric tube or parenteral feedings, as prescribed, if altered LOC or dysphagia prevents adequate oral intake. Elevate the head of the bed to 30 degrees to prevent aspiration.
• If the patient's speech is impaired, consult with the speech therapist and follow a specific rehabilitation program. Provide good mouth care.
• Give a mild laxative or stool softener, as ordered, to prevent constipation and minimize the risk of increased ICP resulting from straining during defecation.

Assessment TimeSaver

Quick detection of worsening viral encephalitis

When you are caring for a patient with viral encephalitis, you must be able to quickly detect subtle changes in his baseline status. Prompt recognition of *early* signs that his condition is worsening (usually because of increased intracranial pressure) and early intervention may prevent more serious consequences associated with the illness. Be on the alert for:
• sudden onset of restlessness
• any subtle change in behavior, speech, or orientation

• Glasgow Coma Scale score deterioration of 2 points
• fever higher than 101° F (38.3° C)
• sluggish pupillary reaction
• unilateral hippus (pupil constricts but then redilates in response to light)
• onset of seizures
• increased motor resistance to passive movement or worsening motor deficit
• inability to maintain arms in outstretched position or arm trembling when outstretched.

• Maintain a quiet environment. Encourage normal sleep and rest patterns.
• Remember that the patient and his family are likely to be frightened by his illness and by frequent diagnostic tests. Provide emotional support.

Patient teaching

🔧 **Timesaving tip:** Because of the patient's often-limited attention span, keep teaching sessions brief and free of extraneous noise and activity. Schedule teaching when the family can be present.
• Teach the patient and his family about the disease and its effects.
• Explain diagnostic tests and treatment measures, including prescribed medications. Explain procedures to the patient even if he's comatose.
• Explain to the patient and his family that some behavioral changes caused by viral encephalitis may be permanent. If a neurologic deficit is severe and appears permanent, refer the patient to a rehabilitation pro-

gram as soon as the acute phase has passed. (See *Ensuring continued care for the patient with viral encephalitis,* page 224.)

EVALUATION

To evaluate the patient's response to your care, gather reassessment data and compare this information with the patient outcomes specified in your plan of care.

Teaching and counseling

When evaluating the patient's response to your teaching, consider the following questions:
• Do the patient and his family understand the disease and its treatments and complications?
• Can the patient communicate his needs, participate in the decision-making process, and interact with others in a socially appropriate manner?

Discharge TimeSaver

Ensuring continued care for the patient with viral encephalitis

Review the following teaching topics, referrals, and follow-up appointments to make sure that your patient is adequately prepared for discharge.

Teaching topics
Make sure that the following topics have been covered and that your patient's learning has been evaluated:
☐ explanation of the disease and its management
☐ medications, including dosage and adverse effects
☐ need for follow-up evaluation
☐ rehabilitation measures.

Referrals
Make sure that the patient has been provided with necessary referrals to:

☐ social service agencies for consultation regarding discharge arrangements
☐ rehabilitation facility for physical therapy, occupational therapy, or speech therapy.

Follow-up appointments
Make sure that the necessary follow-up appointments have been scheduled and that the patient has been notified:
☐ neurologist
☐ physical therapist, if needed.

Physical condition

Conclude your evaluation by reassessing the patient's physical condition. Consider your nursing care effective if your patient:
• maintains a normal body temperature, pupillary response, respiratory pattern, and pulse rate
• scores 11 to 15 on the Glasgow Coma Scale
• shows improved thought processes
• maintains maximum mobility
• experiences no complications related to immobility
• has an ICP that's 15 mm Hg or less
• doesn't demonstrate signs and symptoms of increased ICP or increasing motor deficits
• records systolic blood pressure that's within 20 mm Hg of an acceptable baseline level
• experiences no vomiting or seizures
• remains free of injury.

CHAPTER 10

Caring for patients with bacterial and chlamydial infections

Toxic shock syndrome   226

Gonorrhea   231

Syphilis   237

Chlamydial infection   242

Pelvic inflammatory disease   245

Lyme disease   251

Tuberculosis   255

Helicobacter pylori *infection*   266

Acute pyelonephritis   269

Single-cell microorganisms with well-defined cell walls, bacteria can cause disease in almost every organ and body system. Bacterial infection can range from a relatively simple localized problem, to more serious visceral organ involvement, to a systemic, life-threatening disseminated infection.

In developing countries, where poor sanitation raises the risk of infection, bacterial diseases are a common cause of death and disability. Even in industrialized countries, bacteria are still the most common cause of fatal infectious disease.

Disease-causing bacterial mechanisms comprise three categories: toxicity without invasiveness, invasiveness without toxicity, and a combination of local invasiveness and local toxicity. (See *How bacteria cause disease.*)

Classifying bacteria

Bacteria are commonly classified by shape. Those with a spherical shape are called cocci. Those shaped like a rod are called bacilli. And spiral-shaped bacteria are called spirilla.

They can also be classified by:
- response to staining (gram-positive, gram-negative, or acid-fast)
- tendency toward capsulation (encapsulated or nonencapsulated)
- capacity to form spores (sporulating or nonsporulating)
- oxygen requirements (aerobic bacteria need oxygen to grow; anaerobic don't).

Some bacteria have specialized structures, such as fimbriae or pili, that enhance adherence to the host cell. In at least some cases, the bacterial cell's tendency to adhere to the host cell correlates with its pathogenicity.

Developing pathogenicity

Traditionally, bacteria have been considered pathogenic (disease-producing) or nonpathogenic (not disease-producing). But bacteria long assumed to be nonpathogenic are now causing infection and disease in immunocompromised patients. Today, it is more accurate to view all bacteria as potentially disease-producing and to focus on reinforcing the strength of the patient's defense mechanisms.

Toxic shock syndrome

An acute multisystem illness, toxic shock syndrome (TSS) has a mortality of 15% when not treated promptly. TSS typically strikes 15- to 19-year-old menstruating women who use tampons, particularly high-absorbency tampons. In fact, incidence of TSS has declined since 1985, when certain higher absorbency tampons were removed from the market. (See *Preventing TSS,* page 228.)

Although more than 9 in 10 cases of TSS occur in women, TSS may develop in anyone infected with certain strains of *Staphylococcus.* When not linked to menstruation, TSS is most often associated with a traumatic or surgical wound that's become infected with *S. aureus.* TSS also may be associated with postpartum infection, influenza, or use of contraceptive devices such as the diaphragm or vaginal sponge.

TSS may lead to adult respiratory distress syndrome, acute renal failure, hepatic necrosis, disseminated intravascular coagulation, metabolic acidosis, electrolyte imbalances, cardiomyopathy, and encephalomyopathy. Later complications may include

How bacteria cause disease

Three mechanisms of bacterial infection stimulate corresponding immune responses.

Bacteria can cause disease without invading host tissues. Some — such as *Corynebacterium diphtheriae* and *Clostridium tetani* — release a toxin; others — such as pharyngitis-producing group A streptococci — attach to the epithelial surface. Antibodies that neutralize either function may be sufficient to provide immunity to these bacteria.

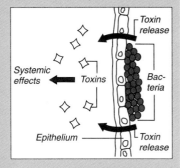

Other types of bacteria are not toxic, but cause disease by invading host tissues. In this case, damage results from the volume of pathogens or from damage caused by the infection, as in lepromatous leprosy. The body's cell-mediated immune response has to destroy and degrade organisms in this category.

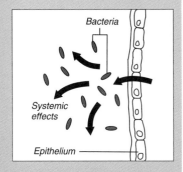

Most bacteria fall somewhere between the two extremes mentioned above. They are locally invasive, aided by local toxicity and enzymes that degrade the extracellular matrix. Examples include *Staphylococcus aureus* and *Clostridium perfringens*. Resistance to these bacteria requires both antibodies and the cell-mediated response.

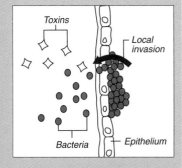

Teaching TimeSaver
Preventing TSS

Use the following guidelines when educating patients on how to avoid toxic shock syndrome (TSS).

Using contraceptive devices
Educate the patient about the use of a diaphragm or vaginal sponge. Explain that she should wash her hands before inserting one of these contraceptive devices. Tell her to wash and rinse a diaphragm thoroughly before use and to clean it immediately after use. Tell her not to use a vaginal sponge if dirty and to wet the sponge with clean tap water before insertion.

Instruct the patient to be careful when inserting the device to avoid injuring vaginal tissue. A diaphragm or vaginal sponge should not remain in place longer than the time limit recommended by the doctor and should not be used during menses.

Using tampons
The patient should wash her hands before inserting a tampon. A tampon should be changed at least every 6 hours. Tell her not to use super-absorbent tampons and not to use tampons overnight while she sleeps. If she's had TSS, she shouldn't use tampons.

chronic renal failure and neuropsychological problems.

Following an episode of TSS, most patients recover fully but remain at increased risk for recurrence. Women who continue to use tampons face the highest risk of recurrence.

CDC definition
The following diagnostic characteristics of TSS have been identified by the Centers for Disease Control and Prevention (CDC):
• fever of at least 103.8° F (38.9° C)
• diffuse macular erythroderma followed by desquamation, particularly on the toes and palms, 1 to 2 weeks after the onset of illness
• hypotension (systolic pressure below 90 mm Hg) or syncope resulting from orthostatic hypotension

• involvement of three or more organ systems (such as GI, renal, hepatic, hematologic, or central nervous systems) and mucous membranes
• negative test results for other likely diagnoses, such as Rocky Mountain spotted fever, measles, leptospirosis, and scarlet fever.

Causes
Most experts now believe that TSS is caused by strains of *S. aureus* that produce a substance known as toxic shock syndrome toxin-1. Bacterial strains that produce this substance are usually resistant to penicillin and ampicillin but susceptible to other antistaphylococcal antibiotics.

ASSESSMENT

In most cases, assessment is straightforward and treatment can begin right away. Your assessment should include a careful consideration of the patient's health history, physical examination findings, and diagnostic test results.

Health history

The patient will report the abrupt onset of a high fever (possibly over 104° F [40° C]), intense myalgia, vomiting, diarrhea, rash, and headache.

Most likely, the patient will be menstruating or will be 2 or 3 days past the end of her menses. Her recent history will almost certainly include tampon use. If not, be sure to ask about a history of using vaginal contraceptive devices. Also ask about recent surgery, childbirth, or influenza.

Physical examination

Inspection may reveal rigors, conjunctival hyperemia, vaginal hyperemia, and vaginal discharge. You may see a deep-red macular rash, especially on the patient's palms and soles. The rash appears within a few hours of the onset of infection (and desquamates about 10 days later). The patient may seem listless and confused.

Timesaving tip: To avoid losing time later trying to evaluate whether the patient's level of consciousness has worsened, use a standard assessment tool — such as the Glasgow Coma Scale — when establishing baseline parameters.

When you assess the patient's vital signs, you'll find fever and possible signs of shock, such as a rapid, thready pulse and hypotension. If the patient is in a critical care unit, hemodynamic monitoring shows decreased central venous pressure and decreased pulmonary artery wedge pressure.

Diagnostic test results

Often, diagnosis of TSS is established clinically based on the case definition put forth by the CDC.

Isolation of toxin-producing *S. aureus* from vaginal discharge or lesions helps support the diagnosis. Rarely, *S. aureus* may be isolated from blood or cerebrospinal fluid.

NURSING DIAGNOSIS

Common nursing diagnoses for a patient with TSS include:
• Hyperthermia related to infection
• Pain (headache, myalgia) related to infection
• Diarrhea related to infection
• Fluid volume deficit related to diarrhea and decreased cardiac output
• Knowledge deficit related to the disease and its risk factors.

PLANNING

Based on the nursing diagnosis *hyperthermia,* develop appropriate patient outcomes. For example, your patient will:
• demonstrate decreased fever following therapy with an antipyretic and an antibiotic
• regain and maintain a normal temperature after TSS has resolved
• avoid complications associated with hyperthermia.

Based on the nursing diagnosis *pain,* develop appropriate patient outcomes. For example, your patient will:
• notify a caregiver immediately when pain occurs
• rate pain on a scale of 1 to 10

Treatments

Medical care of the patient with TSS

Treatment for toxic shock syndrome (TSS) includes the following:
• I.V. antistaphylococcal antibiotics that are beta-lactamase resistant, such as oxacillin, nafcillin, and methicillin
• removal of foreign bodies that might be foci for infection
• drainage of infected areas.
  Administer I.V. 0.9% sodium chloride solution and colloids to replace fluids, and medications to combat shock. Other measures may include supportive treatment for diarrhea, nausea, and vomiting.

• report that pain has decreased or disappeared within 45 minutes after the start of comfort measures.
  Based on the nursing diagnosis *diarrhea,* develop appropriate patient outcomes. For example, your patient will:
• achieve control of diarrhea with medication
• show no signs or symptoms of complications associated with diarrhea, such as skin breakdown or electrolyte imbalance.
  Based on the nursing diagnosis *fluid volume deficit,* develop appropriate patient outcomes. For example, your patient will:
• regain and maintain normal vital signs
• regain and maintain normal fluid balance
• void at least 50 ml/hour each day
• not show clinical signs of dehydration, such as dry mucous membranes or tongue furrows.

Based on the nursing diagnosis *knowledge deficit,* develop appropriate patient outcomes. For example, your patient will:
• verbalize knowledge of the disease and its causes
• explain treatment measures
• identify personal risk factors for TSS and relate plans to eliminate or reduce them.

IMPLEMENTATION

Rapid and accurate treatment of TSS is crucial for achieving a full, prompt recovery. (See *Medical care of the patient with TSS.*)

Nursing interventions
• Administer prescribed I.V. antibiotics over a 15-minute period to ensure peak levels. Monitor for adverse reactions, especially an allergic reaction.
• Replace fluids and electrolytes intravenously, as ordered.
• Reorient the patient as needed. Use appropriate safety measures to prevent injury.
• Follow universal precautions.
• Administer analgesics cautiously because of the risk of hypotension and liver failure.
• Monitor the patient's hemodynamic status.
• Offer emotional support to the patient and family.

Patient teaching
• Explain the nature of TSS.
• Explain all interventions and procedures.
• Advise the patient to avoid using tampons, particularly superabsorbent tampons, because of the risk of recurrence.
• Teach the patient about precautions related to use of the contraceptive diaphragm or vaginal sponge.

Discharge TimeSaver

Ensuring continued care for the patient with TSS

Review the following teaching topics, referrals, and follow-up appointments to make sure that your patient is adequately prepared for discharge.

Teaching topics
Make sure that the following topics have been covered and that your patient's learning has been evaluated:
☐ nature of the disorder and possible complications
☐ antibiotic therapy
☐ methods for reducing the risk of toxic shock syndrome (TSS) recurrence
☐ signs of TSS recurrence to report immediately.

Referrals
Make sure that the patient has been provided with necessary referrals to:
☐ family planning (if warranted).

Follow-up appointments
Make sure that the necessary follow-up appointments have been scheduled and that the patient has been notified:
☐ doctor.

(See *Ensuring continued care for the patient with TSS.*)

EVALUATION

When evaluating the patient's response to your nursing care, gather reassessment data and compare this information with the patient outcomes specified in your plan of care.

Teaching and counseling
Begin by determining the effectiveness of your teaching and counseling. Consider the following question:
• Can the patient explain the nature of the disease, its treatment, and measures that reduce risk?

Physical condition
If treatment has been successful, you should note the following outcomes:
• The patient has resumed a normal bowel elimination pattern.
• She has regained fluid balance.

• She has demonstrated adequate organ perfusion.

Gonorrhea

Gonorrhea is a common sexually transmitted disease (STD), which usually starts as an infection of the genitourinary tract, especially the urethra and cervix. It also can begin in the rectum, pharynx, or eyes. Left untreated, gonorrhea spreads through the blood to the joints, tendons, meninges, and endocardium. It can lead to acute epididymitis, septic arthritis, dermatitis, and hepatitis. In women, it also can lead to chronic pelvic inflammatory disease (PID) and sterility. Severe gonococcal conjunctivitis can lead to corneal ulceration and, possibly, blindness. Rare complications include meningitis, osteo-

Teaching TimeSaver

Preventing sexually transmitted disease

To help prevent sexual transmission of gonorrhea, syphilis, and chlamydial infection, explain the following:

• The most effective way to prevent transmission of sexually transmitted diseases (STDs) is to avoid sexual intercourse with an infected partner.

• If the choice is made to have sexual intercourse with a partner who is or may be infected with an STD, men should use a fresh latex condom with each act of intercourse. Consistent and correct use of a condom is crucial to prevent STDs.

• When a male condom cannot be used, couples should consider using a female condom. Laboratory studies indicate that the female condom — a lubricated polyurethane sheath that is inserted into the vagina — is an effective physical barrier to viruses. However, no clinical studies have been completed to show protection from human immunodeficiency virus infection, gonorrhea, syphilis, or chlamydial infection.

• Sexual partners of patients infected with an STD should be examined, tested, and, when indicated, treated for infection.

• Infected patients need to complete the entire course of antibiotic therapy and should refrain from sexual intercourse until cultures are negative.

myelitis, pneumonia, and adult respiratory distress syndrome.

With proper treatment, the prognosis is usually excellent. However, recurrence is common. (See *Preventing sexually transmitted disease*.)

Although the overall reported incidence of gonorrhea in North America has been decreasing since the 1970s, antimicrobial resistance to the causative organism has increased during the same time period.

Causes
Gonorrhea is caused by the organism *Neisseria gonorrhoeae*. Transmission occurs almost exclusively through sexual contact with an infected person. A child born of an infected mother, however, can contract gonococcal ophthalmia neonatorum during passage through the birth canal. Also, a patient with gonorrhea can contract gonococcal conjunctivitis by touching his eyes with a contaminated hand.

ASSESSMENT

Your assessment should include a careful consideration of the patient's health history, physical examination findings, and diagnostic test results.

Health history
The patient may report unprotected sexual contact (vaginal, oral, or anal) with an infected person, an unknown partner, or multiple partners. He also may have a history of STD.

The patient may be asymptomatic. After a 3- to 6-day incubation period, a male patient may complain of dysuria. A patient with a rectal infection may complain of anal itching, burning, and tenesmus and pain with defecation. A patient with a pharyngeal infection may complain of a sore throat.

Physical examination

Assessment of a patient with gonorrhea reveals a low-grade fever. If the disease has become systemic or if the patient has developed PID or acute epididymitis, the fever will be higher.

Inspection of a male patient's urethral meatus reveals a purulent discharge. In a female patient, this discharge may be expressed from the urethra, and the meatus may appear red and edematous. Inspection of the cervix with a speculum discloses a greenish yellow discharge, the most common sign of infection in females. Vaginal inspection reveals engorgement, redness, swelling, and a profuse purulent discharge.

If the patient has a rectal infection, inspection may reveal a purulent discharge or rectal bleeding. In an ocular infection, inspection may reveal a purulent discharge from the conjunctiva. In a pharyngeal infection, you'll see redness and a purulent discharge.

If the infection has become systemic, papillary skin lesions — possibly pustular, hemorrhagic, or necrotic — may appear on the patient's hands and feet.

Palpation of the patient with PID reveals tenderness over the lower quadrant, abdominal rigidity and distention, and adnexal tenderness (usually bilateral). In a patient with hepatitis, palpation discloses right upper quadrant tenderness.

Examination of a patient with systemic infection may reveal pain and a cracking noise when moving an involved joint. Asymmetrical involvement of only a few joints — typically the knees, ankles, and elbows — may differentiate gonococcal arthritis from other forms of arthritis.

Diagnostic test results

• A culture from the infection site (the urethra, cervix, rectum, or pharynx) grown on a Thayer-Martin medium usually establishes the diagnosis.

• A culture of conjunctival scrapings confirms gonococcal conjunctivitis.

• In a male patient, a Gram stain that shows gram-negative diplococci may confirm gonorrhea.

• Diagnosis of gonococcal arthritis requires identification of gram-negative diplococci on smears made from joint fluid and skin lesions.

• Complement fixation and immunofluorescent assays of serum reveal antibody titers four times the normal rate.

NURSING DIAGNOSIS

Common nursing diagnoses for a patient with gonorrhea include:

• Altered sexuality patterns related to the need for abstinence during the treatment regimen

• Altered urinary elimination related to dysuria and infection

• High risk for infection related to frequency of recurrence and incidence of conjunctivitis

• Pain related to infection.

PLANNING

Based on the nursing diagnosis *altered sexuality patterns,* develop appropriate patient outcomes. For example, your patient will:

• state the need to abstain from sexual activity until therapy is complete and cultures are negative

• resume normal protected sexual activity when gonorrhea has been eradicated.

Based on the nursing diagnosis *altered urinary elimination,* develop ap-

Treatments

Medical care of the patient with gonorrhea

Drug therapy for the patient with gonorrhea will include one or more of the following regimens, depending on the nature of the infection.

Uncomplicated gonorrhea
Medical treatment for the adult patient with uncomplicated gonorrhea typically includes 250 mg of ceftriaxone given I.M. in a single dose, plus 100 mg of doxycycline given twice daily by mouth for 7 days.

As an alternative to doxycycline, the patient may receive 500 mg of oral tetracycline four times daily for 7 days. Tetracycline also treats coexistent chlamydial or mycoplasmal infection.

For patients who can't take doxycycline or tetracycline, such as pregnant women, treatment consists of 500 mg of oral erythromycin for 7 days.

Non-penicillinase-producing gonorrhea
If the infection was acquired from a person proven to have susceptible non-penicillinase-producing gonorrhea, the patient can receive 1 g of probenecid by mouth (to block penicillin excretion) plus 3 g of ampicillin by mouth in a single dose. This therapy is followed by a 7-day course of doxycycline.

Disseminated gonococcal infection
Disseminated gonococcal infection requires 1 g of ceftriaxone given I.M. or I.V. every 24 hours for 7 days. Adult gonococcal ophthalmia requires 1 g of ceftriaxone given I.M. in a single dose.

Follow-up and neonatal considerations
Because there are many strains of antibiotic-resistant gonococci, follow-up cultures are necessary 4 to 7 days after treatment and again in 6 months. (For a pregnant patient, final follow-up must occur before delivery.)

Routine instillation of 1% silver nitrate drops or erythromycin ointment into the eyes of neonates has greatly reduced the incidence of gonococcal ophthalmia neonatorum.

propriate patient outcomes. For example, your patient will:
• void at least 50 ml/hour each day
• return to normal urinary elimination patterns when gonorrhea subsides.

Based on the nursing diagnosis *high risk for infection,* develop appropriate patient outcomes. For example, your patient will:

• describe how gonorrhea is contracted
• state his intention to take precautions during sexual activity to prevent reinfection.

Based on the nursing diagnosis *pain,* develop appropriate patient outcomes. For example, your patient will:

• notify a caregiver when he has pain

Discharge TimeSaver

Ensuring continued care for the patient with gonorrhea

Review the following teaching topics, referrals, and follow-up appointments to make sure that your patient is adequately prepared for discharge.

Teaching topics
Make sure that the following topics have been covered and that your patient's learning has been evaluated:
□ treatment therapy
□ explanation of gonorrheal infection, including its causes and potential complications
□ pain relief
□ prevention of reinfection.

Referrals
Make sure that the patient has been provided with necessary referrals to:
□ public health authorities.

Follow-up appointments
Make sure that the necessary follow-up appointments have been scheduled and that the patient has been notified:
□ doctor or clinic
□ diagnostic tests for reevaluation.

• rate his pain on a scale of 1 to 10
• state that his pain has decreased or stopped after starting therapy, initiating comfort measures, or both.

IMPLEMENTATION

Adapt your nursing interventions to suit your patient's condition. (See *Medical care of the patient with gonorrhea.*)

Nursing interventions
• Use universal precautions when obtaining specimens for laboratory examination and when caring for the patient. Carefully contain all soiled articles and dispose of them according to hospital policy.
• If the patient has gonococcal arthritis, apply moist heat to ease pain in affected joints. Administer prescribed analgesics.
• Before treatment, determine if the patient has any drug sensitivities.

During treatment, watch closely for signs of a drug reaction.
• Monitor the patient for complications.

Patient teaching
• Tell the patient that until culture results are negative, he's still infectious and should abstain from sexual contact. (See *Ensuring continued care for the patient with gonorrhea.*)
• Urge the patient to inform his sexual partners of his infection so that they can seek treatment.
• Advise the partner of an infected person to receive treatment even if she doesn't have a positive culture. Also advise her to abstain from sexual contact with anyone until treatment is complete because reinfection is extremely common.
• Counsel the patient and his sexual partners to be tested for human immunodeficiency virus and hepatitis B infection. Also explain that the pa-

Evaluation TimeSaver

Assessing failure to respond to therapy in gonorrhea

If your patient fails to respond to nursing interventions, this checklist can help you evaluate the reasons why. During your evaluation, consult with the patient, doctor, and members of the health care team to discover possible reasons. Keep in mind that even with optimum treatment and full compliance, flare-ups and complications are still possible.

Factors that may interfere with compliance
☐ Unclear instructions
☐ Failure to provide written instructions
☐ Inadequate patient teaching
☐ Language barrier
☐ Illiteracy
☐ Emotional instability
☐ Inability to afford medication
☐ Inability to tolerate adverse effects of medication
☐ Inconvenient schedule of medication administration

Factors that may interfere with drug therapy
☐ Drug resistance
☐ Insufficient time period for effective drug therapy
☐ Ineffective drug regimen
☐ Renal involvement that interferes with drug elimination
☐ Hypersensitivity to medications

Conditions that may interfere with treatment
☐ Failure to treat partner
☐ Unwillingness to abstain from sexual activity while infected or failure to use condoms

tient should be tested for chlamydial infection.
• Instruct the patient to be careful when coming into contact with his bodily discharges so that he doesn't contaminate his eyes.
• Tell the patient to take anti-infective drugs for the full length of time prescribed.
• Teach the patient ways to prevent reinfection.
• Advise the patient to return for follow-up tests.

EVALUATION

When evaluating the patient's response to your nursing care, gather reassessment data and compare this information with the patient outcomes specified in your plan of care.

Teaching and counseling
Begin by determining the effectiveness of your teaching and counseling. Consider the following questions:
• Has the patient communicated his intention to abstain from sexual activity until the infection clears up?
• Does he know that he can resume protected sexual activity when his infection has been eradicated?
• Does he understand the nature of gonorrhea, how it is contracted, and precautions for preventing infection?

• Does he understand the need to comply with prescribed therapy? (See *Assessing failure to respond to therapy in gonorrhea.*)

Physical condition
If treatment has been successful, you should note the following outcomes:
• The patient reports a reduction or cessation of pain.
• He resumes normal urinary elimination patterns.

Syphilis

A chronic, infectious disease, syphilis begins in the mucous membranes and quickly becomes systemic, spreading to nearby lymph nodes and into the bloodstream. Left untreated, the disease progresses in four stages: primary, secondary, latent, and late (formerly called tertiary). Advanced syphilis can cause aortic insufficiency or aneurysm, meningitis, and widespread damage to the central nervous system. Untreated syphilis can lead to crippling or death. However, with early treatment, the prognosis is excellent.

Causes
Syphilis is caused by a spirochete known as *Treponema pallidum*. Transmission occurs primarily through sexual contact during the primary, secondary, and early latent stages of infection. Prenatal transmission (from an infected mother to the fetus) also is possible. Transmission by way of a fresh blood transfusion is rare. After 96 hours in stored blood, the *T. pallidum* spirochete dies.

ASSESSMENT
Your assessment should include a careful consideration of the patient's health history, physical examination findings, and diagnostic test results. When gathering your assessment data, keep in mind that signs and symptoms of syphilis vary with its stage, as described below.

Health history
The typical patient history includes unprotected sexual contact with an infected person, an anonymous partner, or multiple partners.

Physical examination
If the patient has primary syphilis, you may observe one or more chancres (small, fluid-filled lesions) on the genitalia and possibly others on the anus, fingers, lips, tongue, nipples, tonsils, or eyelids. (See *Syphilitic chancre and rash,* page 238.) In female patients, chancres may develop on the cervix or the vaginal wall. These usually painless lesions start as papules and then erode. They have indurated, raised edges and clear bases and typically heal after 3 to 6 weeks, even when untreated. Palpation of the lymph nodes may reveal enlarged unilateral or bilateral regional adenopathy.

Secondary syphilis
In secondary syphilis (beginning within a few days or up to 8 weeks after the initial chancres appear), the patient may complain of headache, nausea, vomiting, malaise, anorexia, weight loss, sore throat, and a slight fever. On inspection, you may see symmetrical mucocutaneous lesions. The rash of secondary syphilis may appear macular, papular, pustular, or nodular. Lesions are uniform, well defined, and generalized. Macules

Syphilitic chancre and rash

This illustration shows a penile chancre, which appears about 3 to 4 weeks after the initial infection, during the primary syphilis stage.

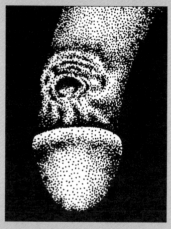

During the secondary syphilis stage, a papular rash may develop with lesions typically covering the palms and soles.

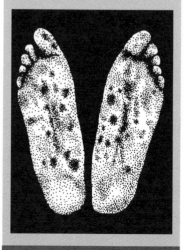

typically erupt between rolls of fat on the trunk and, proximally, on the arms, palms, soles, face, and scalp. In warm, moist body areas (the perineum, scrotum, or vulva, for example), the lesions enlarge and erode, producing highly contagious, pink or grayish white lesions (condylomata lata). Alopecia, which usually is temporary, may occur with or without treatment. The patient also may complain of brittle, pitted nails. Palpation may reveal generalized adenopathy.

Latent syphilis
In latent syphilis, physical signs and symptoms are absent except for a possible recurrence of mucocutaneous lesions that resemble those of secondary syphilis.

Late syphilis
In late syphilis, the patient's complaints will vary with the involved organ. Late syphilis has three subtypes: neurosyphilis, late benign syphilis, and cardiovascular syphilis.

Neurosyphilis
If neurosyphilis affects meningovascular tissues, the patient may report headache, vertigo, insomnia, hemiplegia, seizures, and psychological difficulties. If neurosyphilis affects parenchymal tissue, he may report paresis, alteration in intellect, paranoia, illusions, and hallucinations. Inspection may reveal Argyll Robertson pupil (a small, irregular pupil that does not react to light but does accommodate for vision), ataxia, slurred speech, trophic joint changes, positive Romberg's sign, and a facial tremor.

Late benign syphilis
If the patient has late benign syphilis, he may complain of gummas — lesions that develop between 1 and 10

years after infection. A single gumma may be a chronic, superficial nodule or a deep, granulomatous lesion that's solitary, asymmetrical, painless, indurated, and large or small. Visible on the skin and mucocutaneous tissues, gummas commonly affect bones and can develop in any organ. If they involve the nasal septum or palate, they may perforate and cause disfigurement.

Cardiovascular syphilis
In cardiovascular syphilis, decreased cardiac output may cause decreased urine output and decreased sensorium related to hypoxia. Auscultation may reveal pulmonary congestion.

Diagnostic test results
The following tests may reveal factors that point to a diagnosis of syphilis.
• Darkfield microscopy can identify spiral-shaped *T. pallidum* from lesional exudate and provides an immediate diagnosis.
• Nontreponemal serologic tests include the Venereal Disease Research Laboratory (VDRL) slide test, the rapid plasma reagin (RPR) test, and the automated reagin test. These tests can detect nonspecific antibodies, which become reactive 1 to 2 weeks after the primary syphilis lesion appears or 4 to 5 weeks after the infection begins.
• Treponemal serologic studies include the fluorescent treponemal antibody absorption test, *Treponema pallidum* hemagglutination assay, and microhemagglutination assay-*Treponema pallidum*. These tests detect the specific antitreponemal antibody and can confirm positive screening results. Once reactive, a patient's blood samples will always be reactive.

• Cerebrospinal fluid examination identifies neurosyphilis when the total protein level is above 40 mg/dl, the VDRL slide test is reactive, and the white blood cell (WBC) count exceeds 5 WBCs/mm^3.

NURSING DIAGNOSIS
Common nursing diagnoses for a patient with syphilis include:
• Altered sexuality patterns related to the need for abstinence during the treatment regimen
• Impaired skin integrity related to infection
• Knowledge deficit related to the disease and its transmission, treatment, and prevention.

PLANNING
Based on the nursing diagnosis *altered sexuality patterns,* develop appropriate patient outcomes. For example, your patient will:
• communicate the need to abstain from sexual activity during treatment for syphilis
• state his intention to comply with restrictions on sexual activity until VDRL and RPR test results are normal
• resume normal protected sexual activity when syphilis subsides.
   Based on the nursing diagnosis, *impaired skin integrity,* develop appropriate patient outcomes. For example, your patient will:
• verbalize the importance of skin care measures
• demonstrate skill in performing requisite skin care
• reestablish skin integrity, as evidenced by the eradication of lesions.
   Based on the nursing diagnosis *knowledge deficit,* develop appropriate patient outcomes. For example, your patient will:

Treatments

Medical care of the patient with syphilis

Drug therapy for the patient with syphilis typically involves treatment with antibiotics.

Early-stage syphilis
Antibiotics, including penicillin administered I.M., are the treatment of choice. For early syphilis, treatment may consist of a single I.M. injection of 2.4 million units of penicillin G benzathine.

Advanced illness
Syphilis that is present for more than 1 year may respond to a series of three weekly I.M. injections of 2.4 million units of penicillin G benzathine.

Alternative therapies
Patients allergic to penicillin may be successfully treated with 500 mg of tetracycline by mouth four times daily for 15 days. (Tetracycline is contraindicated during pregnancy.) The preferred alternative therapy is 100 mg of doxycycline by mouth twice daily for 2 weeks.

• seek and obtain information about syphilis from appropriate sources
• describe the disorder
• communicate his understanding of how syphilis is transmitted and prevented
• explain the treatment regimen and state his intention to follow the prescribed therapy.

IMPLEMENTATION

Adapt your nursing interventions to suit the patient's condition, as described below. (See *Medical care of the patient with syphilis.*)

Nursing interventions
• Follow universal precautions when assessing the patient, collecting specimens, and treating lesions.
• Check for a history of drug sensitivity before administering the first dose of medication.

• Promote rest and adequate nutrition.
• In secondary syphilis, keep lesions clean and dry. If they're draining, dispose of contaminated materials properly.
• In late syphilis, provide care to relieve the patient's symptoms during prolonged treatment.
• As needed, consult with physical or occupational therapists. Consult with a social worker to determine home care needs.
• Check lesions for drainage and healing.
• Assess for complications of late syphilis if the patient's infection has lasted longer than 1 year.
• Monitor the patient's compliance with drug therapy.

Patient teaching
• Explain the nature of the disorder and its transmission.

Discharge TimeSaver

Ensuring continued care for the patient with syphilis

Review the following teaching topics, referrals, and follow-up appointments to make sure that your patient is adequately prepared for discharge.

Teaching topics
Make sure that the following topics have been covered and that your patient's learning has been evaluated:
☐ explanation of syphilis, including its causes and complications
☐ drug therapy, including possible adverse reactions
☐ skin care guidelines
☐ prevention methods.

Referrals
Make sure that the patient has been provided with necessary referrals to:

☐ social service agencies
☐ physical therapy
☐ occupational therapy
☐ public health authorities.

Follow-up appointments
Make sure that the necessary follow-up appointments have been scheduled and that the patient has been notified:
☐ doctor
☐ diagnostic tests for reevaluation.

• Make sure that the patient clearly understands his medication and dosage schedule and knows how to obtain the medication.

• Stress the importance of completing the prescribed course of therapy even after symptoms subside. Evaluate the need for home nursing care for selected patients.

• Urge the patient to inform sexual partners of his infection and to encourage them to seek testing and treatment.

• Advise the patient to refrain from sexual activity until he completes treatment and his follow-up VDRL and RPR test results are normal.

• Counsel the patient and his sexual partners about human immunodeficiency virus (HIV) infection. Recommend testing for HIV as well as other sexually transmitted diseases.

• Teach the patient about preventing transmission of syphilis. (See *Preventing sexually transmitted disease,* page 232.)

• Remind the patient to schedule and report for follow-up tests. (See *Ensuring continued care for the patient with syphilis.*)

EVALUATION

When evaluating the patient's response to your nursing care, gather reassessment data and compare this information with the patient outcomes specified in your plan of care.

Teaching and counseling
Begin by determining the effectiveness of your teaching and counseling. Consider the following questions:

• Has the patient verbalized his intention to restrict sexual activity during treatment?
• Has he stated that he plans to resume normal protected sexual activity when syphilis subsides?
• Can he explain appropriate skin care measures?
• Can he explain the nature of the disorder and the means of transmission?
• Can he explain his treatment regimen and has he said that he intends to complete the prescribed therapy?

Physical condition
If treatment has been successful, you should note the following outcomes:
• The patient has regained skin integrity.
• VDRL and RPR test results are normal.
• Complications of syphilis are absent.

Chlamydial infection

Infection with the organism *Chlamydia trachomatis* can cause many complications. For example, men can develop urethritis, women can develop cervicitis and, less commonly, either sex can develop lymphogranuloma venereum.

Complications of lymphogranuloma venereum include urethral and rectal strictures, perirectal abscesses, and rectovesical, rectovaginal, and ischiorectal fistulas. Elephantiasis with enlargement of the penis or vulva develops occasionally.

Left untreated, chlamydial infection can lead to acute epididymitis, salpingitis, pelvic inflammatory disease and, eventually, sterility. In pregnant women, chlamydial infection appears to be associated with spontaneous abortion, premature rupture of membranes, premature delivery, and neonatal death.

Children born to infected mothers may contract associated otitis media, pneumonia, trachoma, and inclusion conjunctivitis while passing through the birth canal. Although trachoma inclusion conjunctivitis seldom occurs in North America, it's a leading cause of blindness in Third World countries.

Chlamydial infection is probably the most common sexually transmitted bacterial disease in developed countries. It affects large numbers of adolescents. In the United States, precise data concerning the prevalence and incidence of chlamydial infection are not available. One reason is that reporting is not mandatory in all states. However, the number of states requiring health care professionals to report chlamydial infections is increasing.

Causes
Transmission of *C. trachomatis,* an intracellular obligate bacterium, typically occurs during vaginal or rectal intercourse or oral-genital contact with an infected individual. Because signs and symptoms of chlamydial infection commonly appear late in the course of the disease, sexual transmission of the organism usually occurs unknowingly.

ASSESSMENT

Your assessment should include a careful consideration of the patient's health history, physical examination findings, and diagnostic test results. When gathering your assessment data, keep in mind that symptoms — if present — vary with the specific type of chlamydial infection and that most women are asymptomatic.

Health history

The patient may have a history of unprotected sexual contact with an infected person, an anonymous partner, or multiple partners. He also may have another sexually transmitted disease (STD) or have had one in the past.

If a woman develops cervicitis, she may complain of mucopurulent discharge, pelvic pain, and dyspareunia. A woman with urethral syndrome may experience dysuria and urinary frequency.

A male patient with urethritis may complain of dysuria, urinary frequency, and a mucoid discharge.

If the infection involves the rectum, the patient may complain of diarrhea, tenesmus, and pruritus.

A patient with lymphogranuloma venereum may have systemic signs and symptoms, such as myalgia, headache, weight loss, backache, fever, and chills.

Physical examination

Inspection by speculum of the patient with cervicitis may reveal cervical erosion and mucopurulent discharge. Inspection of a male patient with urethritis may disclose urethral discharge and erythema of the meatus.

Inspection of a patient with lymphogranuloma venereum may reveal a primary lesion — a painless vesicle or nonindurated ulcer. Such an ulcer usually is 2 to 3 mm in diameter and occurs on the glans or shaft of the penis; on the labia, vagina, or cervix; or in the rectum. It commonly goes unnoticed.

Diagnostic test results

Laboratory tests provide definitive diagnosis of chlamydial infection.

• A swab culture from the infection site (urethra, cervix, or rectum) usually establishes urethritis, cervicitis, salpingitis, endometritis, or proctitis.

• Culture of aspirated blood, pus, or cerebrospinal fluid establishes epididymitis, prostatitis, or lymphogranuloma venereum.

If the infection site is accessible, the doctor may first attempt direct visualization of cell scrapings or exudate with Giemsa stain or fluorescein-conjugated monoclonal antibodies. However, tissue cell cultures are more sensitive and specific.

NURSING DIAGNOSIS

Common nursing diagnoses for a patient with chlamydial infection include:

• Altered urinary elimination related to dysuria and inflammation secondary to infection

• Pain related to infection

• Knowledge deficit related to the nature of the disorder and its transmission, treatment, and prevention.

PLANNING

Based on the nursing diagnosis *altered urinary elimination,* develop appropriate patient outcomes. For example, your patient will:

• not incur complications associated with urethritis

• reestablish a normal urinary elimination pattern when infection subsides.

Based on the nursing diagnosis *pain,* develop appropriate patient outcomes. For example, your patient will:

• notify a caregiver when pain occurs

• rate the pain on a scale of 1 to 10

• verbalize relief from pain following administration of analgesics.

Based on the nursing diagnosis *knowledge deficit,* develop appropri-

ate patient outcomes. For example, your patient will:
• seek and obtain information about chlamydial infections
• describe the treatment regimen and state his intention to adhere to his prescribed therapy
• identify measures effective in preventing chlamydial infection and state his intention to follow recommendations for prevention.

IMPLEMENTATION

Adjust your nursing interventions to suit the patient's condition. (See *Medical care in chlamydial infection.*)

Nursing interventions
• Use universal precautions when examining the patient, giving patient care, and handling contaminated material. Properly dispose of all soiled dressings and contaminated instruments according to your hospital's policy.
• Check the newborn infant of an infected mother for signs of infection. Take specimens for culture from the infant's eyes, nasopharynx, and rectum. Positive rectal cultures will peak about 5 to 6 weeks postpartum.
• Monitor the patient for complications.
• Monitor the patient's compliance with treatment and evaluate the effectiveness of treatment.

Patient teaching
• Teach the patient about chlamydial infection and its risk factors.
• Explain the dosage requirements of his prescribed medication. Stress the importance of taking all of his medication, even after symptoms subside.
• Teach the patient to follow proper hygiene measures.
• To prevent eye contamination, tell the patient to avoid touching any discharge and to wash his hands before touching his eyes.
• Explain measures that prevent chlamydial infection. (See *Preventing sexually transmitted disease,* page 232.)
• Urge the patient to inform sexual partners of his infection so that they can seek treatment also. Explain that they should receive treatment regardless of their test results.
• Suggest that the patient and his sexual partners receive testing for other STDs, including the human immunodeficiency virus.
• Tell the patient to return for followup testing. (See *Ensuring continued care for the patient with chlamydial infection.*)

EVALUATION

When evaluating the patient's response to your nursing care, gather reassessment data and compare this information with the patient outcomes specified in your plan of care.

Discharge TimeSaver
Ensuring continued care for the patient with chlamydial infection

Review the following teaching topics, referrals, and follow-up appointments to make sure that your patient is adequately prepared for discharge.

Patient teaching
Make sure that the following topics have been covered and that your patient's learning has been evaluated:
☐ nature of the disorder and its complications
☐ risk factors
☐ treatment
☐ prevention of reinfection.

Referrals
Make sure that the patient has been provided with necessary referrals to:
☐ state or local health agencies, as required.

Follow-up appointments
Make sure that the necessary follow-up appointments have been scheduled and that the patient has been notified:
☐ doctor or clinic
☐ diagnostic tests for reevaluation.

Teaching and counseling
Begin by determining the effectiveness of your teaching and counseling. Consider the following questions:
• Has the patient verbalized his intention to restrict sexual activity during treatment?
• Has he said that he plans to resume normal protected sexual activity when chlamydial infection subsides?
• Can he explain the disorder and the means by which the disease is spread and prevented?
• Can he explain his treatment regimen and has he said that he intends to complete the prescribed therapy?

Physical condition
If treatment has been successful, you should note the following outcomes:
• The patient has avoided complications associated with urethritis and has reestablished a normal elimination pattern.
• He reports relief from pain.

Pelvic inflammatory disease

An umbrella term, pelvic inflammatory disease (PID) refers to an infection of one or more of the female pelvic structures. (See *What happens in PID,* page 246.)

More than half of PID cases result from overgrowth of one or more of the common bacteria found in cervical mucus. PID is a major problem among women and is the most common serious complication of the current epidemic of sexually transmitted diseases (STDs).

Possible acute complications of PID include potentially fatal septicemia from a ruptured pelvic abscess, pulmonary emboli, and shock. Long-term sequelae are common, affecting one in four women and including ectopic pregnancy, infertility, chronic

What happens in PID

In pelvic inflammatory disease (PID), infection spreads from the lower genital tract to upper reproductive structures by direct mucosal contact or by way of the fimbriated end of the fallopian tubes to the ovaries, parametrium, and peritoneal cavity. Resulting tissue damage, adhesions, and strictures may lead to infertility. This illustration shows specific infections that may result from three causative organisms.

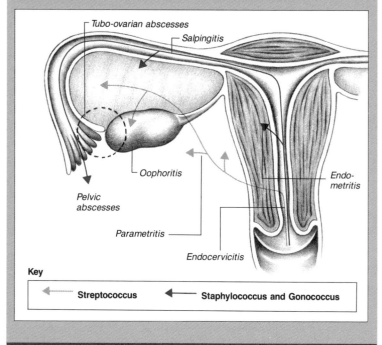

Key

← - - - **Streptococcus**   ◀━━ **Staphylococcus and Gonococcus**

pelvic pain, pelvic adhesions, tubo-ovarian abscess, and pyosalpinx.

Causes

PID can result from infection with aerobic or anaerobic organisms. The organisms *Neisseria gonorrhoeae* and *Chlamydia trachomatis* are the most common causes because they most readily penetrate the bacteriostatic barrier of cervical mucus.

Common bacteria found in cervical mucus include staphylococci, streptococci, diphtheroids, chlamydiae, and coliforms, including *Pseudomonas* and *Escherichia coli.*

Uterine infection can result from any one or several of these organisms or may follow the multiplication of normally nonpathogenic bacteria in an altered endometrial environment. Bacterial multiplication is most common during parturition because the endometrium is atrophic, quiescent, and not stimulated by estrogen.

ASSESSMENT

Your assessment should include a careful consideration of the patient's health history, physical examination findings, and diagnostic test results. Keep in mind that untreated PID may be fatal. Early diagnosis and treatment help prevent damage to the reproductive system.

Health history
The patient with PID may complain of profuse, purulent vaginal discharge, sometimes accompanied by low-grade fever and malaise (particularly if gonorrhea is the cause). She may also report lower abdominal pain and vaginal bleeding. Be sure to ask about the presence of any risk factors. (See *Risk factors for PID*.)

Physical examination
Examination may reveal lower abdominal pain with rigidity or rebound pain. Vaginal examination may reveal pain when the cervix is moved or the adnexa is palpated. (See *Clinical signs of PID,* page 248.)

Diagnostic test results
• Gram stain of secretions from the endocervix or Douglas' cul-de-sac determines the causative agent.
• Culture and sensitivity testing aids selection of the appropriate antibiotic. Urethral and rectal secretions may also be cultured.
• Ultrasonography, computed tomography scan, and magnetic resonance imaging may help to identify and locate an adnexal or uterine mass.

FactFinder

Risk factors for PID

The risk factors for pelvic inflammatory disease (PID) include:
• any sexually transmitted disease
• multiple sexual partners
• conditions or procedures that alter or destroy cervical mucus (such as conization or cauterization of the cervix), allowing bacteria to ascend into the uterine cavity
• any procedure that risks transfer of contaminated cervical mucus into the endometrial cavity by an instrument (such as a biopsy curette or an irrigation catheter) or by tubal insufflation or abortion
• use of an intrauterine device
• infection during or after pregnancy
• infectious foci within the body, such as drainage from a chronically infected fallopian tube, a pelvic abscess, a ruptured appendix, or diverticulitis of the sigmoid colon
• history of PID.

• Culdocentesis obtains peritoneal fluid or pus for culture and sensitivity testing.

NURSING DIAGNOSIS

Common nursing diagnoses for a patient with PID include:
• High risk for injury related to inflammation of and damage to reproductive structures
• Altered sexuality patterns related to pain and discharge secondary to infection of the reproductive system
• Pain related to inflammation secondary to infection

Assessment TimeSaver

Clinical signs of PID

The following list describes clinical features and diagnostic findings for three pelvic inflammatory diseases (PIDs).

Salpingo-oophoritis
• *Acute:* Signs include the sudden onset of lower abdominal and pelvic pain, usually following menses; increased vaginal discharge; fever; malaise; lower abdominal pressure and tenderness; tachycardia; and pelvic peritonitis.
• *Chronic:* Blood studies show leukocytosis or a normal white blood cell (WBC) count. X-rays may show ileus. Pelvic examination reveals extreme tenderness.

Smear of cervical or periurethral gland exudate shows gram-negative intracellular diplococci.

Cervicitis
• *Acute:* Signs include purulent, foul-smelling vaginal discharge; vulvovaginitis with itching or burning; red, edematous cervix; pelvic discomfort; sexual dysfunction; metrorrhagia; infertility; and spontaneous abortion. Cervical palpation reveals tenderness.
• *Chronic:* Signs include cervical dystocia; laceration or eversion of the cervix; and ulcerative vesicular lesions (when cervicitis results from herpes simplex virus 2). Causative or-

ganism is are usually staphylococcus or streptococcus.

Cultures for *Neisseria gonorrhoeae* are positive in more than 90% of patients. Cytologic smears may reveal severe inflammation. If cervicitis isn't complicated by salpingitis, WBC count is normal or slightly elevated and erythrocyte sedimentation rate (ESR) is elevated.

Endometritis
• *Acute:* Signs include mucopurulent or purulent vaginal discharge oozing from the cervix; edematous, hyperemic endometrium, possibly leading to ulceration and necrosis (with virulent organisms); lower abdominal pain and tenderness; fever; rebound pain; abdominal muscle spasm; and thrombophlebitis of uterine and pelvic vessels (in severe forms).
• *Chronic:* In severe infection, palpation may reveal a boggy uterus. Uterine and blood samples are positive for causative organism, usually staphylococcus. WBC count and ESR are elevated. Chronic endometritis is increasingly common due to widespread use of intrauterine devices.

• High risk for impaired skin integrity related to irritating vaginal discharge.

PLANNING

Based on the nursing diagnosis *high risk for injury,* develop appropriate patient outcomes. For example, your patient will:

Medical care of the patient with PID

To prevent progression of pelvic inflammatory disease (PID), antibiotic therapy should begin immediately after culture specimens are obtained. Such therapy can be reevaluated as soon as laboratory results are available (usually after 24 to 48 hours). Infection may become chronic if treated inadequately.

Inpatient therapy
The preferred inpatient antibiotic therapy for PID includes I.V. doxycycline and cefoxitin for 4 to 6 days (alternative therapy includes clindamycin and gentamicin), followed by oral doxycycline for another 10 to 14 days.

Outpatient therapy
Outpatient therapy may consist of I.M. ceftriaxone in one dose, plus oral doxycycline for 10 to 14 days.

Supplemental treatment
Supplemental treatment of PID may include bed rest, analgesics, and I.V. fluids as needed. Nonsteroidal anti-inflammatory agents or narcotics may be prescribed for pain.

Pelvic abscess
Development of a pelvic abscess requires adequate drainage because a ruptured pelvic abscess can be life-threatening. If this complication develops, the patient may need a total abdominal hysterectomy, with bilateral salpingo-oophorectomy.

• comply with the prescribed therapy to minimize the risk of permanent damage to reproductive structures
• demonstrate normal reproductive function following PID.

Based on the nursing diagnosis *altered sexuality patterns,* develop appropriate patient outcomes. For example, your patient will:
• abstain from sexual activity until the infection is eradicated
• identify and avoid sexual activities that increase the chance of reinfection
• resume normal protected sexual activity when the infection subsides.

Based on the nursing diagnosis *pain,* develop appropriate patient outcomes. For example, your patient will:

• express feelings of comfort following analgesic and antibiotic therapy
• use activities and other diversions to minimize her perception of pain.

Based on the nursing diagnosis *high risk for impaired skin integrity,* develop appropriate patient outcomes. For example, your patient will:
• demonstrate recommended skin care measures
• avoid skin breakdown throughout the infection.

IMPLEMENTATION

Adjust your nursing interventions to suit the patient's condition. (See *Medical care of the patient with PID.*)

Discharge TimeSaver

Ensuring continued care for the patient with PID

Review the following teaching topics, referrals, and follow-up appointments to make sure that your patient is adequately prepared for discharge.

Teaching topics
Make sure that the following topics have been covered and that your patient's learning has been evaluated:
□ nature of the disorder and its complications
□ risk factors for PID
□ treatment
□ prevention of reinfection
□ surgery, if warranted
□ signs of recurrence.

Referrals
Make sure that the patient has been provided with necessary referrals to:
□ public health authorities, if needed
□ infertility specialist or support group, if warranted.

Follow-up appointments
Make sure that the necessary follow-up appointments have been scheduled and that the patient has been notified:
□ doctor
□ diagnostic tests for reevaluation.

Nursing interventions

• After establishing that the patient has no drug allergies, administer antibiotics and analgesics, as prescribed. Apply heat to the lower abdomen or back, if prescribed, to help relieve pain.

• Keep the patient's bed in semi-Fowler's position to promote drainage.

• Follow universal precautions. Provide frequent perineal care if the patient has vaginal drainage. Keep the patient's skin dry.

• Monitor vital signs for fever. Watch fluid intake and output for signs of dehydration. Check for abdominal rigidity and distention, which may be signs of developing peritonitis.

• Track the patient's level of pain and the effectiveness of analgesics.

• Assess the patient for adverse reactions to administered medications and other complications of PID.

Patient teaching
• Encourage the patient to discuss her feelings. Offer her emotional support and help her develop effective coping strategies.

• Explain the nature of the disorder and its possible complications.

• If the patient is being treated on an outpatient basis, advise her to return for evaluation 48 to 72 hours after she initiates antibiotic therapy. (See *Ensuring continued care for the patient with PID.*)

• Inform the patient about prescribed drug therapy. Stress the importance of compliance with treatment.

• Stress the need for the patient's sexual partner to be examined and, if necessary, treated for infection.

• Discuss the use of condoms to prevent the spread of STDs.

• Because PID may cause dyspareunia, advise the patient to consult with her doctor about sexual activity.

• If surgery is warranted to remove an abscess or a pelvic mass, explain preoperative and postoperative care measures.

• Inform the patient about signs and symptoms of recurrence and the need to report them at once.

EVALUATION

When evaluating the patient's response to your nursing care, gather reassessment data and compare this information with the patient outcomes specified in your plan of care.

Teaching and counseling

Begin by determining the effectiveness of your teaching. Consider the following questions:

• Has the patient demonstrated compliance with the treatment regimen?

• Can she identify risk factors for PID and state plans to reduce or avoid them?

• Does she know that she can resume sexual activity without discomfort when the infection is eradicated?

Physical condition

If treatment has been successful, you should note the following outcomes:

• The patient reports that her pain has diminished or disappeared.

• She has maintained or regained skin integrity.

Lyme disease

Named for the small Connecticut town in which it was first recognized in 1975, Lyme disease affects multiple body systems. The illness is transmitted by a tick and typically begins in summer or early fall with a classic skin lesion called erythema chronicum migrans. Weeks or months later, cardiac, neurologic, or joint abnormalities develop, possibly followed by arthritis. The highest incidence occurs in eastern and northeastern states.

Known complications of Lyme disease include myocarditis, pericarditis, arrhythmias, heart block, meningitis, encephalitis, cranial or peripheral neuropathies, and arthritis.

Causes

Lyme disease is caused by the spirochete *Borrelia burgdorferi,* which travels on ticks. It occurs only in areas inhabited by the whitetail deer, which is the preferred host of the mature tick that carries the spirochete. The spirochete's life cycle is incompletely understood; it may survive for years in the joints or die after triggering an inflammatory response in the recipient.

ASSESSMENT

Your assessment should include a careful consideration of the patient's health history, physical examination findings, and diagnostic test results. Patient complaints vary in frequency and severity, probably because the illness typically occurs in stages. Always be aware that your assessment findings can be misleading. In many stages of Lyme disease, symptoms closely resemble the symptoms of other musculoskeletal disorders, such as rheumatoid arthritis.

Health history

The patient's history may reveal recent exposure to ticks. However, he may not recall a tick bite, especially if he lives, works, or plays in wooded areas where Lyme disease is endemic.

The patient may report the onset of symptoms in warmer months. Commonly reported symptoms include fatigue, malaise, and migratory myalgia and arthralgia. Nearly 10% of patients report cardiac symptoms, such as palpitations and mild dyspnea, especially in the early stage. Severe headache and stiff neck, suggestive of meningeal irritation, also may occur in the early stage when the rash erupts. At a later stage, the patient may report neurologic symptoms, such as memory loss.

Physical examination

Typically, you may see erythema chronicum migrans, which begins as a red macule or papule at the tick bite site and may grow as large as 2″ (5 cm) in diameter. The patient may describe the lesion as hot and itchy. When characteristic lesions are present, they have bright red outer rims and white centers. They usually appear on the axillae, thighs, and groin. Within a few days, other lesions may erupt, along with a migratory, ring-like rash and conjunctivitis. In 3 to 4 weeks, the lesions fade to small red blotches, which persist for several more weeks.

After several weeks or even months, many patients may develop neurologic manifestations, such as Bell's palsy, meningitis, neuritis, chorea, or myelitis (which can occur alone). In the later stage, inspection may disclose signs and symptoms of intermittent arthritis: joint swelling, redness, and limited movement. Typically, the disease affects one or only a few joints, especially large ones such as the knee.

Palpation of the pulse may detect bradycardia, tachycardia, or an irregular heartbeat, which can indicate some degree of heart block. During the first or second stage, you may detect regional lymphadenopathy as well. The patient may complain of tenderness at the skin lesion site or the posterior cervical area. Less commonly, you may note generalized lymphadenopathy.

If the patient has neurologic involvement, Kernig's and Brudzinski's signs usually aren't positive and neck stiffness typically occurs only with extreme flexion.

Diagnostic test results

• Blood tests, including antibody titers to identify *B. burgdorferi,* are the most practical diagnostic tests. Or the doctor may order an enzyme-linked immunosorbent assay because of the test's greater sensitivity and specificity. However, serologic test results don't always confirm the diagnosis, especially in the disease's early stages before the body produces antibodies. And they may not show seropositivity for *B. burgdorferi.* Also, the validity of test results depends on laboratory techniques and interpretation.
• Mild anemia coupled with elevated erythrocyte sedimentation rate, white blood cell count, serum immunoglobulin-M levels, and aspartate aminotransferase (formerly SGOT) levels support the diagnosis.
• A lumbar puncture may be ordered if the disease involves the central nervous system. Analysis of cerebrospinal fluid may detect antibodies to *B. burgdorferi.*

NURSING DIAGNOSIS

Common nursing diagnoses for the patient with Lyme disease include:
• Fatigue related to infection
• Pain (headache, myalgia, arthralgia) related to effects of the disorder

• Altered thought processes related to meningeal irritation secondary to infection
• Hyperthermia related to infection.

PLANNING

Based on the nursing diagnosis *fatigue,* develop appropriate patient outcomes. For example, your patient will:
• state measures to prevent or minimize fatigue
• incorporate into his daily routine measures necessary to modify fatigue
• regain his normal energy level.
  Based on the nursing diagnosis *pain,* develop appropriate patient outcomes. For example, your patient will:
• notify a caregiver immediately when pain occurs
• rate the pain on a scale of 1 to 10
• report improved comfort after administration of analgesics or other treatments.
  Based on the nursing diagnosis *altered thought processes,* develop appropriate patient outcomes. For example, your patient will:
• remain safe in his environment
• regain normal thought processes.
  Based on the nursing diagnosis *hyperthermia,* develop appropriate patient outcomes. For example, your patient will:
• regain and maintain a normal temperature
• not develop complications associated with hyperthermia, such as seizures and dehydration.

IMPLEMENTATION

Adjust your nursing interventions to suit the patient's condition. (See *Medical care in Lyme disease.*)

Treatments

Medical care in Lyme disease

A three-week course of antibiotics is the treatment of choice for Lyme disease. Adults typically receive tetracycline or doxycycline; alternatives include penicillin and erythromycin. Children usually receive oral penicillin. Administered early in the disease, these medications can minimize later complications. In later stages, high-dose penicillin (administered I.V.) or ceftriaxone (administered I.V. or I.M.) may produce good results.

Nursing interventions

• Plan your care to encourage adequate rest. Instruct the patient to take frequent rest periods throughout the day and help him plan periods of rest.
• Ask the patient about possible drug allergies before administering antibiotics.
• Administer analgesics and antipyretics, if necessary. Monitor temperature and response to analgesics.
• Monitor the effectiveness of all medications administered and observe for any adverse effects.
• If the patient has arthritis, help him with range-of-motion and strengthening exercises, but avoid overexerting him.
• Protect the patient from sensory overload, and reorient him if needed. Also encourage him to express his feelings and concerns about memory loss, if appropriate. Encourage any questions and answer them clearly to his satisfaction.

Teaching TimeSaver
Preventing Lyme disease

The only way to prevent Lyme disease is to completely avoid wooded areas where the spirochete-carrying ticks live. However, the risk of infection is greatly reduced by following some precautions when in wooded areas.

• Advise the patient to wear light-colored long pants tucked into his socks and long-sleeved shirts to help prevent bites. Light-colored clothes may make it easier to see a tick, so it can be brushed off.

• Tell him to apply an insect repellent containing diethyltoluamide to his clothes and to any exposed skin before going into the woods.

• Caution him to wash his clothing immediately after returning from a possibly infested area. Also tell him to inspect his body, especially arms, legs, and hairline, for signs of attached ticks. They are black and about the size of a pinhead or slightly larger after engorgement.

• If your patient finds any ticks, he should remove them with tweezers, being careful to remove the entire tick, including the head, and then flush them down the toilet.

• If he begins to notice flulike symptoms after being in an infested area, he should notify his doctor.

block, he may need a temporary pacemaker; you'll need to prepare him for this procedure.

• Watch for signs and symptoms of other complications, such as cardiovascular or neurologic dysfunction and arthritis.

• All states require that health officials be notified of cases of Lyme disease. Check to make sure this report has been filed by the appropriate person at your hospital, often the infection-control nurse or the patient's doctor.

Patient teaching

• Teach the patient about the disease and the course of illness. You should also instruct him on precautions to take to prevent future incidents. (See *Preventing Lyme disease.*)

• Teach the patient about his medications, including adverse effects. Tell him that it's important to take antibiotic medications exactly as prescribed for optimal absorption and to keep blood levels at a therapeutic level.

• Urge the patient to return for follow-up care and to report recurrent or new symptoms to the doctor.

• Provide rest and activity guidelines and teach energy conservation techniques.

• Inform the patient of the signs and symptoms to watch for as the disease progresses through its stages. (See *Ensuring continued care for the patient with Lyme disease.*)

EVALUATION

When evaluating the patient's response to your nursing care, gather reassessment data and compare this information with the patient outcomes specified in your plan of care. Consider the following questions:

• Protect the patient from injury if the disease has caused changes in his mental status.

• Monitor the patient's vital signs, especially heart rate and rhythm. If the patient develops complete heart

Discharge TimeSaver
Ensuring continued care for the patient with Lyme disease

Review the following teaching topics, referrals, and follow-up appointments to make sure that your patient is adequately prepared for discharge.

Teaching topics
Make sure that the following topics have been covered and that your patient's learning has been evaluated:
☐ nature of the disorder, including its cause
☐ prescribed medications
☐ warning signs and symptoms
☐ prevention guidelines.

Referrals
Make sure that the patient has been provided with necessary referrals to:
☐ rheumatologist, if needed, for arthritis
☐ neurologist, if neurologic manifestations are apparent.

Follow-up appointments
Make sure that the necessary follow-up appointments have been scheduled and that the patient has been notified:
☐ doctor.

• Has the patient gradually increased his energy level?
• Does he show signs of increased daily activities without undue fatigue?
• Does he report pain relief?
• Is he able to maintain normal mental and emotional functioning without lapses, confusion, or disorientation?
• Has he maintained a normal temperature?

Tuberculosis

Most individuals who are infected with the microorganism that causes tuberculosis (TB) do not develop the disease itself. When disease occurs, however, it takes a chronic form because of a delayed (type IV) hypersensitivity reaction.

TB that affects the lungs (pulmonary TB) is characterized by pulmonary infiltrations, formation of granulomas (tubercles) with caseation, fibrosis, and calcification. Necrosis and cavitation may be widespread in advanced TB. Although the primary focus of infection is the lungs, the bacteria responsible for TB may spread to other parts of the body. Possible sites of extrapulmonary TB include the pleurae, meninges, joints, peritoneum, genitourinary tract, bowel, and lymph nodes.

Pulmonary TB may cause many complications, including massive damage to pulmonary tissue with inflammation and necrosis eventually leading to respiratory failure. Bronchopleural fistulas may develop and result in pneumothorax. TB may also result in hemorrhage, pleural effusion, and pneumonia.

Causes

TB is caused by *Mycobacterium tuberculosis*. The bacilli are transmitted from one host to another in droplet nuclei, which are ejected when an infected individual coughs, sneezes, laughs, speaks, or sings. Inhaled bacilli lodge in the pulmonary alveoli of the noninfected individual. Cell-mediated immunity to the mycobacteria develops in 3 to 6 weeks and usually contains the infection, arresting the disease.

In most instances, the host's immune system kills the bacilli or contains them in nodules that are called *tubercles* — hallmarks of TB. Although approximately 5% of infected individuals develop active disease within 1 year, latent infection is more common. The bacilli may lie dormant within the tubercle for years and then reactivate and spread, causing active infection (commonly called reactivation TB).

Tubercle bacilli in the infected patient can exist in three different bacterial settings. (See *Three types of tubercle bacilli.*) After reactivation, characteristic caseation of necrotic tissue results in debris that may spread throughout the lungs.

ASSESSMENT

Your assessment should include a careful consideration of the patient's health history, physical examination findings, and diagnostic test results.

Health history

TB has an insidious onset. The patient with an active infection may complain of progressive weakness and fatigue, anorexia, weight loss, low-grade fever, and night sweats, occurring over a period ranging from weeks to months. The patient may also report a cough, possibly producing sputum streaked with blood. Pain or tightness in the chest may accompany the cough. A patient with laryngeal TB will report hoarseness.

During the health history, determine the patient's risk for TB and investigate possible exposure to TB (especially drug-resistant strains) and human immunodeficiency virus (HIV). (See *Identifying high-risk patients,* page 258.)

Physical examination

During the initial physical examination, look for signs of active TB. Physical findings may vary greatly depending on the severity of pulmonary involvement. Percussion may reveal dullness over the affected area of the lung, signifying consolidation or the presence of pleural fluid. Auscultation may reveal crepitant crackles, bronchial breath sounds, wheezes, and whispered pectoriloquy.

Diagnostic test results

• Tuberculin skin testing, the primary screening tool, may reveal that the patient has been infected with TB at some point; however, it doesn't indicate active disease. (Multipuncture, or tine, tests are usually used only when the probability of infection is low.)

Intradermal tuberculin skin testing using the Mantoux method (Aplisol, Tubersol) is preferred. This test involves an intradermal injection (forearm) of 0.1 ml of intermediate-strength purified protein derivative (PPD) containing 5 tuberculin units. Results are interpreted 48 to 72 hours later by an experienced professional. (See *Interpreting results of the Mantoux test,* page 259.)

Patients with immune system impairment may require anergy testing to verify results of the Mantoux test.

Three types of tubercle bacilli

Tubercle bacilli in the patient with tuberculosis can exist in three different bacterial settings: in extracellular cavities, in closed caseous lesions, and within intracellular macrophages.

Mycobacteria rapidly proliferate in open cavities because of the high oxygen tension. In closed caseous lesions and in macrophages, bacterial growth is slower because oxygen tension is reduced.

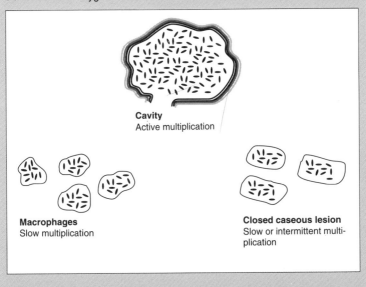

Cavity
Active multiplication

Macrophages
Slow multiplication

Closed caseous lesion
Slow or intermittent multiplication

Companion skin tests (controls) are administered at least once, usually for candidiasis, mumps, or tetanus, to which most people have been exposed. Positive reactions to one or more of these tests indicate that the patient can mount a cell-mediated immune response. Thus, a negative reaction to PPD would most likely be a true negative reaction.

• Chest X-rays may prove inconclusive in distinguishing between active and inactive TB, and they do not confirm the diagnosis. A negative chest X-ray will usually rule out pulmonary TB, but not active disease in other organs. Lesions, with or without cavitation, may appear anywhere in the lungs and may vary in size, shape, and density, especially in HIV-positive and other immunocompromised patients. Classic findings show upper lobe infiltrates; cavitation may be present in advanced disease. Also, scar tissue and calcium deposits may be present in infected individuals without evidence of active disease.

Assessment TimeSaver

Identifying high-risk patients

The incidence of tuberculosis (TB) in North America has increased dramatically since the mid-1980s and once again poses a significant health threat. The spread of acquired immunodeficiency syndrome, a growing homeless population, poverty, drug abuse, prison overcrowding, immigration from countries with high TB rates, cuts in public health funding, and increasingly drug-resistant strains of TB contribute to the problem.

Epidemiology
The greatest incidence of TB occurs in individuals between the ages of 25 and 44. This age-group also has the highest incidence of human immunodeficiency virus (HIV) infection. Incidence of TB is also high in children under age 15 and Black and Hispanic peoples. TB is twice as common in men as in women and four times more likely to affect nonwhites than whites.

High-risk groups
Arrange TB testing and place the patient on acid-fast bacilli isolation if your assessment leads you to suspect TB and your patient falls into one or more of the following high-risk groups:
• HIV-infected individuals (and those at risk for HIV infection)
• individuals in close contact with those who have active infectious TB
• individuals with conditions that increase the risk of active TB after infection, such as silicosis, diabetes mellitus, chronic renal failure, gastrectomy cancers (especially bronchogenic carcinoma, Hodgkin's disease, and leukemia), weight that's 10% below ideal, prolonged corticosteroid or other immunosuppressive therapy, some hematologic disorders (such as leukemia and lymphomas), and other cancers
• substance abusers, such as alcoholics, I.V. drug users, and cocaine or crack cocaine users
• residents of long-term care facilities, nursing homes, prisons, mental institutions, homeless shelters, or other congregate housing settings
• medically underserved, low-income populations, such as racial and ethnic minorities, homeless people, and migrant workers
• health care workers and others who provide services to any high-risk group.

High-risk groups for drug-resistant TB
The following groups are at high risk for drug-resistant strains of TB:
• individuals with a history of preventive treatment or treatment for active TB
• individuals born in countries in Africa, Asia, Central America, or South America
• residents of areas in North America with high rates of drug-resistant TB
• patients with *Mycobacterium tuberculosis* in their sputum specimens after 3 months of drug therapy.

Interpretation

Interpreting results of the Mantoux test

When interpreting the results of the Mantoux test, consider the patient's risk for tuberculosis (TB).

An induration of **5 mm or more** may be considered a positive test if the patient:
• has had recent, close contact with a person with active infectious TB
• has a chest X-ray showing pulmonary fibrotic lesions that might be old, healed TB lesions
• is infected with human immunodeficiency virus (HIV) or has a high risk of HIV infection.

An induration of **10 mm or more** may be considered a positive test if the patient fails to meet the above criteria but meets one or more of the following risk factors for TB:
• a medical condition that increases the risk of active disease after infection has occurred

• birthplace in Asia, Africa, Central America, or South America
• Black, Native American, or Hispanic *and* a member of a low socioeconomic, medically underserved group
• I.V. drug user
• resident or staff member of a congregate living arrangement (such as a long-term care facility, prison, or nursing home)
• health care worker exposed to TB
• very young or very old.

An induration of **15 mm or more** may be considered a positive test in all other patients with no risk factors.

Note: A positive skin test indicates that the patient has been infected with *Mycobacterium tuberculosis*. It does not necessarily indicate active disease.

Induration indicating absence of infection in nonimmunosuppressed patient

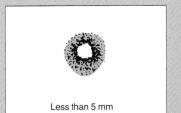

Less than 5 mm

Induration suggesting infection

Greater than 10 mm

• Sputum smear for acid-fast bacilli (AFB), if positive, provides a presumptive diagnosis of TB. Sputum culture is used to confirm the diagnosis of TB because the AFB detected in the smear may be a nontuberculous mycobacteria. However, culture testing, which can identify *M. tuberculosis* colonies, takes much longer (2 to 12 weeks). If you suspect TB, expect to obtain at least three sputum specimens on consecutive days for smear and culture.

• Due to the increased incidence of drug-resistant strains of *M. tuberculosis,* drug-sensitivity testing on initial sputum specimens is essential. Other specimens may be cultured when nonpulmonary TB is suspected.

• Computed tomography or magnetic resonance imaging scans may be used to evaluate lung damage or confirm a difficult diagnosis.

• Bronchoscopy may be performed if the patient has trouble producing an adequate sputum specimen spontaneously or by induced sputum collection.

Several of these diagnostic tests may be necessary to distinguish TB from diseases that may mimic it, such as lung cancer, lung abscess, pneumoconiosis, and bronchiectasis.

NURSING DIAGNOSIS

Common nursing diagnoses for the patient with TB include:

• Ineffective management of therapeutic regimen related to a lack of understanding of the importance of drug therapy or follow-up care

• Altered nutrition: Less than body requirements, related to anorexia, infection, or adverse effects of drug therapy

• Ineffective airway clearance related to copious, viscous sputum production

• Fatigue related to infection and associated weight loss

• Social isolation related to stigma associated with the disease and need for isolation precautions.

PLANNING

Based on the nursing diagnosis *ineffective management of therapeutic regimen,* develop appropriate patient

outcomes. For example, your patient will:

• complete an entire course of drug therapy

• report for scheduled follow-up appointments and obtain sputum specimens regularly

• cover mouth and nose when laughing, coughing, or sneezing.

Based on the nursing diagnosis *altered nutrition: less than body requirements,* develop appropriate patient outcomes. For example, your patient will:

• consume at least 2,000 calories per day, including foods rich in iron, protein, and vitamin C

• stabilize his weight within 2 weeks after the start of therapy

• maintain a normal weight, based on age and sex, within 6 months.

Based on the nursing diagnosis *ineffective airway clearance,* develop appropriate patient outcomes. For example, your patient will:

• exhibit clear breath sounds

• cough and expectorate thin mucus

• have arterial blood gas (ABG) levels within the normal range.

Based on the nursing diagnosis *fatigue,* develop appropriate patient outcomes. For example, your patient will:

• incorporate rest periods into his daily routine

• practice energy conservation techniques when performing activities

• report experiencing less fatigue

• resume usual activities gradually

• return to his normal level of activity before treatment ends, except in very advanced disease.

Based on the nursing diagnosis social isolation, develop appropriate patient outcomes. For example, your patient will:

• verbalize feelings associated with isolation

Treatments

Medical care of the patient with TB

Antitubercular therapy involving daily oral doses of isoniazid or rifampin (occasionally with pyrazinamide or ethambutol) for 6 to 9 months usually cures tuberculosis (TB). In most cases, the patient is no longer infectious after 2 to 4 weeks of therapy and can resume normal activities while continuing to take medication.

Multiple-drug regimens
Newer regimens typically include multiple drugs to which the organisms are susceptible. Multiple-drug regimens are designed to destroy the organism quickly while preventing the emergence of drug-resistant organisms.

Initial regimens currently employ four drugs — typically, isoniazid, rifampin, pyrazinamide, and ethambutol or streptomycin. After 2 months, when susceptibilities are known, the pyrazinamide and ethambutol or streptomycin are discontinued. This regimen is one of a number of possi-ble drug combinations and schedules. The regimen selected may depend on the patient's human immunodeficiency virus status and the likelihood that he's been exposed to drug-resistant *Mycobacterium tuberculosis*.

Treating drug-resistant strains
Patients with drug-resistant TB may require second-line drugs, such as cycloserine, ethionamide, or para-aminosalicylic acid (PAS). Other alternative drugs include kanamycin, amikacin, capreomycin, ciprofloxacin, ofloxacin, and clofazimine.

Surgical intervention
Although not common, surgery may be performed to remove as much of the disease as possible. It's considered if the patient has localized disease and the infecting organism is resistant to several drugs. In most instances, surgery is combined with aggressive antibiotic therapy.

• communicate with caregivers, family, and friends
• participate in at least one activity he prefers each day
• report decreased feelings of isolation.

IMPLEMENTATION
Treatment for TB seeks to reduce the patient's discomfort, destroy the infectious organism as quickly as possible, and avoid promoting drug-resis-tant organisms. (See *Medical care of the patient with TB.*)

Nursing interventions
Patients with TB require immediate care to combat the disease and ongoing care to prevent the emergence of drug-resistant organisms.

Initial care
Your first priority is to institute precautions to prevent the transmission of TB. Precautions will vary depending on the clinical setting.

• To protect yourself, other health care workers, and other patients, obtain sputum specimens in a small room or booth containing an exhaust fan, high-efficiency particulate air filters, or ultraviolet air disinfection (ideally, all three). If this is impossible, wear a particulate respirator and collect the specimen in a private room.

• Patients with suspected TB and suspicious signs and symptoms lasting 3 weeks or more should be placed on AFB isolation precautions — don't wait for confirmation of the diagnosis. AFB isolation precautions include the use of an isolation room with negative air pressure and exhaust ventilation to the outside. Upper room irradiation is preferred if other environmental controls are not available.

• Make sure that all visitors and hospital staff members wear a particulate respirator or a tightly fitting submicron filtering mask while in the patient's room. Standard masks are not considered effective because the AFB particles can pass through the mask material. The patient should wear a mask if he is transported outside his room.

• Place a covered trash can near the patient's bed, or tape a lined bag to the bedside for the patient's used tissues.

• Keep all doors to the room closed while the patient is on AFB precautions.

• Keep the infection-control nurse informed of all developments, including the patient's degree of compliance with therapy.

Additional interventions
After precautionary measures have been taken, you may continue with other interventions.

• Provide the patient with appropriate diversions and activities. Check on him frequently and make sure that the call button is conveniently located.

• Listen to the patient's concerns and fears and provide emotional support. Encourage communication with friends and relatives, especially while AFB isolation precautions are in effect.

• Administer prescribed medications. Observe the patient for adverse reactions and take steps to prevent them. For example, isoniazid and ethambutol, which may cause nausea, could be given with food.

Ongoing care
• Make sure that the patient gets plenty of rest. Schedule alternating periods of rest and light activity to promote health, conserve energy, and reduce oxygen demand. Explain that fatigue will fade as treatment progresses.

• Provide the patient with a nutritious, high-calorie diet. Encourage small, frequent meals to help him conserve energy. If the patient asks for supplements, consult with the dietitian.

• Provide supportive care and help the patient adjust to any necessary lifestyle changes.

• Include the patient in decisions about his care. Encourage family members to participate in his care whenever possible.

• Monitor the patient's respiratory status. Auscultate breath sounds frequently.

• Monitor the patient's weight at least weekly. Report any weight loss of 2 lb (0.9 kg) or more.

• Begin discharge planning early. Consult with the social services department about evaluating the patient's living conditions. Arrange for

follow-up home care visits, if appropriate.
• It's essential to monitor the patient's compliance with therapy after discharge. If noncompliance is a continuing problem, the patient may be required to take medication under the direct supervision of a health care professional.
• Refer the patient to sources of information and support in the community, for example, the American Lung Association or a local health department.
• If the patient reports having a problem with alcohol or drugs, refer him for appropriate counseling and treatment, and recommend that he attend a self-help group, such as Alcoholics Anonymous.
• If the patient is at high risk for HIV infection, refer him to appropriate counseling and testing.

Patient teaching
• Explain the nature of the disease, how it spreads, and how it's prevented.
• Teach the patient to cover his mouth and nose when laughing, coughing, or sneezing, even when he's alone in a room.
• Teach him how to obtain a good sputum specimen. Explain that the sputum must come from his lungs. Tell him to inhale and exhale deeply three times; then inhale swiftly and cough forcefully; and, finally, expectorate into the sputum container. If these efforts fail, he may need the help of a hypertonic saline aerosol mist. Instruct him to take several normal breaths of the aerosol mist and then inhale deeply, cough, and expectorate into the sputum container.
• If ordered, explain the use of bronchoscopy to obtain bronchial washings, brushings, and biopsy specimens.

• Show the patient and his family how to perform postural drainage and percussion to loosen secretions.
• Teach the patient the importance of strict compliance to the medication regimen for the entire prescribed period. Describe possible adverse effects. Tell the patient to report any adverse reactions immediately.
• Teach the patient and his family the signs and symptoms of recurring TB.
• Advise the family that anyone exposed to the patient should receive a tuberculin test and, if necessary, a chest X-ray and prophylactic drug therapy (typically, isoniazid for 6 months unless the organism is isoniazid-resistant or the patient is HIV positive).
• If your patient is taking rifampin, explain that the drug will temporarily make bodily secretions appear orange. Reassure him that this is harmless. If your patient is female and taking oral contraceptives, warn her that rifampin may make the contraceptive less effective. If your patient is also receiving methadone, the dose may need to be adjusted while he's taking rifampin.
• Explain the importance of rest and teach the patient energy conservation techniques. Advise a gradual return to normal activities as he starts to feel better.
• Discuss the signs and symptoms that require medical assessment, including increased bouts of coughing, hemoptysis, unexplained weight loss, fever, and night sweats.
• Stress the importance of adopting a balanced diet that is high in calories and protein.
• Explain respiratory and universal precautions. Tell the patient to take precautions against spreading the disease until the doctor tells him that he's no longer contagious (usually after three consecutive sputum smears

Discharge TimeSaver

Ensuring continued care for the patient with TB

Review the following teaching topics, referrals, and follow-up appointments to make sure that your patient is adequately prepared for discharge.

Teaching topics
Make sure that the following topics have been covered and that your patient's learning has been evaluated:
☐ nature of TB, including symptoms, complications, management, and prevention
☐ guidelines for activity and rest
☐ drug therapy, including adverse effects, precautions, and the importance of compliance
☐ importance of a high-calorie, balanced diet
☐ warning signs and symptoms
☐ infection-control measures
☐ postural drainage and percussion
☐ importance of follow-up care and testing
☐ need for close contacts to be tested
☐ sources of information and support.

Referrals
Make sure that the patient has been provided with necessary referrals to:
☐ social service agencies
☐ public health nurse
☐ dietitian
☐ alcohol or drug treatment program (if indicated).

Follow-up appointments
Make sure that the necessary follow-up appointments have been scheduled and that the patient has been notified:
☐ doctor
☐ home health care agency
☐ community outreach worker
☐ diagnostic tests for reevaluation.

---

return negative results). Explain the need to notify health care providers, such as his dentist or eye doctor, of his condition so that they can institute infection-control precautions.

• Teach the patient precautionary measures that will help him avoid spreading the infection, such as coughing and sneezing into tissues and then disposing of the tissues properly. Stress the importance of washing his hands after handling soiled tissues.

• Emphasize the importance of scheduling and keeping follow-up appointments. Monthly (or more frequent) sputum testing is critical to monitor his response to therapy and determine the duration of therapy. If sputum tests continue to be positive after 3 months, suspect drug resistance or noncompliance with drug therapy. (See *Ensuring continued care for the patient with TB.*)

EVALUATION

When evaluating the patient's response to your nursing care, gather reassessment data and compare this information to the patient outcomes in your plan of care.

Evaluation TimeSaver

Assessing failure to respond to antitubercular therapy

If your patient fails to respond to interventions, this checklist can help you evaluate the reasons why. When performing evaluation, consult with the patient, doctor, and members of the health care team. Remember, even with optimum treatment and full compliance, flare-ups and complications are still possible.

Nursing factors
☐ Unclear instructions
☐ Failure to provide written instructions
☐ Inadequate patient teaching

Patient factors
☐ Language barrier
☐ Illiteracy
☐ Emotional instability
☐ Inability to afford medication
☐ Inability to tolerate adverse effects of medication
☐ Inconvenient schedule of medication administration
☐ Homelessness
☐ Drug abuse

Drug therapy factors
☐ Drug resistance
☐ Insufficient dosage
☐ Insufficient time period for effective drug therapy
☐ Inadequate antitubercular drug regimen
☐ Renal involvement interfering with drug elimination

Interfering conditions
☐ Human immunodeficiency virus infection
☐ Liver disease
☐ Alcohol consumption
☐ Hypersensitivity to medications
☐ Infection with organism resistant to many drugs

Teaching and counseling

Begin by determining the effectiveness of your teaching and counseling. Consider the following questions:
• Does the patient understand the nature of TB and its treatment and prevention?
• Is he willing to follow the treatment plan, institute infection-control measures, and complete the medication regimen? (See *Assessing failure to respond to antitubercular therapy.*)
• Does the patient understand the possible adverse effects of the medications?
• Is he able to expectorate sputum?

• Does the patient know the signs and symptoms of recurring tuberculosis?
• Does he verbalize a reduction in his feelings of isolation?
• Does the patient understand the importance of keeping follow-up appointments?
• Has the patient identified individuals who may have been exposed to his illness?
• Do family members who may have been exposed to active infectious tuberculosis know what steps to take?

Physical condition

If treatment has been successful, you should note the following:
• stable body weight at or near the desired target weight
• clear breath sounds
• a productive cough with thin mucus
• less fatigue
• a return to his normal level of activity
• normal ABG values for his age
• negative results of sputum specimen tests.

Helicobacter pylori infection

Helicobacter pylori infection is difficult to cure and usually exists for years, possibly for life. Antimicrobial therapy typically stops *H. pylori* infection for a time, but the infection and its associated tissue changes usually return after therapy ends. There is no known way to prevent *H. pylori* infection.

Causes

Infection is caused by *H. pylori,* a gram-negative bacteria first isolated in 1982 and formerly called *Campylobacter pylori.* This extremely common human pathogen lives unscathed in gastric epithelial cells; its strong urease activity and motility seem to protect it from gastric acidity. The organism is a chief cause of type B gastritis and strongly linked with the development of peptic ulcer.

ASSESSMENT

Your assessment should include a careful consideration of the patient's health history, physical examination findings, and diagnostic test results.

Health history

Most patients with *H. pylori* infection develop chronic, persistent type B gastritis, but have no symptoms. The patient may have had an acute episode of gastritis in the past, with severe epigastric pain, nausea, and vomiting that resolved in 1 to 2 weeks.

Many patients complain of dyspepsia, a commonly associated problem. Symptoms mirror those of peptic ulcer disease and include aching, burning, or cramping epigastric pain.

Depending on what symptoms the patient reports, assess how they affect nutritional intake, weight, sleep, occupation, recreation, and family life.

Physical examination

Inspection may reveal signs of discomfort caused by an ulcer or gastritis. Auscultation may reveal hyperactive bowel sounds.

Diagnostic test results

The following tests can help confirm the diagnosis:
• GI endoscopy can be used to gather mucosal biopsy specimens. Isolation of *H. pylori* from these specimens confirms the diagnosis. Or the diagnosis can be presumed through direct microscopic examination of stained biopsy specimens.
• Serologic testing can help diagnose *H. pylori* infection, based on the ability to detect antibodies to *H. pylori* antigens.
• A noninvasive procedure called the urea breath test can also aid diagnosis. The test uses orally administered urea that contains carbon-13 or carbon-14. The enzyme urease in *H. pylori* breaks down the urea, and the patient exhales high levels of labeled carbon dioxide.

Treatments

Medical care of the patient with *H. pylori* infection

Because *Helicobacter pylori* is resistant to the usual agents for treating ulcer disease (including histamine$_2$-receptor blockers and sucralfate), a precise treatment regimen hasn't been established.

Drug therapy
The recommended treatment for patients who have dyspepsia (but no ulcer) caused by *H. pylori* infection that doesn't respond to conventional therapy includes the administration of bismuth salts and two antimicrobial agents, usually tetracycline or amoxicillin and metronidazole, for 1 to 4 weeks. The bismuth salts are given before antibiotic therapy to lower bacterial load and lessen the likelihood of resistance.

NURSING DIAGNOSIS

Common nursing diagnoses for the patient with *H. pylori* infection include:
• Altered nutrition: Less than body requirements, related to gastric pain, dyspepsia, nausea, and vomiting
• Knowledge deficit related to the infection and its treatment
• Pain related to gastric or duodenal inflammation secondary to *H. pylori* infection.

PLANNING

Based on the nursing diagnosis *altered nutrition: less than body requirements,* develop appropriate patient outcomes. For example, your patient will:
• regain and maintain weight within the normal range for his height, age, and sex
• consume and tolerate a well-balanced, 2,000-calorie diet daily
• not develop signs and symptoms of nutritional deficiencies.

Based on the nursing diagnosis knowledge deficit, develop appropriate patient outcomes. For example, your patient will:
• obtain information about *H. pylori* infection and treatment
• describe the relationship among *H. pylori* infection, gastritis or peptic ulcer, and prescribed treatment.

Based on the nursing diagnosis *pain,* develop appropriate patient outcomes. For example, your patient will:
• identify factors that aggravate or reduce pain
• verbalize reduced or absent pain after initiation of comfort measures.

IMPLEMENTATION

Adjust your nursing interventions to suit your patient's condition. (See *Medical care of the patient with* H. pylori *infection.*)

Nursing interventions
• Administer prescribed medications, monitor their effectiveness, and watch for adverse reactions.
• Ask about the effectiveness of medications for pain. Help the patient identify factors that increase or reduce the pain.

Teaching TimeSaver
Avoiding gastric irritants

Instruct your patient to avoid the following agents to prevent irritation of the gastric mucosa, which could worsen his condition:
• drugs containing aspirin
• reserpine
• nonsteroidal anti-inflammatory drugs, such as ibuprofen
• indomethacin
• phenylbutazone
• corticosteroids, such as prednisone
• excessive intake of caffeine-containing and alcoholic beverages during flare-ups (moderate alcohol intake is acceptable during remission).

Notifying others
Tell the patient that when he buys over-the-counter drugs he should ask the pharmacist whether they contain any of these agents. He should also notify doctors and dentists of his illness before they prescribe new medications for him. Advise the patient to use other analgesics, such as acetaminophen, to relieve pain.

• Provide six small meals daily or hourly meals, as ordered. Advise the patient to eat slowly, chew thoroughly, and have modest snacks between meals. Help ensure a relaxed and comfortable atmosphere during meals.
• Assess the patient's nutritional status and the effectiveness of measures used to maintain it. Weigh him regularly.
• Schedule care so that the patient gets plenty of rest.

• Assess the patient for indications of GI bleeding.

Patient teaching
• Teach the patient about *H. pylori* infection and its relationship to gastritis and peptic ulcer disease.
• Explain scheduled diagnostic tests and prescribed therapies.
• Review symptoms associated with complications, and urge the patient to notify the doctor if any of these occurs. Emphasize the importance of complying with treatment even after his symptoms disappear.
• Review the proper use of prescribed medications, discussing the desired actions and possible adverse effects of each drug.
• Instruct the patient to avoid substances that can irritate the gastric mucosa. (See *Avoiding gastric irritants*.)
• Also caution him to avoid systemic antacids, such as sodium bicarbonate, because they can cause an acid-base imbalance.
• If the patient smokes, urge him to quit, because smoking stimulates gastric acid secretion. Refer him to a smoking cessation program in your community. (See *Ensuring continued care for the patient with* H. pylori *infection.*)

EVALUATION
When evaluating the patient's response to your nursing care, gather reassessment data and compare this information with the patient outcomes specified in your plan of care.

Teaching and counseling
Begin by determining the effectiveness of your teaching and counseling. Consider the following questions:
• Can the patient describe the relationship between *H. pylori* infection and gastritis or peptic ulcer?

Discharge TimeSaver

Ensuring continued care for the patient with *H. pylori* infection

Review the following teaching topics, referrals, and follow-up appointments to make sure that your patient is adequately prepared for discharge.

Teaching topics
Make sure that the following topics have been covered and that your patient's learning has been evaluated:
☐ nature of the disorder and its complications
☐ pain-relief measures
☐ importance of adequate nourishment
☐ medications, including any adverse effects.

Referrals
Make sure that the patient has been provided with necessary referrals to:
☐ dietitian, as needed.

Follow-up appointments
Make sure that the necessary follow-up appointments have been scheduled and that the patient has been notified:
☐ doctor
☐ diagnostic tests for reevaluation.

• Does he understand the prescribed treatment?

Physical condition

If treatment has been successful, you should note the following outcomes:
• The patient's weight is within normal range for his height, age, and sex.
• The patient reports reduced or absent pain.

Acute pyelonephritis

Acute pyelonephritis is one of the most common renal diseases. In this disorder, bacterial invasion causes a sudden inflammation, mainly in the interstitial tissue and renal pelvis and occasionally in the renal tubules. (See *What happens in acute pyelonephritis,* page 270.) It may affect one or both kidneys. With treatment and continued follow-up care, the prognosis is

good and extensive permanent damage is rare.

Associated complications include calculus formation, further renal damage, renal abscesses with possible metastasis to other organs, septic shock, and chronic pyelonephritis.

Chronic pyelonephritis is a persistent kidney inflammation that can scar the kidneys and lead to chronic renal failure. Its etiology may be bacterial, metastatic, or urogenous. This disease most frequently occurs in patients who are predisposed to recurrent acute pyelonephritis — for instance, those with urinary obstructions or vesicoureteral reflux.

Causes

Most often, infecting bacteria are normal intestinal and fecal flora that grow readily in urine. The most common causative organism is *Escherichia coli,* but *Proteus, Pseudomonas, Staphylococcus aureus,* and *Entero-*

What happens in acute pyelonephritis

Urine produced in nephron units drains into collecting ducts in the renal cali-
ces and then into the renal pelvis, a small collecting basin in the kidney. In
acute pyelonephritis, microorganisms reach the renal pelvis and cause an inflammatory reaction. Inflammation begins in tissues near the papillae but may
reach into the renal cortex.

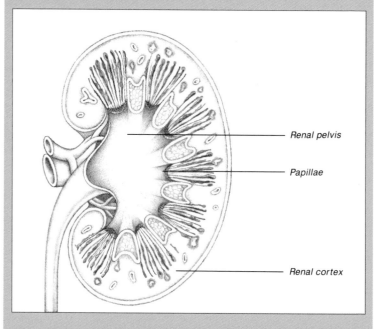

Renal pelvis

Papillae

Renal cortex

coccus faecalis also may cause such
infections. Nosocomial infections are
caused by a wider spectrum of microorganisms; they often are resistant to
multiple antimicrobials and conse-
quently are more difficult to treat.

Most often, acute pyelonephritis
results from an ascending infection.
Typically, the infection spreads from
the bladder to the ureters and then to
the kidneys. Bacteria may also invade
the kidneys by hematogenous spread

from a distant infection, such as endocarditis. They can also be introduced by instruments, such as a cys-
toscope, or through urologic surgery.
(See *Risk factors for acute pyelonephritis.*)

ASSESSMENT

Your assessment should include a
careful consideration of the patient's

FactFinder

Risk factors for acute pyelonephritis

Factors that increase susceptibility to acute pyelonephritis include:
• urinary stasis resulting from an obstruction caused by tumors, strictures, or benign prostatic hyperplasia; congenital or acquired vesicoureteral reflux; or neurogenic bladder (as seen in diabetes, spinal cord injury, multiple sclerosis, and tabes dorsalis)
• the presence of a foreign body, such as a calculus or catheter, that serves as a nidus for infecting microorganisms
• trauma, including trauma from sexual activity or surgical instruments

• systemic disease or compromised immune function, such as with diabetes mellitus or malnutrition
• glycosuria, which may support bacterial growth in urine
• other renal diseases, in which compromised renal function increases susceptibility to acute pyelonephritis
• pregnancy (about 5% of all pregnancies are associated with asymptomatic bacteriuria). If untreated, approximately 40% of these women develop pyelonephritis.

---

health history, physical examination findings, and diagnostic test results.

Health history
The patient usually complains of unilateral or bilateral flank or abdominal pain. Other common symptoms include fever, shaking chills, anorexia, and general fatigue. The patient may also report urinary frequency, burning, and urgency. Hematuria (usually microscopic but possibly gross) may be reported as well. The patient usually states that the symptoms developed rapidly over a few hours or a few days.

Physical examination
A patient with acute pyelonephritis commonly looks very ill. Costovertebral angle tenderness is usually noted on palpation. Urine may appear cloudy and have an ammonia-like or fishy odor. Vital signs may reveal a fever of 102° F (38.9° C) or higher.

Diagnostic test results
Diagnosis requires urinalysis and culture and sensitivity testing. Typical findings include:
• Pyuria. A test of urine sediment reveals leukocytes singly, in clumps, and in casts — and possibly a few red blood cells.
• Significant bacteriuria. Urine culture reveals more than 100,000 organisms/mm^3 of urine.
• Low specific gravity and osmolality.
• Slightly alkaline urine pH.
• Proteinuria, glycosuria, and ketonuria.

Blood tests and X-rays also help in evaluating acute pyelonephritis. A complete blood count shows an elevated white blood cell count (up to 40,000/mm^3), neutrophil count, and erythrocyte sedimentation rate.

Kidney-ureter-bladder radiography may reveal calculi, tumors, or cysts in the kidneys and urinary tract.

Excretory urography may show asymmetrical kidneys.

The presence of fluorescent bacteria indicates antibody coating that appears only on bacteria of renal origin. Bacteria from the bladder don't have an antibody coating and therefore will not fluoresce.

NURSING DIAGNOSIS

Common nursing diagnoses for the patient with acute pyelonephritis include:
• Altered urinary elimination related to bladder spasm, dysuria, and inflammation
• Hyperthermia related to infection
• Pain related to infection.

PLANNING

Based on the nursing diagnosis *altered urinary elimination,* develop appropriate patient outcomes. For example, your patient will:
• void at least 50 ml/hour daily
• avoid related complications, such as urine retention or fluid retention
• regain and maintain normal urinary elimination with eradication of pyelonephritis.

Based on the nursing diagnosis *hyperthermia,* develop appropriate patient outcomes. For example, your patient will:
• reestablish a normal body temperature with antipyretic and antibiotic therapy
• avoid complications associated with hyperthermia, such as seizures and dehydration.

Based on the nursing diagnosis *pain,* develop appropriate patient outcomes. For example, your patient will:
• state and carry out appropriate interventions for pain relief

• express feelings of comfort and relief from pain when pyelonephritis subsides.

IMPLEMENTATION

Adjust your interventions to suit the patient's condition. Most patients are hospitalized for parenteral administration of fluids and antibiotic therapy. Some patients are treated on an outpatient basis. (See *Medical care of the patient with acute pyelonephritis.*)

Nursing interventions
• Administer antipyretics for fever; use additional cooling methods, such as a hypothermia blanket, as prescribed for high fever.
• Assess the patient's temperature regularly to determine his response to interventions.
• Administer prescribed antimicrobial therapy and analgesics, and monitor for therapeutic and adverse reactions.
• Force fluids or administer prescribed parenteral fluids, or both, to achieve a urine output of more than 2,000 ml/day. This helps empty the bladder of contaminated urine and is the best way to prevent calculus formation.
• Be sure to refrigerate or culture a urine specimen within 30 minutes of collection to prevent overgrowth of bacteria.
• Check the patient's voiding pattern and urine characteristics for evidence of improvement or complications. Measure his intake and output.
• Prepare the patient for surgery, if warranted, to correct underlying structural abnormality or to remove a source of repeated infection.

Patient teaching
• Explain acute pyelonephritis and its treatment.

Treatments

Medical care of the patient with acute pyelonephritis

Treatment of acute pyelonephritis focuses on antibiotic therapy.

Drug therapy
• *Enterococcus* infections require treatment with ampicillin, penicillin G, or vancomycin.
• *Staphylococcus* infections require treatment with penicillin G or, if the bacterium is resistant, a semisynthetic penicillin such as nafcillin or a cephalosporin.
• *Escherichia coli* may be treated with sulfisoxazole, nalidixic acid, or nitrofurantoin.
• *Proteus* infections require treatment with ampicillin, sulfisoxazole, nalidixic acid, or a cephalosporin.
• *Pseudomonas* infections may be treated with gentamicin, tobramycin, or carbenicillin.

When the infecting organism can't be identified, therapy usually consists of a broad-spectrum antibiotic, such as ampicillin or cephalexin.

Drug precautions
Antibiotics must be prescribed cautiously for older patients and pregnant patients. In these patients, urinary analgesics, such as phenazopyridine, can help relieve pain.

Recovery
Symptoms may disappear after several days of antibiotic therapy. Although urine usually becomes sterile within 48 to 72 hours, the course of drug therapy typically ranges from 10 to 14 days.

Follow-up treatment
Follow-up treatment includes reculturing urine 1 week after drug therapy stops and then periodically for the next year. A patient with an uncomplicated infection usually responds well to therapy and doesn't experience reinfection. A patient at high risk for recurring urinary tract and kidney infections — such as a patient with a long-term indwelling urinary catheter or on maintenance antibiotic therapy — requires lengthy follow-up care.

Surgery
If infection results from obstruction or vesicoureteral reflux, antibiotics may be less effective and surgery may be necessary to relieve the obstruction or correct the anomaly.

• Teach proper technique for collecting a clean-catch urine specimen (midstream).
• Stress the need to complete the prescribed antibiotic regimen even after symptoms subside. Tell the patient to report adverse reactions rather than discontinue drug therapy.

• Advise the patient to force fluids (unless contraindicated) and to eat a balanced diet.
• Stress the need to balance rest with activity.
• Advise routine checkups for a patient with a history of urinary tract infections. Explain the signs and symptoms of reinfection, such as cloudy

Discharge TimeSaver

Ensuring continued care for the patient with acute pyelonephritis

Review the following teaching topics, referrals, and follow-up appointments to make sure that your patient is adequately prepared for discharge.

Teaching topics
Make sure that the following topics have been covered and that your patient's learning has been evaluated:
☐ explanation of acute pyelonephritis, including its causes, symptoms, and complications
☐ medications, including dosage and adverse effects
☐ importance of follow-up care
☐ importance of taking medication.

Referrals
Make sure that the patient has been provided with necessary referrals to:
☐ urologist, if needed, for obstruction or recurring problems.

Follow-up appointments
Make sure that the necessary follow-up appointments have been scheduled and that the patient has been notified:
☐ doctor
☐ diagnostic tests for reevaluation.

urine, burning on urination, and urinary urgency and frequency, especially when accompanied by a low-grade fever and back pain.
• If surgery is planned, reinforce the doctor's explanation and teach the patient about preoperative and postoperative care measures. (See *Ensuring continued care for the patient with acute pyelonephritis.*)

EVALUATION

When evaluating the patient's response to your nursing care, gather reassessment data and compare this information with the patient outcomes specified in your plan of care.

Teaching and counseling
Begin by determining the effectiveness of your teaching and counseling. Consider the following questions:

• Can the patient explain acute pyelonephritis and its treatment?
• Does he understand the need to complete the full course of therapy?

Physical condition
If treatment has been successful, you should note the following outcomes:
• The patient maintains an adequate output of urine and a normal pattern of elimination.
• His fever has subsided.
• The patient is free of complications associated with hyperthermia.
• The patient reports pain reduction or relief.

CHAPTER 11

Caring for patients with infections of varying etiology

Pneumonia   276

Wound infection   287

Meningitis   292

Lower urinary tract infection   299

Gastroenteritis   304

Sepsis   310

Osteomyelitis   318

The increase in resistant infectious strains, changes in the epidemiology of community-acquired infections (for example, the rise in sexually transmitted diseases), and the increase in nosocomial infections have created new health care challenges. Hospital infection-control procedures vary greatly, which makes it especially important to be familiar with your hospital's specific infection-control policies.

Nosocomial infection

Four of the disorders discussed in this chapter — pneumonia, wound infection, urinary tract infection, and laboratory-confirmed bloodstream infection (described under sepsis) — represent the most common nosocomial infections. In the United States, 2 million nosocomial infections are estimated to occur in 1 year, resulting in approximately 20,000 deaths. (See *Risk factors for nosocomial infection.*)

Pneumonia

Pneumonia is an acute infection of the lung parenchyma, usually accompanied by exudate in the bronchioli and alveoli. Depending on the lung area affected, the infection is classified as bronchopneumonia (distal airways and alveoli), lobular pneumonia (part of a lobe), or lobar pneumonia (entire lobe). Cytomegalovirus and *Pneumocystis carinii* pneumonia are increasingly common among high-risk populations.

Causes

Pneumonia is caused by viruses, bacteria, mycoplasmas, fungi, or protozoa. (See *Key points about pneumonia,* page 278, and *Assessing types of pneumonia,* pages 279 to 282.)

ASSESSMENT

Because of the potential severity of pneumonia, you'll need to obtain a timely and thorough history from the patient and family members. Support your findings by performing a physical examination and reviewing diagnostic test results.

Health history

The patient may report pleuritic chest pain, cough, sputum production, dyspnea, fever, or chills.

Physical examination

Your patient may be shaking and appear flushed, dyspneic, anxious, and uncomfortable. Note the characteristics of his sputum, keeping in mind the following:

• Creamy yellow sputum suggests staphylococcal pneumonia.
• Green sputum suggests a *Pseudomonas* organism.
• Sputum that looks like currant jelly indicates *Klebsiella* infection.
• Rust-colored sputum indicates pneumococcal pneumonia.
• Clear sputum suggests atypical pneumonia, lack of infection, or a poor specimen.

In advanced cases of pneumonia, percussion of the affected lung area reveals dullness. Auscultation may disclose crackles or rhonchi over the affected lung area. Bronchial breath sounds are usually present over areas of consolidation, but wheezing is uncommon. Vocal and tactile fremitus are increased with lung consolidation; vital signs reveal fever, tachycardia, and tachypnea.

Diagnostic test results

The following tests can confirm a diagnosis of pneumonia and identify its cause.

• A chest X-ray may reveal infiltrates.

• Gram stain and culture and sensitivity tests of sputum specimens may show acute inflammatory cells and help identify the causative bacteria.

• White blood cell (WBC) count may reveal leukocytosis in bacterial pneumonia; a normal or low WBC count may indicate viral or mycoplasmal pneumonia.

• Blood cultures and pleural fluid specimens may reveal bacteremia and the causative organism.

• Pulse oximetry may reveal a reduced arterial oxygen saturation (SaO_2) level.

Other tests include bronchoscopy, bronchoalveolar lavage, or transtracheal aspiration to collect specimens of respiratory secretions for culture or to identify causative factors.

NURSING DIAGNOSIS

Common nursing diagnoses for a patient with pneumonia include:

• Ineffective breathing pattern related to thoracic pain and hypoxemia

• Impaired gas exchange related to impaired ventilation and perfusion secondary to pneumonia

• Ineffective airway clearance related to thick sputum production secondary to pneumonia

• Hyperthermia related to inflammation and infection.

PLANNING

Based on the nursing diagnosis *ineffective breathing pattern*, develop appropriate outcomes. For example, your patient will:

FactFinder

Risk factors for nosocomial infection

The following factors place your patient at high risk for nosocomial infection:

• anesthesia

• burns

• circulatory stasis associated with immobility or pressure

• depressed cough reflex

• endotracheal intubation

• hypovolemia

• immunocompromised status secondary to such factors as human immunodeficiency virus infection, chemotherapy, radiation therapy, or corticosteroid therapy

• intravascular lines

• invasive diagnostic studies

• large-volume nebulizers

• nasogastric intubation

• neurologic deficits

• oropharyngeal bacterial colonization

• oxygen therapy

• pulmonary impairment due to illness, such as obstructions

• recent surgery

• smoking

• tracheostomy

• urinary tract catheterization (intermittent and indwelling)

• urinary tract disease, such as obstructions

• urologic instrumentation

• vascular impairment due to disease

• vascular shunts.

• maintain a respiratory rate that's within 5 breaths/minute of baseline

• exhibit symmetrical chest expansion

FactFinder
Key points about pneumonia

- *Complications:* Pneumonia can lead to septic shock, hypoxemia, and respiratory failure. The infection can also spread within the patient's lungs or pleural space, causing lung abscess or empyema. It may also spread via the bloodstream and infect other parts of the body, causing endocarditis, pericarditis, and meningitis. Pneumonia is the leading cause of infection-related death in North America.
- *Transmission:* The causative organism is usually inhaled but can spread from another site within the host's body. The inhalation of foreign matter, such as vomitus or food particles, can cause aspiration or noninfectious pneumonia.
- *Risk factors:* The patient's risk of developing pneumonia is increased by advanced age (over 65), tracheostomy or nasogastric tube feedings, chronic disease (such as cancer, chronic obstructive pulmonary disease, sickle cell disease, diabetes mellitus, heart disease, alcoholism, kidney disease, and liver disease). Other risk factors include immunosuppressive disorders or therapies (such as human immunodeficiency virus or chemotherapy), recent upper abdominal or thoracic surgery, exposure to noxious gases, atelectasis, influenza, and prolonged bed rest.

- demonstrate clear, bilateral breath sounds.

Based on the nursing diagnosis *impaired gas exchange*, develop appropriate outcomes. For example, your patient will:
- maintain partial pressure of arterial oxygen of 80 to 100 mm Hg
- maintain partial pressure of arterial carbon dioxide ($PaCO_2$) of 35 to 45 mm Hg or return to acceptable baseline status
- maintain SaO_2 of 93% to 97% or return to acceptable baseline status (above 82%).

Based on the nursing diagnosis *ineffective airway clearance*, develop appropriate outcomes. For example, your patient will:
- cough and expectorate thin mucus
- demonstrate clear or baseline breath sounds
- exhibit arterial blood gas (ABG) values that are normal or baseline.

Based on the nursing diagnosis *hyperthermia*, develop appropriate outcomes. For example, your patient will:
- exhibit a normal temperature
- avoid complications of hyperthermia
- state the importance of completing his course of medication.

IMPLEMENTATION

Focus your nursing care on minimizing patient discomfort and eradicating the infection. Treatment may consist of drug therapy, bed rest, fluid increase, and dietary modifications. (See *Medical care of the patient with pneumonia*, page 283.)

Nursing interventions
- Administer antimicrobial medications as prescribed.
- Maintain a patent airway. Encourage the patient to practice effective coughing and deep-breathing exercises at least every 2 hours. If chest pain inhibits coughing, administer or-

(Text continues on page 282.)

Assessing types of pneumonia

Below you'll find a quick review of different types of pneumonia to help you plan your nursing care.

Viral pneumonias
Types of viral pneumonias include adenovirus, varicella, cytomegalovirus, influenza, measles, and respiratory syncytial virus.

Adenovirus
This type of pneumonia has an insidious onset, and it typically affects young adults. The prognosis is good: The condition usually clears with no residual effects. Mortality is low.
• *Signs and symptoms:* These include sore throat, fever, cough, chills, malaise, small amounts of mucoid sputum, retrosternal chest pain, anorexia, rhinitis, adenopathy, scattered crackles, and rhonchi.
• *Diagnostic test results:* Chest X-ray shows patchy distribution of pneumonia, more severe than indicated by physical examination. White blood cell (WBC) count is normal to slightly elevated.

Chicken pox (varicella)
Pneumonia with chicken pox is uncommon in children but is present in 30% of adults with varicella.
• *Signs and symptoms:* These include a characteristic rash, cough, dyspnea, cyanosis, tachypnea, pleuritic chest pain, hemoptysis, and rhonchi 1 to 6 days after onset of rash.
• *Diagnostic test results:* Chest X-ray shows more extensive pneumonia than indicated by physical examination and bilateral, patchy, diffuse nod-

ular infiltrates. Sputum analysis shows predominant mononuclear cells and characteristic intranuclear inclusion bodies.

Cytomegalovirus
In adults with healthy lung tissue, this pneumonia resembles mononucleosis and is generally benign. In neonates, it occurs as a devastating multisystemic infection. In immunocompromised patients, the effect of cytomegalovirus varies from clinically inapparent to fatal infection.
• *Signs and symptoms:* This viral pneumonia is difficult to distinguish from other nonbacterial pneumonias. Symptoms include fever, cough, shaking chills, dyspnea, cyanosis, weakness, and diffuse crackles.
• *Diagnostic test results:* Chest X-ray in early stages shows variable patchy infiltrates; later, bilateral, nodular infiltrates that are more predominant in lower lobes. Percutaneous aspiration of lung tissue, transbronchial biopsy, or open lung biopsy shows typical intranuclear and cytoplasmic inclusions on microscopic examination; the virus can be cultured from lung tissue.

Influenza
Severe disease and death occur more commonly in older or debilitated patients. The prognosis is poor even with treatment; 50% of deaths result from cardiopulmonary collapse.

(continued)

Assessing types of pneumonia *(continued)*

- *Signs and symptoms:* These include cough (initially nonproductive; later, purulent sputum), marked cyanosis, dyspnea, high fever, chills, substernal pain and discomfort, moist crackles, frontal headache, and myalgia.
- *Diagnostic test results:* Chest X-ray shows diffuse bilateral bronchopneumonia radiating from the hilus. WBC count will be normal to slightly elevated. Sputum smear shows no specific organisms.

Measles (rubeola)
An acute, highly contagious infection that causes a characteristic rash, measles is one of the most common and serious communicable childhood diseases.
- *Signs and symptoms:* Signs are fever, dyspnea, cough, small amounts of sputum, coryza, rash, and cervical adenopathy.
- *Diagnostic test results:* Chest X-ray shows reticular infiltrates, sometimes with hilar lymph node enlargement. Lung tissue specimen shows characteristic giant cells.

Respiratory syncytial virus
This is most prevalent in infants and children. Complete recovery may take 1 to 3 weeks.
- *Signs and symptoms:* These include listlessness, irritability, tachypnea with retraction of intercostal muscles, slight sputum production, fine moist crackles, fever, severe malaise and, possibly, cough or croup.
- *Diagnostic test results:* Chest X-ray shows patchy bilateral consolidation.

WBC count is normal to slightly elevated.

Bacterial pneumonias
This category includes pneumonia caused by *Klebsiella, Legionella pneumophila, Pseudomonas aeruginosa, Staphylococcus,* and *Streptococcus.*

Klebsiella
Pneumonia caused by *Klebsiella* is more common among patients with chronic alcoholism, pulmonary disease, or diabetes mellitus. It is often acquired while in the hospital but may be seen in the community.
- *Signs and symptoms:* Signs include fever and recurrent chills; cough producing rusty, bloody, viscous sputum (like currant jelly); cyanosis of lips and nail beds from hypoxemia; and shallow, grunting respirations.
- *Diagnostic test results:* Chest X-ray usually shows consolidation in the upper lobe that causes bulging of fissures. WBC count is elevated. Sputum culture and Gram stain may show gram-negative cocci, *Klebsiella.*

Legionella pneumophila
The cause of Legionnaires' disease, this bacterium is associated with contaminated water distribution systems.
- *Signs and symptoms:* These include malaise, anorexia, headache, diarrhea, and myalgia, followed by cough, dyspnea, chest pain, bradycardia, fever higher than 102° F (38.9° C), and altered level of consciousness (LOC).

• *Diagnostic test results:* Chest X-ray reveals multilobar consolidation. Direct immunofluorescent antibody staining of sputum, bronchial washings or brushings, or pleural fluid may provide rapid diagnosis. Deoxyribonucleic acid probe is newly available, fast, and accurate. Sputum culture identifies the causative organism but takes much longer.

Pseudomonas aeruginosa

The prognosis is poor, with high mortality. Occurrence is more common among hospitalized patients, especially those who are immunocompromised, are using respiratory equipment, or have tracheostomies.
• *Signs and symptoms:* These include a productive cough with green, foul-smelling sputum; bradycardia; cyanosis; and altered LOC.
• *Diagnostic test results:* Chest X-ray reveals multiple infiltrates.

Staphylococcus

This infection is most often acquired during hospitalization. It should be suspected if the patient has cystic fibrosis or a viral illness, such as influenza or measles; is undergoing dialysis; has recently undergone surgery; or has a history of drug abuse.
• *Signs and symptoms:* Staphylococcal pneumonia is characterized by a temperature of 102° to 104° F (38.9° to 40° C), recurrent shaking chills, bloody sputum, dyspnea, tachypnea, and hypoxemia.
• *Diagnostic test results:* Chest X-ray shows multiple abscesses and infiltrates; frequently empyema. WBC

count is elevated. Sputum culture and Gram stain may show gram-positive staphylococci.

Streptococcus (pneumococcal pneumonia)

This is the most common of all pneumonias that are acquired outside the hospital.
• *Signs and symptoms:* This pneumonia starts with a sudden onset of a single, shaking chill and sustained temperature of 102° to 104° F (38.9° to 40° C), tachypnea, shortness of breath, and chest pain. These symptoms are often preceded by an upper respiratory tract infection.
• *Diagnostic test results:* Chest X-ray shows areas of consolidation, often lobar. WBC count is elevated. Sputum culture may show gram-positive *Streptococcus pneumoniae*.

Mycoplasmal pneumonia

In young adults, *Mycoplasma pneumoniae* is the most common form of pneumonia acquired outside the hospital. It is also associated with mild respiratory infection in children.
• *Signs and symptoms:* Signs and symptoms include a hacking cough (often unproductive), fever below 102° F (38.9° C), sore throat, headache, and malaise.
• *Diagnostic test results:* Chest X-ray reveals peripheral infiltrates. Erythrocyte sedimentation rate and WBC count are elevated. Cold agglutinins may be positive, but the test is not specific for this disease. Complement fixation and culture of sputum will confirm the diagnosis, but results

(continued)

Assessing types of pneumonia *(continued)*

are usually not available until after the patient has recovered.

Protozoan pneumonia
Pneumocystis carinii pneumonia is currently categorized as a protozoan pneumonia.

Pneumocystis carinii
The incidence of *Pneumocystis carinii* pneumonia (PCP), an opportunistic infection, has increased significantly since the 1980s. Immunocompromised patients have the highest risk. PCP is especially prevalent in patients infected with human immunodeficiency virus; up to 90% of these patients contract PCP during their lifetime.
• *Signs and symptoms:* The onset of signs and symptoms is abrupt. Mild fever, shortness of breath, and nonproductive cough may be accompanied by anorexia, fatigue, and weight loss, and may progress to respiratory failure.

• *Diagnostic test results:* Histologic tests reveal the causative organism by staining of cells obtained from bronchoalveolar lavage or, occasionally, induced sputum. Chest X-ray may show slowly progressive infiltrates and occasional nodular lesions or a spontaneous pneumothorax.

Fungal pneumonia
This category includes *Aspergillus fumigatus* (aspergillosis), *Candida albicans* (candidiasis), *Histoplasma capsulatum* (histoplasmosis). The occurrence of these fungal pneumonias is most common in immunocompromised patients.
• *Signs and symptoms:* These include persistent fever, dyspnea, tachypnea, cough, pleuritic chest pain, and pleural friction rub.
• *Diagnostic test results:* Chest X-ray may reveal nodular cavity formation. Sputum smear may reveal a fungal organism; however, its presence doesn't confirm the diagnosis. A needle or open-lung biopsy of lung tissue

dered analgesics and splint the painful area while the patient is coughing. An incentive spirometer may be necessary.
• If auscultation reveals that excessive secretions are not mobilized by coughing, perform postural drainage and chest percussion.

Timesaving tip: When you need to make a quick, focused assessment, take the following steps: Check skin color for cyanosis or flushing; look for rapid, irregular, or labored respiration; ask the patient to

cough and note effectiveness as well as characteristics of the expectorant. Ask about chest pain.
• For the patient receiving antibiotic therapy, the best time to obtain a sputum specimen is in the morning after he awakes and before his first dose of antibiotics. Obtaining the specimen first will prevent it from being affected by the medication.
• Administer supplemental oxygen by Venturi mask or nasal cannula as ordered. (See *How to use a Venturi mask and nasal cannula.*)

Treatments

Medical care of the patient with pneumonia

Treatment includes drug therapy and supportive measures.

Drug therapy

Drug therapy is based on the identified organism from a sputum culture. A broad-spectrum antibiotic is used until a specific cause is identified. Viral pneumonias are treated with antibiotics until the diagnosis is certain and it's clear that no complicating bacterial infection is present.

Antibiotic sensitivity studies are also obtained from the sputum culture. Antibiotic-resistant organisms are an increasing problem, particularly in immunocompromised patients with frequent infections who receive multiple courses of antibiotics. Treatment should be reevaluated early, especially when treating immunocompromised patients.

Types of pneumonia and their common pharmacologic treatments include:

- Streptococcal pneumonia: penicillin G (or erythromycin if the patient is allergic to penicillin)
- *Klebsiella pneumoniae* pneumonia: third-generation cephalosporin
- Staphylococcal pneumonia: prompt treatment with nafcillin or oxacillin, or vancomycin if organism is methicillin-resistant
- *Legionella pneumophila* pneumonia: prompt treatment with erythromycin (rifampin may be given in conjunction with the antibiotic)
- *Mycoplasma pneumoniae* pneumonia: erythromycin or, alternatively, doxycycline
- *Pneumocystis carinii* pneumonia: Co-trimoxazole (treatment of choice) or pentamidine (alternative) may be administered to patients with acquired immunodeficiency syndrome. Corticosteroids may be used in severe illness.
- Viral pneumonias: If influenza A virus is the cause, amantadine may be used; antiviral agents, such as acyclovir, may prove effective for some patients. Otherwise, treatment focuses on symptoms with antipyretics used for fever and analgesics for headache.

Supportive care

Treatment of all types of pneumonia also involves supportive care. Common interventions include:

- bed rest
- high-calorie diet with foods that are easy to chew and swallow
- adequate fluid
- humidified oxygen therapy for hypoxemia
- bronchodilator therapy
- chest physiotherapy to help mobilize secretions, if necessary
- antitussives for cough
- analgesics to relieve pleuritic chest pain.

If the patient has severe pneumonia with respiratory failure, mechanical ventilation and, possibly, positive end-expiratory pressure are used to maintain adequate oxygenation.

• If the patient has an underlying chronic lung disease, monitor his ABG levels and SaO_2 carefully. A rising $PaCO_2$ and decreasing pH are signs of impending respiratory failure. If respiratory failure occurs, expect to assist with endotracheal intubation and mechanical ventilation.

• Give 3,000 ml/day of oral or parenteral fluids to prevent dehydration due to fever and infection and to help liquefy secretions. Monitor intake and output.

• If the patient has excessive secretions but is unable to cough effectively, perform nasotracheal suctioning as ordered. If the patient is hypoxemic, be sure to hyperoxygenate before, during, and after suctioning.

Timesaving tip: To dispose of a used suction catheter quickly and aseptically, wrap the catheter around your gloved hand, disconnect the catheter from the connecting tube, and then pull the glove off over the catheter. The catheter will be safely contained inside the disposable glove. Then pull your other glove over the catheter and first glove, and discard all in a suitable receptacle.

• Place the patient in semi-Fowler's position to make breathing easier.

• Give the patient disposable tissues, and tape a lined bag to the side of the bed for tissue disposal.

• If the patient is able to perform activities of daily living (ADLs), encourage him to work slowly, rest often, and use supplemental oxygen if necessary. Monitor for signs of cyanosis.

• Take the patient's temperature at least every 4 hours. Administer antipyretics as ordered. If fever is high, assess the patient's level of consciousness. If necessary, provide a hypothermia blanket.

• Prevent aspiration during nasogastric tube feedings by elevating the patient's head, checking the tube position, and administering the feeding slowly. Large volumes may cause vomiting.

Patient teaching

• Explain pneumonia and its risk factors. Emphasize that adequate rest is crucial for full recovery and preventing relapse. Teach energy-conserving techniques, and explain that the patient must resume ADLs gradually.

• Emphasize that the patient must take the entire course of his medication — even if he feels better — because he's susceptible to recurrent respiratory infection. However, warn against the indiscriminate use of antibiotics.

• Teach the patient diaphragmatic breathing exercises, effective coughing techniques, chest physiotherapy, and proper use of the incentive spirometer, if warranted. Encourage him to practice breathing exercises and effective coughing four times a day (or more) for 8 weeks. Explain that postural drainage, percussion, and vibration help mobilize mucus in the lungs for removal.

• If the patient will require home oxygen therapy, teach him how to use equipment safely and effectively.

• Encourage the patient to drink 2 to 3 quarts (liters) of fluid each day (unless contraindicated) to maintain adequate hydration and to keep mucous secretions thin and easier to remove.

• Tell the patient to notify the doctor if he experiences signs and symptoms of relapse, such as chest pain, fever, chills, shortness of breath, hemoptysis, or increased fatigue.

• Tell the patient to avoid cigarette smoke, dust, significant environmental pollution (by staying inside on smoggy days), and other bronchial irritants. If appropriate, refer the pa-

How to use a Venturi mask and nasal cannula

Oxygen delivery system	Advantages	Disadvantages	Nursing checklist
Nasal cannula (low-flow system) 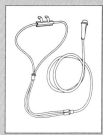	• Comfortable; easily tolerated • Nasal prongs can be shaped to fit facial contour. • Effective for delivering low oxygen concentrations • Allows freedom of movement; doesn't impede eating or talking • Inexpensive; disposable	• Contraindicated in complete nasal obstruction, for example, mucosal edema or polyps • May cause headaches or dry mucous membranes if flow rate exceeds 6 liters/minute • May cause pressure ulcer on ear pinna if adjusted too tightly or if friction exists between strap and ear tissue • Can dislodge easily • Strap may pinch chin if too tight. • Patient must be alert and cooperative to help keep cannula in place.	• Remove and clean cannula every 8 hours with a wet cloth. • Provide good mouth and nose care. • See if your patient is restless. If so, explore other methods of oxygen delivery. • Check for reddened areas under the nose and over the ears. If reddened areas are present, apply gauze padding. • Moisten the lips and nose with water-soluble jelly, but avoid occluding the cannula.
Venturi mask (high-flow system) 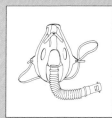	• Delivers exact oxygen concentration despite patient's respiratory pattern or if flowmeter knob is bumped • Has adjustable diluter jets that enable oxygen concentration to be changed with a turn of a dial • Doesn't dry mucous membranes • Can be used to deliver humidity or aerosol therapy	• Possible lowered fraction of inspired oxygen if air intake ports are blocked • Interferes with eating and talking • Condensate may collect and drain on patient if humidification is being used.	• Apply petroleum jelly to skin around mouth. • Remove and clean the mask every 8 hours.

Discharge TimeSaver
Ensuring continued care for the patient with pneumonia

Review the following teaching topics, referrals, and follow-up appointments to make sure that your patient is adequately prepared for discharge.

Teaching topics
Make sure that the following topics have been covered and that your patient's learning has been evaluated:
☐ the nature of pneumonia, including risk factors and complications
☐ diagnostic studies
☐ energy conservation techniques
☐ need for adequate fluid intake
☐ medications, including their purpose, dosage, adverse effects, and the importance of completing the course of therapy
☐ procedure for coughing effectively
☐ warning signs and symptoms of a worsening condition
☐ sources of additional information and support.

Referrals
Make sure that the patient has been provided with necessary referrals to:
☐ social service agencies
☐ home health care agency
☐ medical equipment supplier (oxygen equipment)
☐ smoking cessation program (if appropriate).

Follow-up appointments
Make sure that the necessary follow-up appointments have been scheduled and that the patient has been notified:
☐ doctor
☐ diagnostic tests for reevaluation.

tient to a local smoking cessation program.
• Discuss how to avoid spreading infection. Remind the patient to cover a sneeze or cough and to dispose of used tissues in a plastic bag. Tell him to wash his hands thoroughly after sneezing, coughing, or handling contaminated tissues.
• Encourage the patient to perform self-care measures, such as recording input and output and performing deep-breathing and coughing exercises. Offer frequent reassurance and point out signs of progress whenever possible. (See *Ensuring continued care for the patient with pneumonia*.)

EVALUATION

When evaluating the patient's response to your nursing care, gather reassessment data and compare this information with the patient outcomes specified in your plan of care.

Teaching and counseling
Determine the effectiveness of your teaching and counseling by considering the following questions:
• Does the patient understand how to prevent pneumonia from recurring and from spreading to others?
• Can he demonstrate diaphragmatic breathing exercises, effective coughing techniques, chest physiotherapy, incentive spirometry, and home oxy-

gen therapy techniques (if necessary)?
• Does he understand the importance of bed rest, increased fluid intake, and gradual, moderate exercise?

Physical condition
A physical examination and diagnostic tests will provide additional information. To evaluate the success of treatment, consider the following questions:
• Has the patient's respiratory rate returned to within 5 breaths/minute of baseline?
• Does his chest expand symmetrically?
• Are breath sounds clear and equal bilaterally?
• Does he expectorate clear mucus?
• Has his temperature returned to normal?
• Does he report that pain is decreased or absent?
• Can he tolerate increased activity without fatigue, dyspnea, or changes in vital signs?

Wound infection

Wound infection may result from neglect of a wound or from vascular impairment secondary to peripheral vascular disease or uncontrolled diabetes mellitus. It may also occur as a complication of surgery.

Causes
Wound infection usually results from invasion by bacteria. (See *Key points about wound infection.*)

ASSESSMENT

Your assessment should include consideration of the patient's health his-

---

FactFinder

Key points about wound infection

• *Risk factors:* Obesity, extremes of age, malnutrition, immunocompromise (related to illness or treatment), shock, anemia, and renal failure all increase the risk of wound infection.
• *Complications:* Wound infection may lead to osteomyelitis, secondary systemic infection, deep abscess, septic shock, or dehiscent peritonitis. It may also cause inflammation or infection of an adjacent organ, such as endocarditis, endometritis, empyema, or suppurative arthritis.
• *Causes: Staphylococcus aureus,* a gram-positive nonmotile organism, is the most common cause of wound infections. One type of *S. aureus* is methicillin-resistant *S. aureus* (MRSA). MRSA is universally susceptible only to vancomycin. As with other infectious organisms, hospital personnel may become colonized with MSRA and further an outbreak, greatly endangering immunocompromised patients. In most cases, MRSA infection is spread on the hands of caregivers because of inadequate hand washing.
• Other common causes of surgical wound infection include coagulase-negative staphylococci, enterococci, *Escherichia coli, Pseudomonas aeruginosa,* and *Enterobacter* species.

tory, physical examination findings, and diagnostic test results.

Health history

The patient with a surgical wound infection may complain of pain and purulent drainage or inflammation. He may also report a recent surgical procedure, usually within the last month (although infection may appear up to 1 year after an implant). Patients with nonsurgical wound infections may report a history of traumatic injury, pressure ulcer associated with immobility, or stasis ulcer associated with diabetes mellitus or peripheral vascular disease.

Physical examination

You may note purulent drainage, odor, erythema and warmth, or a fever. Measure the wound to establish a baseline. To measure depth, insert a sterile cotton swab at the deepest point of the wound; then hold the swab against a centimeter measuring guide. Next, document the wound's appearance, measurement, and drainage to allow comparison and evaluation of the wound by the entire staff. Make a sketch of the wound if needed.

Timesaving tip: To remember the six areas you need to address when describing a wound — **M**easurement, **P**ain, **W**armth, **R**edness, **S**welling, and **D**rainage — use the mnemonic "**M**y **P**atient's **W**ound **R**equires **S**ome **D**escription."

Timesaving tip: A recent trend in wound description is to photograph the wound (using color film and a camera that produces pictures instantly) during the initial assessment and then daily. Longer intervals may be adequate for long-term management. This supplement to your description is helpful for medical or legal purposes and elimi-

nates the difficulty of trying to determine from another nurse's description whether or not wounds have changed.

Diagnostic test results

A wound culture and sensitivity test may provide information about the nature of the infection, the appropriate antimicrobial therapy, and the causative organism, such as methicillin-resistant *Staphylococcus aureus* (MRSA) or other superresistant organisms. All wounds are contaminated to some degree. If sepsis occurs, the wound culture must match the blood culture before the wound infection can be deemed the cause of the sepsis. X-rays and scanning techniques may also be used to diagnose deep infections.

NURSING DIAGNOSIS

Common nursing diagnoses for a patient with a surgical wound infection include:
• High risk for infection (secondary) related to inadequate secondary defenses or effects of chronic disease
• Fluid volume deficit related to copious wound drainage and decreased fluid intake
• High risk for impaired skin integrity related to maceration secondary to wound drainage.

PLANNING

Based on the nursing diagnosis *high risk for infection,* develop appropriate patient outcomes. For example, your patient will:
• show no evidence of secondary infection while his wound heals
• have a normal temperature within 72 hours
• have a normal white blood cell (WBC) count within 72 hours

• show no signs of dehiscence
• have normal vital signs within 72 hours.

Based on the nursing diagnosis *fluid volume deficit,* develop appropriate patient outcomes. For example, your patient will:
• drink at least 3,000 ml of fluid every day
• maintain fluid intake that exceeds output plus insensible loss
• maintain normal urine output
• have electrolyte values remain within normal range.

Based on the nursing diagnosis *high risk for impaired skin integrity,* develop appropriate patient outcomes. For example, your patient will:
• show no evidence of skin breakdown in areas surrounding the wound
• show a decrease in wound size of 0.5 cm within 1 week
• demonstrate skill in care of wound or incision
• communicate feelings about change in body image.

IMPLEMENTATION

Treatment of wound infection requires vigorous antimicrobial therapy, removal of necrotic tissue, and drainage of abscessed cavities. (See *Medical care of the patient with wound infection,* page 290.)

Nursing interventions
• Follow appropriate infection-control precautions, such as body substance isolation or your hospital's established infection-control policy regarding wound infection.
• Never place an immunocompromised patient in the same room as a patient with a wound infection. Place a patient whose drainage cannot be contained in a private room.

• Assess the wound characteristics for indications of healing, such as reduction in purulent exudate, absence of slough, and increasing red, healthy granulation tissue. Monitor and record the size of the wound daily, and check that the wound is neither dry nor excessively moist from exudate.
• Check the surrounding skin for signs of irritation or breakdown, and prevent skin maceration near the wound site with moisture barriers if necessary.
• For difficult wounds, consult the enterostomal therapy nurse, clinical nurse specialist, or wound care specialist for the best course of action or type of dressings.
• Watch for signs and symptoms of secondary infection; notify the doctor if such signs and symptoms develop.
• Monitor vital signs, noting whether the patient's fever decreases with therapy.
• Review WBC count daily.
• Provide a diet high in protein, calories, vitamins, and minerals. Provide snacks as needed. Monitor serum albumin levels. Request a nutritional consultation if the results are borderline or low.
• Monitor the patient's hydration status. Record fluid intake and output, and observe for clinical signs and symptoms of dehydration, such as decreased skin turgor, oliguria, thirst, and sunken eyes.
• Notify the doctor or enterostomal specialist if the wound does not show signs of healing within a week (or sooner if you detect signs of worsening infection).

Patient teaching
• Review risk factors for developing wound infection, and teach the patient how to eliminate or reduce them.

Treatments

Medical care of the patient with wound infection

The patient with a wound infection requires treatment with an appropriate antimicrobial agent. Selection of the agent depends upon causative organisms and sensitivity testing. Follow-up testing is important because resistance may develop. To promote healing and to protect the surrounding skin from damage, keep the wound moist, clean, and free of exudate.

Cleaning the wound
Before inspecting and cleaning the wound, you should refer to your hospital's policy on the care of an infected wound or administer care as ordered. If the wound is filled with exudate, this care may include irrigating with 0.9% sodium chloride solution, using an 18G or 19G angiocath and a 30- or 35-ml syringe, and then covering the wound with a moist dressing.

If the wound has copious exudate, your hospital's policy on caring for an infected wound may include the use of an exudate-absorbing product to keep the wound clean or calcium alginates, copolymer starches, foams, or hypertonic saline dressings.

Applying a dressing
For a nonexudative infected wound, use a wet-to-moist dressing and hydrogel, which will provide moisture to the wound. Hydrocolloids are contraindicated in nonexudative infected wounds.

Moisture barriers for heavily exudative wounds include aloe vera, Hollihesive, Stomahesive, or Critic-Aid (for draining bowel wounds or pancreatic fluid).

With extensive drainage, a pouch may be more effective. Although a pouch may take longer to apply than a dressing, it needs to be changed less frequently (every 1 to 2 days).

Debriding the wound
Debridement of necrotic tissue is essential for proper wound healing. Surgical debridement to remove loose avascular tissue and slough can convert a chronic wound to an acute wound. If the patient is a poor surgical candidate, a doctor or specially trained nurse may debride the wound. A newer technique, enzymatic ointment debridement, is available by doctor's order only. Other newer debriding agents include chemical debriding agents and autolysis. Carefully follow manufacturer's guidelines for application.

• Teach wound care management to the patient and caregiver, stressing cleanliness and especially hand washing.
• Tell the patient to promptly report warning signs of worsening infection (fever, increased or sudden pain, increased malodorous or purulent drainage at the wound site, widened wound incision, or pressure or tightness within the wound). (See *Ensuring continued care for the patient with wound infection*.)

Discharge TimeSaver

Ensuring continued care for the patient with wound infection

Review the following teaching topics, referrals, and follow-up appointments to make sure that your patient is adequately prepared for discharge.

Teaching topics
Make sure that the following topics have been covered and that your patient's learning has been evaluated:
☐ explanation of wound infection, associated risk factors, and potential complications
☐ wound care management guidelines, especially cleanliness
☐ drug therapy, including precautions and possible adverse effects
☐ need for a diet high in protein, calories, vitamins, and minerals
☐ need for adequate hydration, including the amount of liquid that should be consumed daily
☐ warning signs of secondary infection that should be reported to the doctor
☐ sources of information and support.

Referrals
Make sure that the patient has been provided with necessary referrals to:
☐ social service agencies
☐ home health care services
☐ enterostomal therapist
☐ dietitian
☐ physical therapist.

Follow-up appointments
Make sure that the necessary follow-up appointments have been scheduled and that the patient has been notified:
☐ doctor
☐ diagnostic tests for reevaluation.

EVALUATION

To evaluate the patient's response to your care, gather reassessment data and compare this information to the patient outcomes specified in your plan of care. (See *Assessing failure to respond to wound infection therapy,* page 292.) Note whether the patient or caregiver can demonstrate effective wound management techniques and consider the following questions:
• Has the patient shown any evidence of secondary infection?
• Have the patient's temperature and vital signs returned to normal?

• Are his WBC count and erythrocyte sedimentation rate within normal limits?
• Does he drink at least 3,000 ml of fluid daily? Does his intake exceed output plus insensible loss?
• Does the skin surrounding the wound show any evidence of breakdown?
• Has the wound size decreased by 0.5 cm within 1 week?
• Does he show skill in caring for his wound?
• Can he discuss his feelings about his body image?

Evaluation TimeSaver

Assessing failure to respond to wound infection therapy

To evaluate a patient's failure to respond to interventions, use this checklist and consult the patient, the doctor, and members of the health care team. The doctor may need to evaluate drug therapy.

Factors interfering with compliance
☐ Unclear instructions
☐ Failure to provide written instructions
☐ Inadequate patient teaching
☐ Cognitive impairment
☐ Emotional instability
☐ Inadequate funds for medication or wound care products
☐ Knowledge deficit related to obtaining wound care products
☐ Inability to tolerate adverse effects of medication
☐ Inconvenient medication schedule
☐ Physical disability interfering with ability to manage wound
☐ Lack of caregiver to provide wound care
☐ Poor sanitary conditions in the home

Factors interfering with drug therapy
☐ Drug resistance

☐ Drug allergy
☐ Inappropriate choice of antimicrobial agent
☐ Renal impairment interfering with drug elimination

Conditions or factors interfering with treatment
☐ Malnutrition
☐ Diabetes mellitus
☐ Impaired blood supply
☐ Immunodeficiency due to disease or treatment
☐ Dehydration
☐ Depression
☐ Excessive moisture accumulation at wound site
☐ Obesity
☐ Corticosteroid therapy
☐ Friction or pressure applied to granulating tissue
☐ Failure to remove devitalized tissue

Meningitis

Meningitis is an inflammation of the meninges surrounding the brain and spinal cord. It may lead to such complications as visual impairment, optic neuritis, cranial nerve palsies, seizures, deafness, paresis or paralysis, hydrocephalus, pneumonia, encephalitis, endocarditis, coma, vasculitis, cerebral infarction, brain abscess, and syndrome of inappropriate secretion of antidiuretic hormone. Other complications, including epilepsy, mental retardation, hydrocephalus, and subdural effusions, occur primarily in children.

Causes

Meningitis is usually caused by bacteria, including *Neisseria meningitidis, Haemophilus influenzae,* and *Streptococcus pneumoniae.* Less frequently, the disorder is caused by viruses (aseptic viral meningitis), protozoa, or fungi. Bacterial meningitis is a medical emergency; failure to treat it promptly can result in death within a few days. Aseptic viral meningitis is typically self-limiting with the patient achieving a full recovery. (See *Meningitis risk factors,* right, and *What happens in meningitis,* page 294.)

ASSESSMENT

Your assessment should include careful consideration of the patient's health history, physical examination findings, and diagnostic test results.

Health history

The patient usually reports a severe headache; other complaints include stiff neck and back, malaise, photophobia, chills and, in some patients, vomiting, twitching, and seizures. The patient or a family member may also report an altered level of consciousness (LOC) with confusion or delirium. Vomiting and fever occur more often in children than in adults. An infant may also be fretful or listless, refuse to eat, and have bulging fontanels. A recent history of head trauma or surgery may also predispose the patient to meningitis.

Physical examination

Physical findings vary, depending on the severity of the meningitis. LOC may be altered. Initially, the patient may have mild symptoms, such as decreased attention span or memory impairment. As the disease progresses, symptoms may worsen, and the

FactFinder

Meningitis risk factors

Risk factors for meningitis include:
• skull fracture
• penetrating head wound
• lumbar puncture
• ventricular shunting procedures
• neurosurgery
• ear or sinus surgery
• bacteremia (especially from pneumonia, empyema, mastoiditis, osteomyelitis, and endocarditis)
• sinusitis or otitis media.

Viral meningitis
The following factors increase the risk of viral meningitis:
• viral infections, such as measles, mumps, infections caused by a herpes virus, and human immunodeficiency virus infection
• immunosuppression secondary to malnourishment, disease, radiation therapy, chemotherapy, or long-term corticosteroid therapy
• crowded living conditions.

patient may become disoriented and possibly comatose.

Timesaving tip: Always establish a sound baseline for LOC by using a standardized assessment tool such as the Glasgow Coma Scale. This will enable you to evaluate the patient more efficiently and avoid confusion over vague or subjective terms used by different caregivers.

Assessment of motor function may reveal muscle hypotonia early in the illness. Paresis or paralysis may occur later. The patient may also exhibit signs of meningeal irritation, such as Brudzinski's and Kernig's signs, ex-

What happens in meningitis

In meningitis, microorganisms invade the central nervous system through the bloodstream, through peripheral nerves, or from adjacent areas. Pathogens in the subarachnoid space then invade the cerebrospinal fluid (CSF) and inflame the pia mater, arachnoidea, and ventricles. Exudate accumulates over the brain and spinal cord and can extend to the cranial and peripheral nerves. Exudate may also block CSF flow and lead to hydrocephalus and increased intracranial pressure (ICP). The meningeal cells may then become edematous, which can further increase ICP, engorge the blood vessels in the meninges, disrupt the blood flow, and possibly cause thrombosis or rupture the vessel walls.

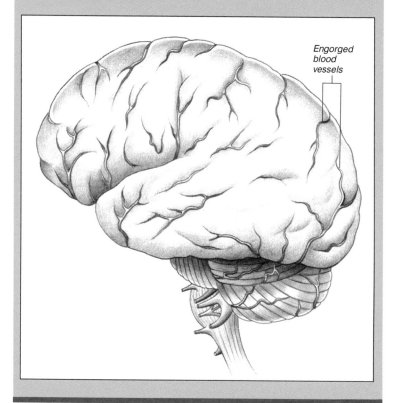

Engorged blood vessels

aggerated and symmetrical deep tendon reflexes, and opisthotonos. *(See Key signs of meningitis, page 296.)*

Cranial nerve assessment may reveal unequal pupils that are sluggish in response to light. If the patient's condition deteriorates, pupils may become fixed and dilated. Major deficits include ocular palsies involving cranial nerves III, IV, and VI; facial paresis involving cranial nerve VII; and deafness and vertigo involving cranial nerve VIII. Findings may also include facial weakness and ptosis. In meningococcal meningitis, inspection of the skin may reveal a petechial, purpuric, or ecchymotic rash on the lower part of the body.

The patient may have a fever (up to 105° F [40.6° C]), especially in viral meningitis. Tachycardia and tachypnea may be present unless intracranial pressure (ICP) is increased.

Diagnostic test results
The following tests may confirm a diagnosis of meningitis and confirm the extent of infection.
• Lumbar puncture shows elevated cerebrospinal fluid (CSF) pressure, cloudy and turbid CSF in bacterial meningitis, and clear and turbid CSF in viral meningitis. In bacterial meningitis, CSF protein level is increased and glucose concentration is usually decreased. In viral meningitis, protein levels are normal or slightly increased, and the glucose concentration is normal. Gram stain and culture can help identify the infecting bacterial organism.
• Blood, urine, and respiratory tract cultures may identify the source of the infection. A blood culture is positive in most patients.
• Chest X-rays may reveal pneumonitis or lung abscess, tubercular lesions, or granulomas secondary to fungal infection.

• White blood cell (WBC) count may indicate leukocytosis.
• Serum electrolyte levels may be abnormal.
• A computed tomography scan can rule out cerebral hematoma, hydrocephalus, hemorrhage, or tumor.

NURSING DIAGNOSIS

Common nursing diagnoses for a patient with meningitis include:
• Pain related to meningeal irritation
• Altered cerebral tissue perfusion related to increased ICP
• Hyperthermia related to infection
• High risk for injury related to altered LOC and seizures.

PLANNING

Based on the nursing diagnosis *pain*, develop appropriate patient outcomes. For example, your patient will:
• report relief from pain.

Based on the nursing diagnosis *altered cerebral tissue perfusion*, develop appropriate patient outcomes. For example, your patient will:
• demonstrate ICP equal to or less than 10 mm Hg
• achieve a Glasgow Coma Scale score of 11 to 15
• exhibit equal and reactive pupils
• exhibit a normal respiratory pattern
• maintain a systolic blood pressure within 20 mm Hg of acceptable baseline
• maintain a normal pulse rate
• experience no vomiting or seizures
• remain free of motor deficits.

Based on the nursing diagnosis *hyperthermia*, develop appropriate patient outcomes. For example, your patient will:
• exhibit a temperature less than 101.5° F (38.6° C)

Assessment TimeSaver

Key signs of meningitis

Eliciting Brudzinski's and Kernig's signs may help establish a diagnosis of meningitis.

Brudzinski's sign
Place the patient in a supine position; then put your hands behind her neck and lift her head toward her chest. If the patient has meningitis, she'll flex her hips and knees in response to passive neck flexion.

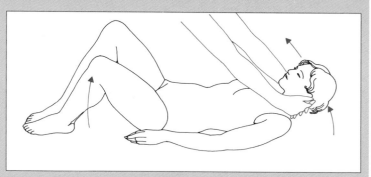

Kernig's sign
With the patient in a supine position, flex her leg at the hip to a 90-degree angle; then straighten her knee. Pain or resistance (caused by inflammation of the meninges and spinal roots) usually indicates meningitis.

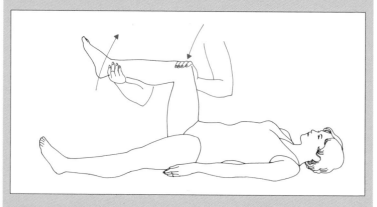

- avoid complications of hyperthermia
- maintain fluid intake approximately equal to output
- indicate increased comfort through verbal reports or behavior.

Based on the nursing diagnosis *high risk for injury,* develop appropriate patient outcomes. For example, your patient will:

- remain injury-free while in the hospital.

IMPLEMENTATION

Focus your nursing care on relieving pain and teaching the patient to cope with the debilitating acute stage of his illness. (See *Medical care of the patient with meningitis.*)

- Follow your hospital's infection-control policy until the causative organism is identified. Initiate appropriate isolation measures, such as respiratory isolation for bacterial meningitis and enteric precautions for viral meningitis.
- Continually assess neurologic function and vital signs, including a full cranial nerve assessment in every neurologic check.
- Monitor for signs of worsening meningitis, including increasing ICP, a deteriorating Glasgow Coma Scale score, temperature increase to above 105° F (40.6° C), pupillary changes, and motor dysfunction.
- Obtain arterial blood gas measurements and administer oxygen, as required. If your patient can't maintain a patent airway or adequate oxygenation, place him on mechanical ventilation.
- Maintain and monitor for adequate fluid intake, as prescribed, to avoid dehydration and control cerebral edema.
- Position the patient carefully to prevent joint stiffness and neck pain.

Treatments

Medical care of the patient with meningitis

Medical management of meningitis includes appropriate drug therapy and vigorous supportive care.

Drug therapy
Usually, meningitis has a bacterial origin and I.V. antibiotics are given for at least 2 weeks, followed by oral antibiotics. Penicillin is the drug of choice; other antibiotics usually include cefotaxime, ceftriaxone, and ampicillin. However, if the patient is allergic to penicillin, co-trimoxazole may be administered.

Other prescribed drugs may include the following:

- mannitol to decrease cerebral edema
- an anticonvulsant (usually given I.V.) or a sedative to reduce restlessness
- acetaminophen to relieve fever
- codeine (which will not mask neurologic symptoms) to relieve pain.

Supportive therapy
Supportive measures consist of bed rest, measures to reduce fever, and fluid therapy to prevent dehydration yet control cerebral edema.

Treatment may also be provided for any coexisting conditions, such as endocarditis or pneumonia. Rehabilitation may be required if neurologic complications develop.

Turn him often and assist him with range-of-motion exercises, but caution him to avoid isometric exercises

Discharge TimeSaver

Ensuring continued care for the patient with meningitis

Review the following teaching topics, referrals, and follow-up appointments to make sure that your patient is adequately prepared for discharge.

Teaching topics
Make sure that the following topics have been covered and that your patient's learning has been evaluated:
☐ explanation of the disorder, its management, and its associated risk factors
☐ medications, including adverse effects and need to complete entire course
☐ need for follow-up evaluation
☐ warning signs and symptoms that should be reported immediately.

Referrals
Make sure that the patient has been provided with necessary referrals to:
☐ social service agencies
☐ physical therapist (if rehabilitation is needed)
☐ occupational therapist.

Follow-up appointments
Make sure that the necessary follow-up appointments have been scheduled and that the patient has been notified:
☐ speech therapist, if necessary
☐ doctor
☐ diagnostic tests for reevaluation.

and hip flexion because these may increase ICP.

• Elevate the head of the bed 30 to 45 degrees to promote venous drainage and reduce ICP.

• Give the patient a mild laxative or stool softener as prescribed to prevent constipation and minimize the risk of increased ICP from straining during defecation.

• Monitor the patient's temperature at least every 2 hours, and administer antipyretic medications as prescribed. Tepid sponge baths or a hypothermia blanket may help control fever.

• Initiate seizure precautions. Pad the bed's side rails and keep them up. Make certain that suction equipment and an airway are on hand.

• Relieve headache with a nonnarcotic analgesic such as acetaminophen. Never flex the patient's neck; this can elevate ICP.

• Provide reassurance and support. The patient may be frightened by his illness and frequent lumbar punctures. Reassure the family that the delirium and behavior changes associated with meningitis usually disappear. If a severe neurologic deficit appears permanent, refer the patient to a rehabilitation program.

Patient teaching
• Explain the nature of the illness to the patient and family and discuss infection-control measures.

• Tell the patient with meningococcal meningitis and his family to notify anyone who had close contact with the patient; they'll need antibiotic prophylaxis and immediate medical attention if fever or other signs of meningitis develop. (See *Ensuring continued care for the patient with meningitis.*)

EVALUATION

Gather reassessment data and compare this information with the patient outcomes specified in your plan of care.

Teaching and counseling
Determine the effectiveness of your teaching and counseling by asking the following questions:
• Can the patient explain measures to control infection?
• Can he describe activities that may elevate ICP?
• Can he list warning signs and symptoms of increased ICP?

Physical condition
A physical examination and diagnostic tests will provide additional information. To evaluate the success of treatment, consider the following questions:
• Is the patient afebrile?
• Are results of CSF analysis and WBC count normal?
• Is the patient free of pain?
• Are his vital signs stable and within normal limits?
• Has his LOC returned to baseline?
• Is he free of neurologic deficits and injury?

Lower urinary tract infection

Cystitis (infection of the bladder) and urethritis (infection of the urethra) affect up to 20% of all women. In men, lower urinary tract infections (UTIs) are associated with anatomic or physiologic abnormalities and require close evaluation.

Although UTIs usually respond readily to treatment, resistance to antimicrobial therapy may cause bacterial flare-ups. Even small amounts of bacteria (10,000/ml or less) in a midstream urine specimen may indicate recurrence. Recurrent lower UTIs may also result from persistent infection (usually associated with renal calculi), chronic bacterial prostatitis, or a structural anomaly. Left untreated, chronic UTI can seriously damage the urinary tract lining or infect adjacent organs and structures. (See *UTI risk factors,* page 300).

Causes
Most UTIs result from ascending infection by a single microorganism in the bladder mucosa. Gram-negative enteric bacterium such as *Escherichia coli* and *Klebsiella* may cause acute cystitis; *Chlamydia trachomatis, Neisseria gonorrhoeae,* and herpes simplex virus may cause acute urethritis. Normal urination does not readily eliminate these bacteria.

Factors that may contribute to lower UTI include a neurogenic bladder, presence of an indwelling urinary catheter, or a fistula between the intestine and bladder due to simultaneous infection with multiple pathogens.

ASSESSMENT

The patient's health history and diagnostic testing usually provide the most important assessment information. Physical examination may yield ambiguous results.

FactFinder
UTI risk factors

A variety of factors can increase a patient's risk for urinary tract infection (UTI).

Natural anatomic variations
The female urethra is shorter than the male urethra (about half the length) and closer to the anus. This proximity allows bacterial entry into the urethra from the vagina, perineum, or rectum or from a sexual partner.

Pregnant women are especially prone to UTIs because of hormonal changes and the pressure of the enlarged uterus on the ureters, which holds urine and bacteria in the urinary tract.

In men, the prostate gland begins to enlarge around age 50. Enlargement may promote urine retention and bacterial growth.

Trauma or invasive procedures
Fecal matter, sexual intercourse, and instruments such as catheters and cystoscopes that are used in invasive procedures can introduce bacteria into the urinary tract.

Obstructions
A narrowed ureter or calculi lodged in the ureters or the bladder can obstruct urine flow. Slowed urine flow allows bacteria to remain and multiply, risking damage to the kidneys.

Reflux
Vesicoureteral reflux results when pressure inside the bladder (caused by coughing or sneezing) pushes a small amount of urine into the urethra. When the pressure returns to normal, the urine flows back into the bladder, bringing bacteria with it. A healthy vesicoureteral valve normally shuts off reflux. However, damage to the valve may allow for contamination.

Other risk factors
Urinary stasis can promote infection, which, if undetected, can spread to the entire urinary system. Because urinary tract bacteria thrive on sugars, diabetes mellitus is a risk factor.

Health history
The patient with a UTI may report urinary urgency and frequency, dysuria, bladder cramps or spasms, itching, a feeling of warmth during urination, or nocturia. A male patient may report urethral discharge. Other complaints include hematuria, low back pain, malaise, nausea, vomiting, pain or tenderness over the bladder, and chills.

Physical examination
Inspection may not reveal any abnormalities. Alternatively, it may show accompanying genital lesions, redness, swelling, or discharge. The patient's urine may be cloudy. In a patient with cystitis, palpation may detect suprapubic tenderness. (See *Comparing acute cystitis and acute urethritis.*)

Assessment TimeSaver

Comparing acute cystitis and acute urethritis

Use the chart below for a quick review of the distinguishing features of two types of urinary tract infection (UTI).

Disorder	Onset	Health history	Signs and symptoms	Physical examination findings
Acute cystitis	Abrupt, often severe symptoms	Recurrent UTIs, diaphragm use	Dysuria, frequency, urgency, possible hematuria	Suprapubic tenderness
Acute urethritis	Gradual, mild symptoms	New sexual partner or multiple partners; in males, may coexist with prostatitis	Dysuria, frequency, urgency, vaginal or urethral discharge	Possible lesions, redness, or discharge

Diagnostic test results

The following tests may help to diagnose lower UTI:

• A microscopic urinalysis may show red blood cell and white blood cell counts greater than 10 per high-power field.

• A clean-catch urinalysis may reveal a bacterial count greater than 100,000/ml, confirming UTI. Lower counts, however, don't necessarily rule out infection, especially if the patient is urinating frequently or has other symptoms.

• Voiding cystoureterography or intravenous pyelography may detect congenital anomalies that predispose the patient to UTIs.

• A blood test, a stained smear of urethral discharge, or a more specific test may be required to rule out a sexually transmitted disease.

NURSING DIAGNOSIS

Common nursing diagnoses for a patient with lower UTI include:

• Altered urinary elimination related to inflammation and infection

• High risk for infection related to recurrent UTIs

• Pain related to bladder spasms and dysuria secondary to the infection.

PLANNING

Based on the nursing diagnosis *altered urinary elimination*, develop appropriate patient outcomes. For example, your patient will:

• report that signs and symptoms of abnormal urine elimination have decreased

• report a return to a normal elimination pattern

• avoid complications.

Based on the nursing diagnosis *high risk for infection*, develop appropriate patient outcomes. For example, your patient will:

• remain free of recurrent UTIs, as evidenced by normal urinalysis results and an absence of signs and symptoms

Treatments

Medical care of the patient with lower UTI

Antimicrobial medications are the treatment of choice for most lower urinary tract infections (UTIs).

Course of therapy
The standard course of therapy is 7 to 10 days, but studies suggest that a larger single dose or a 3- to 5-day regimen may be sufficient to render the urine sterile. (A shorter regimen may not be effective in older patients). If, after 3 days of antimicrobial therapy, a urine culture shows infection, the bacteria is probably resistant and requires a different antimicrobial.

Acute uncomplicated UTI
A single dose of amoxicillin or co-trimoxazole may be effective for females with acute, uncomplicated UTI. A urine culture taken 1 to 2 weeks later will indicate whether the infection has been eradicated.

Infections associated with urinary obstruction
Recurrent infections associated with urinary obstructions, such as renal calculi, chronic prostatitis, or structural abnormalities, may require surgery. Prostatitis also requires long-term antimicrobial therapy.

• communicate an understanding of the need to report signs and symptoms of UTI.

Based on the nursing diagnosis *pain*, develop appropriate patient outcomes. For example, your patient will:
• describe how to use a topical antiseptic for pain relief
• confirm the absence of pain and discomfort as the infection clears.

IMPLEMENTATION

Focus your nursing care on helping the patient avoid reinfection. Emphasize the need to complete the entire course of antibiotics. (See *Medical care of the patient with lower UTI*.)

Nursing interventions
• Carefully collect all urine specimens for culture and sensitivity testing, and promptly take them to the laboratory.
• Administer prescribed antimicrobial therapy. Monitor for therapeutic effectiveness and adverse reactions.
• Assess the patient for complications of UTI, such as fever, flank pain, hematuria, chills, and sweats (may indicate pyelonephritis).
• Evaluate the patient's voiding pattern, any associated discomfort, urine color, and urine output.

Patient teaching
• Explain the nature, purpose, and possible adverse effects of antimicrobial therapy. Emphasize the importance of completing the prescribed course of therapy. If the patient is receiving long-term prophylaxis, encourage him to strictly adhere to the prescribed dosage.
• Explain that an uncontaminated midstream urine specimen is essen-

tial for accurate diagnosis. Before collection, teach the female patient how to clean her perineum properly and how to keep the labia separated during urination.

• Teach the patient how to reduce the risk of recurrent UTI. (See *Preventing UTIs.*)

• Urge the patient, especially the older patient, to drink at least 3,000 ml of fluid each day of treatment. Older patients may resist because it causes frequent trips, possibly up and down stairs, to urinate.

• Explain that fruit juices, especially cranberry juice, and oral doses of vitamin C may help acidify urine and enhance the medication's action. Encourage the patient to drink two glasses of cranberry juice per day. (See *Ensuring continued care for the patient with lower UTI*, page 304.)

EVALUATION

When evaluating the patient's response to your nursing care, gather reassessment data and compare this information to the patient outcomes specified in your plan of care. Consider the following questions.

Teaching and counseling

• Does the patient understand the importance of completing the entire course of antimicrobial therapy?

• Does he understand measures to prevent UTI recurrence?

• Does the patient understand the need to maintain adequate fluid consumption?

Physical condition

A physical examination and diagnostic tests will provide additional information. To evaluate the success of treatment, consider the following questions:

 Teaching TimeSaver
Preventing UTIs

To reduce the risk of repeated urinary tract infections (UTIs), instruct your patient in the following preventive measures:

• Tell the patient to drink 10 glasses of fluid a day to flush out harmful microorganisms. He should try to include two glasses of cranberry juice.

• Tell him to eat foods high in acid content to acidify the urine.

• Warn him to avoid, or at least minimize, the use of caffeine, carbonated beverages, and alcohol. Explain that these substances are bladder irritants.

• Instruct the patient on good hygiene practices. For women, this includes cleansing from front to back after each urination.

• Tell him to change underwear daily and wear cotton, which allows better ventilation.

• Advise a female patient prone to recurrent UTIs to urinate after sexual intercourse.

• Tell the patient to avoid wearing tight jeans and slacks, which can decrease air circulation.

• Recommend taking showers instead of tub baths to avoid microorganisms in the bath water that may enter the urinary tract and lead to infection.

• Tell the patient to urinate as soon as he feels the urge; delaying urination may lead to infection. The bladder should be emptied completely each time.

Discharge TimeSaver

Ensuring continued care for the patient with lower UTI

Review the following teaching topics, referrals, and follow-up appointments to make sure that your patient is adequately prepared for discharge.

Teaching topics
Make sure that the following topics have been covered and that your patient's learning has been evaluated:
☐ explanation of urinary tract infection (UTI)
☐ how to obtain a clean-catch specimen
☐ risk factors associated with UTI
☐ warning signs of recurrence or complications
☐ prevention measures
☐ compliance with medication regimen
☐ follow-up evaluation.

Referrals
Make sure that the patient has been provided with necessary referrals to:
☐ urologist.

Follow-up appointments
Make sure that the necessary follow-up appointments have been scheduled and that the patient has been notified:
☐ doctor
☐ laboratory tests for reevaluation.

• Has the patient reported that his normal urinary elimination pattern has been restored?
• Does he have a normal urinalysis and a negative urine culture?
• Are the signs and symptoms of UTI, including pain and discomfort, absent?

Gastroenteritis

An inflammation of the stomach and small intestine, gastroenteritis causes bowel hypermotility, leading to severe diarrhea and secondary depletion of intracellular fluid.

Gastroenteritis affects persons of all ages. In North America, it's second to the common cold as a cause of lost work time. In most patients, the disorder resolves with no aftereffects. However, persistent or untreated gastroenteritis can cause severe dehydration and loss of crucial electrolytes, which can lead to shock, vascular collapse, renal failure, and death. Mortality risk is greatest in children and older and debilitated patients.

Causes
Possible causes include bacteria (*Staphylococcus aureus, Salmonella, Shigella, Clostridium botulinum, C. perfringens,* and *Escherichia coli*), amoebae (especially *Entamoeba histolytica*), parasites (*Ascaris, Enterobius,* and *Trichinella spiralis*), viruses (adenoviruses, echoviruses, and coxsackieviruses), adverse drug reactions (chiefly to antibiotics), and food allergies. (See *Causes of infectious diarrhea*.)

Causes of infectious diarrhea

Different causes of infectious diarrhea produce distinct signs and symptoms.

***Campylobacter* species**
• *How transmitted:* fecal-oral; food and water; animals, including poultry, waterfowl, sheep, pigs, cattle, horses, cats, dogs, and monkeys, are the predominant source of infection
• *Illness duration:* 7 to 14 days, with 25% of patients experiencing a relapse of symptoms
• *Signs and symptoms:* diarrhea preceded by febrile prodromal period (in half of patients) with headache, malaise, backache, dizziness, fever of 102° to 104° F (38.9° to 40° C), abdominal pain, gross blood in stools (in 10% of patients), occult blood in stools (in almost all patients), and nausea but little vomiting

***Cryptosporidium* species**
• *How transmitted:* fecal-oral; food and water
• *Illness duration:* 36 to 72 hours in immunocompromised patients; can become serious
• *Signs and symptoms:* acute watery diarrhea without blood or mucus

Entamoeba histolytica
• *How transmitted:* fecal-oral; food and water; oral-anal contact
• *Illness duration:* indefinite if untreated
• *Signs and symptoms:* frequent fluid stools, often with blood or mucus

Escherichia coli
• *How transmitted:* fecal-oral
• *Illness duration:* 24 to 36 hours

• *Signs and symptoms:* from enterotoxigenic *E. coli* (traveler's diarrhea), voluminous, watery stools; from enteropathogenic *E. coli,* infant diarrhea; from enteroinvasive *E. coli,* dysenteric diarrhea

Giardia lamblia
• *How transmitted:* fecal-oral; food and water
• *Illness duration:* indefinite if untreated
• *Signs and symptoms:* abdominal distention, gassy diarrhea, and absence of fever, chills, and fecal blood

Norwalk virus
• *How transmitted:* fecal-oral; contaminated water or shellfish
• *Illness duration:* 1 to 2 days
• *Signs and symptoms:* vomiting, diarrhea (either may predominate), abdominal cramps, myalgia and, rarely, fever

Rotavirus
• *How transmitted:* fecal-oral
• *Illness duration:* usually about 7 days; occasionally up to 1 month
• *Signs and symptoms:* vomiting (1 to 5 days), diarrhea (4 to 7 days), fever (below 102° F [38.9° C]), upper respiratory infection (in up to 75% of patients), cough, nasal discharge, otitis media, and erythematous throat

***Salmonella* species**
• *How transmitted:* fecal-oral; contaminated food or water; domestic livestock, poultry in particular

(continued)

Causes of infectious diarrhea *(continued)*

• *Illness duration:* 1 to 7 days; occasionally 2 weeks
• *Signs and symptoms:* diarrhea (predominant symptom; some patients may develop dysentery); headache, malaise, abdominal pain, nausea, vomiting, fever, and chills; bacteremia (in fewer than 10% of patients)

***Shigella* species**
• *How transmitted:* fecal-oral; food and water

• *Illness duration:* 4 to 7 days
• *Signs and symptoms:* mild diarrhea to severe dysentery with tenesmus; biphasic pattern in symptoms; first phase — fever, voluminous liquid stools, abdominal pain; second phase — more frequent, smaller stools (with grossly apparent blood in 40% of patients); respiratory symptoms in either phase; in children, occasionally seizures and other neurologic symptoms with fever above 104° F (40° C)

Sites of infection
The illustration below shows which pathogens occur in the small bowel and which occur in the colon.

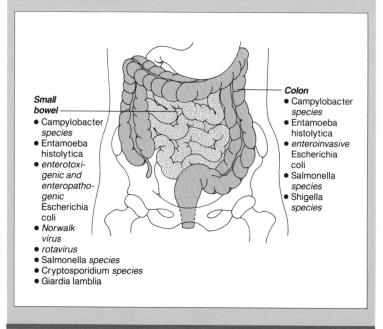

Small bowel
• Campylobacter *species*
• Entamoeba histolytica
• *enterotoxigenic and enteropathogenic* Escherichia coli
• *Norwalk virus*
• *rotavirus*
• Salmonella *species*
• Cryptosporidium *species*
• Giardia lamblia

Colon
• Campylobacter *species*
• Entamoeba histolytica
• *enteroinvasive* Escherichia coli
• Salmonella *species*
• Shigella *species*

ASSESSMENT

Your assessment should include careful consideration of the patient's health history, physical examination findings, and diagnostic test results.

Health history

Typically, the patient reports an acute onset of diarrhea accompanied by abdominal pain and discomfort. He may complain of cramping, nausea, and vomiting. He may also report malaise, fatigue, anorexia, fever, abdominal distention, and rumbling in his lower abdomen. In severe cases, the patient may experience rectal burning, tenesmus, and bloody mucoid stools.

Try to determine if the patient had contaminated food or water. Did people who dined with him experience similar signs and symptoms? Ask the patient to describe recent travels. (See *Gastroenteritis risk factors*.)

Physical examination

Inspection may reveal slight abdominal distention. Auscultation may reveal hyperactive bowel sounds. Temperature may be normal or elevated and signs of dehydration may be present.

Diagnostic test results

Laboratory studies to identify the causative bacteria, parasites, or amoebae include Gram stain, stool culture (by direct rectal swab), and blood culture.

NURSING DIAGNOSIS

Common nursing diagnoses for a patient with gastroenteritis include:
• Fluid volume deficit related to decreased oral intake and excessive flu-

FactFinder

Gastroenteritis risk factors

If the patient's chief complaint is diarrhea, note the presence of the following risk factors:
• recent hiking or camping
• recent travel to underdeveloped regions or tropical climates
• homosexual activity (in men)
• day care center attendance
• ingestion of untreated water
• ingestion of raw or undercooked beef, poultry, or seafood
• ingestion of creamy, unprocessed, or nonrefrigerated items, such as custard, pastry, mayonnaise, salad dressing, milk, or gravy.

id loss secondary to vomiting and diarrhea
• Diarrhea related to effects of inflammation and infection in the GI tract.

PLANNING

Based on the nursing diagnosis *fluid volume deficit*, develop appropriate patient outcomes. For example, your patient will:
• consume at least 3,000 ml of fluid every 24 hours unless contraindicated
• show no signs or symptoms of dehydration
• maintain stable vital signs
• have normal electrolyte levels
• show normal skin turgor and moist mucous membranes
• maintain normal fluid balance.

Based on the nursing diagnosis *diarrhea*, develop appropriate patient

outcomes. For example, your patient will:
• comply with antidiarrheal treatment
• avoid complications of diarrhea, including dehydration and skin breakdown in the anal area
• maintain normal weight
• regain normal bowel patterns before discharge.

IMPLEMENTATION

Treatment focuses on eliminating the causative organism and restoring the patient's fluid status. (See *Medical care of the patient with gastroenteritis.*)

Nursing interventions
Follow your hospital's infection-control policy. The Centers For Disease Control and Prevention recommends enteric precautions for patients with acute infectious diarrhea. If the patient is an infant, a young child, or an adult incapable of practicing proper hygiene, remove him to a private room.
• Plan uninterrupted rest periods for the patient.
• Monitor the patient's fluid status carefully. Assess vital signs at least every 4 hours, weigh him daily, and record intake and output. Check serum electrolyte and hematocrit levels, and look for signs of dehydration.
• If dehydration occurs, administer oral and I.V. fluids as prescribed. If a potassium supplement is added to the I.V. solution, monitor for hyperkalemia.

Timesaving tip: You can quickly evaluate your patient's fluid status by checking for signs of dehydration such as sunken eyes, dry skin and mucous membranes, furrowed tongue, and skin turgor. Inquire about diarrhea and cramping,

and listen for improvement in bowel sounds.
• Replace lost fluids and electrolytes with broth, ginger ale, tea, or diluted fruit juices. Warn the patient to avoid milk and milk products, which may provoke nausea.
• Administer medications as prescribed. Correlate administration with the patient's meals and activities.
• To ease anal irritation caused by diarrhea, clean the area carefully and apply a repellent ointment, such as petroleum jelly. Warm sitz baths and application of witch hazel compresses can soothe irritation.
• Wash your hands thoroughly after caring for the patient.
• If you suspect food poisoning, contact public health authorities to investigate suspected contaminated food.

Patient teaching
• Teach the patient about gastroenteritis, its symptoms and causes. Explain why a stool specimen may be necessary for diagnosis.
• Instruct the patient to wait until his diarrhea subsides and then to start drinking unsweetened fruit juice, tea, bouillon, or other clear broths. Tell him to avoid solid foods for at least 12 hours and then to try eating bland soft foods, such as cooked cereal, rice, or applesauce. Tell him to avoid spicy, greasy, or high-roughage foods, such as whole-grain products, raw fruits, or raw vegetables, which can cause renewed diarrhea.
• Review drug regimens, making sure the patient understands desired effects and possible adverse effects.
• If the patient expects to travel, advise him to pay close attention to what he eats and drinks, especially when visiting developing nations.
• Review proper hygiene measures to prevent recurrence and tell the pa-

Treatments

Medical care of the patient with gastroenteritis

Drug therapy for gastroenteritis may include antidiarrheals, antiemetics, or antibiotics.

Antidiarrheals

Antidiarrheals, such as bismuth subsalicylate, typically are used as the first-line defense against diarrhea. If necessary, other antidiarrheals, such as camphorated opium tincture (paregoric), diphenoxylate with atropine, and loperamide, may be prescribed.

Antiemetics

Antiemetics (oral, I.M., or rectal suppository), such as prochlorperazine or trimethobenzamide, may be prescribed for severe vomiting. However, they should be avoided in patients with viral or bacterial gastroenteritis.

Antibiotics

Specific antibiotic administration is restricted to patients who have bacterial gastroenteritis, as identified by diagnostic tests. Metronidazole usually is prescribed for symptomatic amebiasis. Iodoquinol may be prescribed after the course of metronidazole is completed to eradicate intraluminal cysts.

---

tient to thoroughly cook foods, especially pork. Instruct him to refrigerate perishable foods such as milk, mayonnaise, potato salad, and cream-filled pastry; to always wash his hands with warm water and soap before handling food, especially after using the bathroom; to clean utensils thoroughly; and to eliminate flies and roaches in the home. (See *Ensuring continued care for the patient with gastroenteritis,* page 310.)

EVALUATION

When evaluating the patient's response to nursing care, gather reassessment data and compare this information to the patient outcomes specified in your plan of care.

Teaching and counseling

Begin by evaluating the effectiveness of your teaching and counseling. Consider the following questions:
• Does the patient understand what caused the gastroenteritis?
• Does he understand the importance of maintaining adequate hydration and complying with antidiarrheal treatment?
• Does he understand steps to prevent a recurrence?

Physical condition

A physical examination and diagnostic tests will provide additional information. To evaluate the success of treatment, consider the following questions:
• Is the patient's fluid balance normal?
• Has he avoided complications of diarrhea?

Discharge TimeSaver

Ensuring continued care for the patient with gastroenteritis

Review the following teaching topics, referrals, and follow-up appointments to make sure that your patient is adequately prepared for discharge.

Teaching topics
Make sure that the following topics have been covered and that your patient's learning has been evaluated:
□ medications
□ need for rest and fluids
□ dietary measures
□ warning signs and symptoms that should be reported
□ prevention of recurrence.

Referrals
Make sure that the patient has been provided with necessary referrals to:

□ public health authorities as warranted.

Follow-up appointments
Make sure that the necessary follow-up appointments have been scheduled and that the patient has been notified:
□ doctor
□ entertostomal specialist, if warranted, on reappearance of symptoms (may be antibiotic-related colitis caused by superresistant *Clostridium difficile*).

• Has he regained a normal bowel elimination pattern and bowel sounds?

Sepsis

When microorganisms invade the body, they trigger an inflammatory response. The inflammatory response continuum begins with infection and progresses through sepsis, severe sepsis, and septic shock. Sepsis is characterized by tachycardia, tachypnea, altered temperature, and leukocytosis. (See *Understanding sepsis*.)

Causes

Sepsis occurs secondary to an infection caused by invading microorganisms, including bacteria, fungi, viruses, rickettsiae, mycoplasmas, and chlamydiae.

ASSESSMENT

Since sepsis can result from an infection anywhere in the body, a thorough history and physical examination is needed to pinpoint the source and severity of infection. Findings should be supported by diagnostic test results.

Health history

Usually the patient will report fever, chills, pain, warmth, redness, or swelling. However, the patient's chief complaint may not suggest infection. For example, in an older patient, an episode of confusion may be the only signal of a health problem.

Depending upon the site of infection, other complaints may include rash, headache, photophobia, stiff neck, vomiting, chest pain, diarrhea, frequent or painful urination, cough, and shortness of breath.

Understanding sepsis

Learning the new standard definitions of sepsis, severe sepsis, and septic shock will help you distinguish each stage of illness. (Note that the term septicemia is no longer used to describe systemic disease associated with sepsis.) The diagram below shows the relationship between systemic inflammatory response syndrome (SIRS), sepsis, and infection.

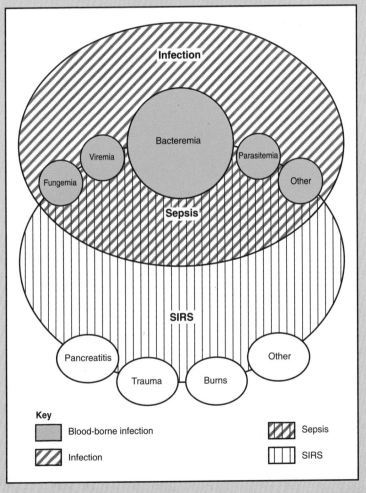

(continued)

Understanding sepsis *(continued)*

Sepsis
In sepsis, infection is accompanied by two or more of the following conditions:
• temperature above 101° F (38° C) or below 97° F (36° C)
• heart rate greater than 90 beats/minute
• respiratory rate greater than 20 breaths/minute or partial pressure of arterial carbon dioxide less than 32 mm Hg
• white blood cell count greater than 12,000 mm³, less than 4,000 mm³, or greater than 10% immature neutrophils (bands).

Severe sepsis
In addition to the symptoms of sepsis, the patient may experience hypoperfusion, hypotension, or major organ-system dysfunction. Hypoperfusion and perfusion abnormalities may include lactic acidosis, oliguria, or an acute alteration in mental status.

Septic shock
The patient in septic shock has hypotension that's unresponsive to fluid resuscitation.

SIRS
SIRS refers to widespread inflammation in patients with infection. It includes sepsis, severe sepsis, and septic shock. SIRS may also result from noninfectious disorders, such as burns, trauma, and pancreatitis.

Neonates, because of their immature immune systems, and older patients, because of chronic illness and a somewhat diminished immune system, are more likely to develop sepsis.

Physical examination
Determining the site and cause of infection requires a review of several body systems. (See *Sepsis assessment and monitoring guide*.)

Diagnostic test results
Smears, cultures, and serologic tests are used to diagnose sepsis. Note that bacteremia is present only in about half of patients with sepsis.

NURSING DIAGNOSIS

Common nursing diagnoses for a patient with sepsis include:
• Altered protection related to decreased immune response, effects of invasive procedures, and medication therapy
• Altered temperature related to infection
• Fluid volume deficit related to decreased fluid intake, systemic inflammatory response syndrome, and persistent hyperthermia.

PLANNING

Based on the nursing diagnosis *altered protection,* develop appropriate

Sepsis assessment and monitoring guide

Since sepsis can result from an infection anywhere in the body, assessment should include a thorough history, physical examination, and review of diagnostic test results.

Health history
Note the presence of the following risk factors:
• chronic diseases such as diabetes mellitus, cirrhosis, and congestive heart failure
• prosthetic valves, grafts, and joints, which are potential infection breeding grounds
• recent surgery, invasive procedures, or dental extractions
• prior antibiotic therapy (may lead to resistant strains of bacteria or an overgrowth of fungal microorganisms)
• corticosteroid use (may mask localized symptoms of infection until sepsis develops)
• immunosuppressive therapy for transplantation or oncologic disorders
• a history of I.V. drug abuse. (Contaminated needles can cause bloodstream infections, and I.V. drug abuse may itself contribute to immune system depression.)

Also ask the patient about diet and lifestyle. Recent food intake may have caused GI bacterial infections, especially in patients with acquired immunodeficiency syndrome and other immunosuppressing conditions. Ask about types of food, time of ingestion, and method of preparation and storage.

Inquire about lifestyle factors, including travel, sports, types of pets, and living arrangements. Note the patient's work setting, such as a hospital, laboratory, pet shop, or construction site. (Different work sites may implicate different pathogens.) Nursing home residents may be exposed to specific colonizing flora.

Physical examination
Your physical examination should include a check of vital signs; inspection of the skin, head, and neck; and assessment of the patient's neurologic, cardiovascular, respiratory, musculoskeletal, and lymphatic systems.

Vital signs
Note the presence of the following clinical findings:
• temperature above 101° F (38° C) or below 97° F (36° C)
• heart rate greater than 90 beats/ minute
• respiratory rate greater than 20 breaths/minute
• systolic blood pressure less than 90 mm Hg or a reduction of 40 mm Hg from baseline (indicates sepsis-induced hypotension in the absence of other causes).

Integumentary system
Inspect the skin for lesions. Skin lesions may be indicative of primary infection, as in cellulitis. Lesions may also result from the cutaneous involvement in mycotic or systemic bacterial infections — for example, petechiae associated with meningococcemia and purpura associated with endocarditis. Lesions from burns,

(continued)

Sepsis assessment and monitoring guide *(continued)*

ulcers, or animal bites may become secondarily infected.

Inspection of the nails may reveal red or brown linear streaks, which are associated with endocarditis. Drainage or redness at the entry sites of vascular access catheters may indicate catheter-related sepsis.

Head and neck

Examine the patient's mouth and teeth for irregularities. Poor dentition and periodontal disease may be an entry point for endocarditis.

Neurologic system

Examine the patient for signs of meningitis and brain abscess. Headache, nuchal rigidity, Brudzinski's sign, and Kernig's sign suggest meningitis. Focal neurologic deficits, such as hemiparesis, suggest brain abscess. Observe for acute changes in mental status, which may be the only readily apparent signs of sepsis, especially in older patients.

Cardiovascular system

Auscultation may reveal a murmur, suggesting endocarditis. Diminished peripheral pulses indicate peripheral vasoconstriction or decreased cardiac output, possible indications of sepsis. Falling central venous pressure may indicate a loss of intravascular volume and consequent fluid volume deficit.

Respiratory system

An early sign of sepsis, hyperventilation may be detected before fever or chills. Other important findings include increased sputum production; changes in sputum color or odor; rales, wheezes, or rhonchi; dullness to percussion; and dyspnea.

Musculoskeletal system

Acute onset of impaired mobility and pain may suggest joint involvement.

Genitourinary system

Cloudy, foul-smelling urine points to a urinary tract infection. Flank tenderness suggests kidney infection. Oliguria (urine output less than 0.5 ml/kg/hour) indicates severe sepsis. Note that the presence of a suprapubic or urinary catheter increases the risk of a urinary tract infection.

Palpate the abdomen. Rebound tenderness and involuntary rigidity may indicate peritoneal inflammation secondary to an abdominal infection.

Lymphatic system

Palpable nodes, especially supraclavicular, preauricular, or postauricular, suggest infection.

Diagnostic test results

• Complete blood count with differential may show a white blood cell count greater than $12,000/mm^3$, less than $4,000 \ mm^3$, or greater than 10% immature (band) forms.
• Arterial blood gas (ABG) analysis may reveal partial pressure of arterial carbon dioxide less than 32 mm Hg, indicating hyperventilation or hypoxia. Blood pH less than 7.45 (venous) or 7.41 (arterial) suggests acidosis.

Sepsis assessment and monitoring guide *(continued)*

Monitoring

Once sepsis has been diagnosed, monitor the patient regularly. Progression to septic shock may be rapid.

• Watch for signs of irritation, restlessness, disorientation, or confusion, which may indicate decreasing cerebral perfusion.

• Palpate peripheral pulses. Note amplitude. Weak pulses may indicate peripheral vasoconstriction or decreased cardiac output.

• Monitor central venous pressure.

• Monitor blood pressure every 2 to 4 hours (more frequently if the patient is hemodynamically unstable). Watch for early indicators of shock, such as normal mean arterial pressure with a widening pulse pressure. Hypotension and tachycardia may accompany severe shock.

• Auscultate for heart sounds at four valvular sites.

• Assess skin color and capillary refill. Note skin that is cool and cyanotic and a capillary refill time longer than 2 seconds.

• Monitor all external invasive sites, such as I.V. lines and indwelling urinary catheters.

• Monitor intake and output. Output less than 30 ml/hour suggests decreased renal perfusion or decreased intravascular volume.

• Measure urine specific gravity. Note increased levels.

• Monitor blood urea nitrogen and creatinine levels for elevations.

• Weigh patient daily.

• Monitor breath sounds. Note crackles, rhonchi, and decreased breath sounds. Note the color, consistency, and amount of pulmonary secretions.

• Monitor respiratory rate, rhythm, and effort. Note tachypnea, hyperventilation, rapid shallow breathing, or respiratory distress.

• Obtain ABG values as ordered. Evaluate for abnormal values.

• Record the patient's temperature every 4 hours.

---

patient outcomes. For example, your patient will:

• show no evidence of secondary infection throughout therapy

• demonstrate use of protective measures, such as conserving energy, maintaining a balanced diet, and receiving adequate rest

• demonstrate personal cleanliness and maintain a clean environment

• show increased strength and resistance

• not develop infectious complications

• list signs and symptoms of complications.

Based on the nursing diagnosis *altered temperature,* develop appropriate patient outcomes. For example, your patient will:

• regain temperature within normal limits within 72 hours

• not develop dehydration or other complications associated with hyperthermia

• state measures to prevent dehydration.

- maintain an intake of at least 3,000 ml of fluid per day
- maintain fluid intake that exceeds output plus insensible loss.

IMPLEMENTATION

Therapy for sepsis is directed toward eliminating the offending microorganisms, blocking the effects of toxins, and supporting major organs affected by the disorder. (See *Medical care of the patient with sepsis.*)

Nursing interventions
- Monitor the patient for indications of improvement or deterioration.
- Administer prescribed I.V. fluids as prescribed. Capillary leak associated with sepsis may necessitate large fluid volume, and hyperthermia increases insensible loss.
- Administer antimicrobial therapy, vasopressors, and positive inotropic agents as prescribed. Monitor for drug effectiveness and adverse reactions.
- Administer antipyretics as prescribed. Note that the doctor may not order an antipyretic because suppression of the patient's temperature may interfere with the body's normal protective mechanisms.
- Turn the patient every 1 to 2 hours to mobilize secretions.
- Monitor nutritional intake. If adequate oral nutrition cannot be maintained, enteral or parenteral nutrition will be necessary. Keep in mind that metabolic demands increase with stress and fever.
- Administer analgesics, as prescribed, for pain relief.
- Provide scrupulous aseptic technique and follow your hospital's policy concerning removal of invasive devices such as a peripheral I.V. line or an indwelling catheter.

Treatments
Medical care of the patient with sepsis

Early detection and diagnosis of sepsis are crucial. Measures may include drug therapy to eliminate infection, surgery, and administration of fluids.

Drug therapy
Antimicrobials are always included in treatment. Specific drug selection is based on the causative organism, if known.

A wide range of experimental drugs may be used to inhibit the mediators of sepsis. These therapies are aimed at interrupting the septic cascade and include inhibitors of inflammation, modulators of coagulation, prostaglandins, and others.

Surgery
Surgical excision or drainage of the nidus of infection may be necessary.

Fluid therapy
Crystalloid fluids are administered as needed to maintain fluid volume.

Additional treatments
Vasopressors and positive inotropic agents may supplement volume expansion. Supplemental oxygen or assisted ventilation may help correct hypoxia and acidosis.

Based on the nursing diagnosis *fluid volume deficit,* develop appropriate patient outcomes. For example, your patient will:

Discharge TimeSaver

Ensuring continued care for the patient with sepsis

Review the following teaching topics, referrals, and follow-up appointments to make sure that your patient is adequately prepared for discharge.

Teaching topics
Make sure that the following topics have been covered and that your patient's learning has been evaluated:
☐ explanation of the disorder, its management, and its associated risk factors
☐ medications, including adverse effects and the need to complete entire course of antimicrobial drugs
☐ dressing changes
☐ need for follow-up evaluation
☐ warning signs and symptoms that should be reported immediately.

Referrals
Make sure that the patient has been provided with necessary referrals to:
☐ social service agencies
☐ physical therapist (if needed)
☐ rehabilitation center (if warranted)
☐ home health care agency.

Follow-up appointments
Make sure that the necessary follow-up appointments have been scheduled and that the patient has been notified:
☐ doctor
☐ diagnostic tests for reevaluation.

Patient teaching
• Inform the patient and caregiver about the nature of the infection, sepsis, and associated treatment.
• Help the patient plan for follow-up care.
• Instruct the patient in the use of an incentive spirometer, if necessary.
• Tell the patient with an indwelling device to immediately report pain, fever, chills, or unusual sensations at the site.
• Teach the patient about the purpose, correct dosage, schedule, and adverse reactions of antimicrobial drugs. Emphasize the need to complete the entire course of antimicrobial therapy.
• Teach the patient discharged with an indwelling medical device about appropriate care techniques.

Timesaving tip: If the patient will require prolonged antibiotic therapy or rehabilitative care, begin planning his discharge and patient teaching as soon as possible. This will prevent a delay in the patient's discharge, dramatically cut your patient-teaching time, and promote compliance. (See *Ensuring continued care for the patient with sepsis.*)

EVALUATION
When evaluating the patient's response to your nursing care, gather reassessment data and compare it with the patient outcomes specified in your plan of care.

Teaching and counseling
Begin by evaluating the effectiveness of your teaching and counseling.

Document statements by the patient indicating:

• understanding of the nature of the infection, sepsis, and associated treatment

• intent to comply with follow-up care

• knowledge of how to use an incentive spirometer, if necessary

• knowledge of how to care for indwelling medical devices, if applicable

• understanding of the need to report pain, fever, chills, or unusual sensations at the site of an indwelling device

• awareness of the importance of protective measures, such as obtaining sufficient rest and maintaining a balanced diet

• willingness to comply with the antibiotic drug regimen and intent to complete the entire course of therapy.

Physical condition

A physical examination and diagnostic tests will provide additional information. Continue your evaluation by reassessing the patient's physical condition. Consider the following questions:

• Did the patient avoid secondary infection throughout the course of therapy?

• Did he experience any complications of therapy during hospitalization?

• Did his temperature return to within normal limits within 72 hours?

• Did he develop complications associated with hyperthermia, such as dehydration?

• Did he maintain fluid intake of at least 3,000 ml/day?

• Has his hemodynamic status remained within normal parameters?

• Has his neurologic status remained within normal parameters?

Osteomyelitis

A pyogenic bone infection, osteomyelitis commonly results from traumatic injury combined with an acute infection originating elsewhere in the body. Although osteomyelitis usually remains a local infection, it can spread through the bone to the marrow, cortex, and periosteum.

Osteomyelitis may be chronic or acute. The prognosis for acute osteomyelitis is good if the patient receives prompt treatment. The prognosis for chronic osteomyelitis is less favorable. (See *Key points about osteomyelitis.*)

Causes

Pyogenic bacteria are the most common agents, but the disease also may result from fungi or viruses. Typically, these organisms find a culture site in a recent hematoma or a weakened area, such as a site of local infection. From there, they spread directly to bone.

ASSESSMENT

Your assessment should include careful consideration of the patient's health history, physical examination findings, and diagnostic test results.

Health history

The patient may report a sudden, severe pain in a bone, accompanied by chills, nausea, or malaise. He may describe the pain as unrelieved by rest and worse with motion. Note whether he has a history of previous injury, surgery, or primary infection.

Usually, chronic osteomyelitis produces similar effects as acute forms of the disorder. However, chronic osteomyelitis can persist intermittently for years, flaring up spontaneously after minor trauma. For some patients, the only sign of chronic infection may be persistent pus drainage from an old pocket in a sinus tract.

Physical examination

Assessment of vital signs may reveal tachycardia and a fever. Inspection may reveal swelling and restricted movement over the infection site. The patient may refuse to use the affected area. Palpation may detect tenderness and warmth over the infection site.

Diagnostic test results

• White blood cell (WBC) count shows leukocytosis.
• Erythrocyte sedimentation rate is increased.
• Blood culture can identify the pathogen.
• X-rays may show bone involvement only after the disease has been active for some time, usually for 2 to 3 weeks.
• Bone scans can detect early infection.

NURSING DIAGNOSIS

Common nursing diagnoses for a patient with osteomyelitis include:
• Activity intolerance related to pain, weakness, and fatigue secondary to infection
• Impaired physical mobility related to pain, bed rest, and immobilization devices
• Pain related to bone necrosis and inflammation.

PLANNING

Based on the nursing diagnosis *activity intolerance*, develop appropriate patient outcomes. For example, your patient will:

FactFinder
Key points about osteomyelitis

• *Infection sites:* In children, the most common disease sites include the lower end of the femur and the upper end of the tibia, humerus, and radius. In adults, the disease commonly localizes in the pelvis and vertebrae.
• *Causative organisms:* The most common causative organism is *Staphylococcus aureus*; others include *Streptococcus pyogenes*, *Pseudomonas aeruginosa*, *Escherichia coli*, and *Proteus vulgaris*.
• *Complications:* Untreated osteomyelitis may lead to chronic infection, skeletal and joint deformities, disturbed bone growth (in children), and impaired mobility.

• seek assistance when performing activities
• adhere to prescribed activity restrictions to minimize tissue damage
• report reduction in fatigue
• regain normal activity level.
    Based on the nursing diagnosis *impaired physical mobility*, develop appropriate patient outcomes. For example, your patient will:
• maintain normal muscle strength and joint range of motion
• avoid complications, such as contractures, venous stasis, and skin breakdown
• state feelings about limitations
• regain normal physical mobility after completion of therapeutic regimen.
    Based on the nursing diagnosis *pain*, develop appropriate patient outcomes. For example, your patient will:

Treatments

Medical care of the patient with osteomyelitis

The treatment regimen depends largely on whether the patient's condition is acute or chronic.

Treating acute conditions

To decrease internal bone pressure and prevent infarction, treatment for acute osteomyelitis begins before confirmation of the diagnosis. Treatment measures may include:
• surgical drainage of the infection site, often by needle aspiration, to relieve pressure and remove sequestrum
• immobilization of the infected bone with a cast or traction
• administration of analgesics and I.V. fluids
• administration of I.V. antibiotics (usually a penicillinase-resistant agent, such as nafcillin or oxacillin; in chronic osteomyelitis, antibiotics may be combined with rifampin), which may be followed by oral administration of antibiotics
• hyperbaric oxygen therapy to increase the activity of naturally occurring white blood cells
• use of free tissue transfers and local muscle flaps to fill dead space and increase blood supply.

Treating chronic conditions

The patient with chronic osteomyelitis may require prolonged hospitalization. He may also undergo surgery — sequestrectomy to remove dead bone and saucerization to promote drainage and decrease pressure. Unrelieved chronic osteomyelitis in an arm or a leg may require amputation.

• notify a caregiver immediately when pain occurs
• rate his pain on a scale of 1 to 10, with 1 being no pain and 10 being severe pain
• express relief from pain.

IMPLEMENTATION

Focus your nursing care on controlling infection, protecting the bone from injury, and providing support. (See *Medical care of the patient with osteomyelitis.*)

Nursing interventions

• Use strict aseptic technique when changing dressings and irrigating wounds.
• If the patient has a cast, check circulation and drainage in the affected limb. If a wet spot appears on the cast, circle it with a marking pen and note the time of its appearance (on the cast). Check the circled spot at least every 4 hours. Assess and report increasing drainage as appropriate.

Timesaving tip: To quickly estimate drainage, keep in mind that one drop of blood will cause a 3″ (7.5-cm) stain on the cast.
• Monitor vital signs to help detect excessive blood loss.
• If the patient is in skeletal traction for compound fractures, cover the pin insertion points with small, dry dressings. Tell him not to touch the skin around the pins and wires.
• Provide a diet high in protein and vitamin C to promote healing.
• Support the affected limb with firm pillows. Keep it level with the body; don't let it sag.
• Provide thorough skin care. Turn the patient gently every 2 hours.
• Provide complete cast care. Support the cast with firm pillows, and petal the edges with pieces of adhe-

Discharge TimeSaver

Ensuring continued care for the patient with osteomyelitis

Review the following teaching topics, referrals, and follow-up appointments to make sure that your patient is adequately prepared for discharge.

Teaching topics
Make sure that the following topics have been covered and that your patient's learning has been evaluated:
□ nature of the disorder, associated risk factors, and potential complications
□ medications, including precautions and possible adverse effects
□ warning signs and symptoms that should be reported to the doctor
□ need for follow-up evaluation
□ rest and activity guidelines.

Referrals
Make sure that the patient has been provided with necessary referrals to:
□ social service department
□ occupational therapist
□ physical therapist
□ home health care nurse
□ community sources of support.

Follow-up appointments
Make sure that the necessary follow-up appointments have been scheduled and that the patient has been notified:
□ doctor
□ physical therapist
□ occupational therapist.

---

sive tape or moleskin to smooth rough edges.
• Protect the patient from falls or other trauma.
• Administer prescribed analgesics for pain.
• Note new pain daily. This symptom may indicate the spread of infection.
• Carefully monitor drainage, including drainage accumulated in suctioning equipment. Keep containers of the prescribed irrigant nearby, and write the date, the time, and your initials on the label when opening one. Monitor the amount of solution instilled and drained during wound care.
• Watch for signs of pressure ulcer formation. Also watch for sudden malpositioning of the affected limb, which may indicate fracture.

Patient teaching
• Explain all test and treatment procedures.
• Review prescribed medications, and instruct the patient to report any adverse reactions to the doctor.
• Tell him to report sudden pain, unusual bone sensations and noises (crepitus), or deformity immediately.
• Before surgery, explain all preoperative and postoperative procedures to the patient and his family.
• Before discharge, teach the patient how to protect and clean the wound site and how to recognize signs of recurring infection. (See *Ensuring continued care for the patient with osteomyelitis.*)
• Instruct and encourage the patient to perform as much self-care as his condition allows. Allow him ade-

quate time to perform these activities at his own pace.
• Urge the patient to schedule follow-up examinations and to seek treatment for possible sources of recurrent infection — blisters, boils, sties, and impetigo.

EVALUATION

When evaluating the patient's response to your nursing care, gather reassessment data and compare this information with the patient outcomes specified in your plan of care.

Teaching and counseling
Determine the effectiveness of your teaching and counseling by asking the following questions:
• Does the patient understand the nature and causes of osteomyelitis?
• Does he acknowledge the necessity of taking the entire course of prescribed medication?
• Can he identify signs and symptoms of hidden or recurrent infection?
• Can he demonstrate proper skin care?
• Does he perform prescribed range-of-motion exercises?
• Does he understand the importance of preventing fractures and other trauma of the affected limb?

Physical condition
A physical examination and diagnostic tests will provide additional information. To evaluate the success of treatment, consider the following questions:
• Has the patient maintained muscle strength and range of motion in unaffected joints?
• Can he function within limitations?
• Has he reported that pain is decreased or absent?
• Has he regained mobility?
• Are complications related to immobility absent?

Appendices and index

Quick reference to treatments for immune
and infectious disorders   324

Quick reference to drugs used in
immune disorders   326

Quick reference to drugs used in
infectious disorders   332

Transmission prevention guidelines   344

Universal precautions   346

Guidelines for minimizing infection   348

Checklist of reportable diseases   352

Index   353

Quick reference to treatments for immune and infectious disorders

Bone marrow transplantation

Bone marrow transplantation (BMT) is the infusion of fresh or stored bone marrow from a donor to a recipient. This treatment replaces diseased bone marrow with healthy bone marrow and may thus enable the recipient to resume normal production of blood cells. Whether a patient receives BMT depends on his age, his health status, the underlying disease, and the availability of a histocompatible donor.

Types of BMT include autologous (procured from the patient and frozen), syngeneic (procured from the patient's identical twin), and allogeneic (procured from a histocompatible donor). Autologous bone marrow must be thawed immediately before infusion. Syngeneic and allogeneic bone marrow are infused immediately after procurement from the donor.

Although autologous BMT poses the least risk of infection, it is not always a viable option for patients with diseased bone marrow. Because it doesn't pose a risk of graft-versus-host disease (GVHD), syngeneic BMT poses a lower risk of infection than allogeneic BMT.

Indications
• To treat aplastic anemia, severe combined immunodeficiency disease, lymphoma, and acute or chronic leukemia
• Under investigation as a possible treatment for other diseases, such as multiple myeloma and selected solid tumors

Complications
• Acute or chronic GVHD (allogeneic BMT)
• Bleeding
• Life-threatening bacterial, viral, and fungal infections

• Hepatic veno-occlusive disease, leading to multisystem organ failure

Plasmapheresis

Also known as therapeutic plasma exchange, plasmapheresis involves the removal of plasma from withdrawn blood and the reinfusion of formed blood elements. Treatment may remove up to 90% of unwanted plasma factors, including autoantibodies, immune complexes, metabolites, toxic substances, and unknown mediators of disease.

Indications
• To treat renal disease, thrombotic thrombocytopenic purpura, autoimmune thrombocytopenic purpura, Guillain-Barré syndrome, multiple sclerosis, or myasthenia gravis

Complications
• Infection around the venipuncture site
• Hypersensitivity reaction to the ingredients of the replacement solution
• Hypocalcemia from excessive binding of circulating calcium to the citrate solution used as an anticoagulant in the replacement solution
• Arrhythmias
• Hypotension and other complications of low blood volume, such as syncope
• Hypomagnesemia leading to severe muscle cramps, tetany, and paresthesia (may follow repeated plasmapheresis)
• Symptoms of myasthenic crisis, such as dysphagia, ptosis, and diplopia, in patients with myasthenia gravis (secondary to removal of antibodies or antimyasthenic drugs from the blood)
• Hemolysis or embolism (rare)

Radiation therapy

Radiation therapy provides high levels of X-rays or gamma rays through a beam of electrons to a targeted area of cells or tissues.

Indications
• To treat cancer through the destruction of neoplastic cells or the curtailment of their growth
• To control pain, bleeding, or obstruction (palliative therapy)
• To treat severe rheumatoid arthritis or lupus nephritis and to prevent kidney transplant rejection (these indications are still under investigation)

Complications
• Interstitial pneumonitis
• Pulmonary fibrosis
• Pulmonary toxicity
• Chronic gastritis or enteritis
• GI bleeding
• Diarrhea
• Intractable nausea
• Vomiting
• Intestinal obstruction
• Oral complications such as stomatitis
• Myelosuppression
• Pericarditis and pericardial effusions
• Cerebral edema with an increased risk of seizures, inflammation, and increased intracranial pressure

Splenectomy

Removal of the spleen (splenectomy) curtails the spleen's role in intercepting antigens or antigenic chemical products that have succeeded in reaching the circulating blood.

Indications
• To treat rupture of the spleen caused by trauma
• To stage Hodgkin's disease
• To treat symptomatic hypersplenism associated with such disorders as autoimmune thrombocytopenic purpura or autoimmune hemolytic anemia

Complications
• Increased susceptibility to infection, especially with encapsulated bacteria such as *Streptococcus pneumoniae;* high incidence of fulminant, rapidly fatal bacteremia

Quick reference to drugs used in immune disorders

Anti-inflammatory drugs

Corticosteroids, gold salts, nonsteroidal anti-inflammatory drugs (NSAIDs), and nonopioid analgesics

Corticosteroids
• *Short-acting:* hydrocortisone, cortisone
• *Intermediate-acting:* prednisone, prednisolone, triamcinolone, methylprednisolone
• *Long-acting:* dexamethasone, betamethasone
• *Mineralocorticoids:* fludrocortisone

Indications
Adrenal insufficiency; systemic or inhalation therapy for respiratory diseases (asthma); relief of inflammation in rheumatoid arthritis and collagen disorders (lupus erythematosus, scleroderma); suppression of inflammatory reactions in asthma, ulcerative colitis, and Crohn's disease; food and drug allergies; emergency treatment of shock and anaphylactic reactions; prevention of rejection in organ and tissue transplants; adjunctive treatment of leukemias, lymphomas, and myelomas; multiple sclerosis; topical treatment of dermatologic and ocular inflammations

Adverse reactions
CNS: *euphoria, insomnia,* psychotic behavior, pseudotumor cerebri
CV: edema, hypertension, ***congestive heart failure***
Endocrine: menstrual irregularities, growth suppression in children, cushingoid signs (moon face, buffalo hump, truncal obesity)
GI: nausea, vomiting, *peptic ulcer,* ***pancreatitis***
Metabolic: hyperglycemia, hypocalcemia, hypokalemia
Other: muscle weakness or myopathy and weakening of the skeletal system

due to loss of calcium from bones; acne, hirsutism, impaired wound healing, emotional instability, ophthalmic changes. ***Abrupt withdrawal of corticosteroids after long-term use can precipitate potentially fatal adrenal crisis.***

Gold salts
Auranofin, aurothioglucose, gold sodium thiomalate

Indications
Progressive rheumatoid arthritis

Adverse reactions
Blood: ***agranulocytosis, aplastic anemia, thrombocytopenia***
GI: stomatitis, metallic taste, *nausea, vomiting, abdominal cramps* (especially with auranofin)
GU: nephrotic syndrome, proteinuria, renal impairment
Hepatic: hepatitis
Respiratory: pneumonitis, pulmonary fibrosis
Skin: *rash, pruritus, dermatitis,* ***exfoliative dermatitis***

Nonsteroidal anti-inflammatory drugs and nonopioid analgesics
NSAIDs, salicylates, acetaminophen

NSAIDs
Diclofenac, etodolac, fenoprofen, flurbiprofen, ibuprofen, indomethacin, ketoprofen, ketorolac, meclofenamate, nabumetone, naproxen, piroxicam, sulindac, tolmetin

Indications
Mild to moderate pain, such as myalgia or arthralgia; inflammation due to rheumatoid arthritis or other inflammatory disorders (used with an opioid analgesic for severe pain); short-term postoperative analgesia (I.M. ketorolac)

Common reactions are in *italics;* life-threatening reactions are in ***bold italics.***

Adverse reactions
Blood: *prolonged bleeding time*
GI: *GI upset, heartburn, nausea, vomiting,* **peptic ulcer,** *bleeding*
GU: acute renal failure
Hepatic: *hepatotoxicity*
Other: *bronchospasm, anaphylaxis* (in aspirin-allergic patients)

Salicylates
Aspirin, choline magnesium trisalicylate, choline salicylate, diflunisal, salsalate, sodium salicylate

Indications
Mild to moderate pain, such as myalgia or arthralgia; inflammation due to rheumatoid arthritis or other inflammatory disorders (used with an opioid analgesic for severe pain)

Adverse reactions
Blood: *prolonged bleeding time,* **blood dyscrasias**
CNS: headache, dizziness, confusion, lassitude, drowsiness (in patients receiving diflunisal)
CV: tachycardia
EENT: *tinnitus, hearing loss,* dim vision
GI: *dyspepsia, heartburn, epigastric distress, nausea, abdominal pain*
Hepatic: *hepatotoxicity*
Respiratory: *bronchospasm* (with or without angiospasm), hyperventilation
Other: sweating, renal damage, **hypersensitivity manifested by anaphylaxis or, as with aspirin, by asthma**

Acetaminophen

Indications
Mild to moderate pain; preferable to aspirin or NSAIDs for pain if patient has a history of GI bleeding, peptic ulcer, or aspirin or NSAID intolerance

Adverse reactions
Hepatic: *hepatic necrosis* (with high doses)
Skin: rash, urticaria
Other: angioedema, *anaphylaxis* (rare)

Immunosuppressants

Azathioprine, cyclophosphamide, cyclosporine, hydroxychloroquine, lymphocyte immune globulin (antithymocyte globulin [ATG]), methotrexate, muromonab-CD3, penicillamine, tacrolimus (Prograf)

Azathioprine

Indications
Inflammatory diseases, such as rheumatoid arthritis, psoriatic arthritis, and systemic lupus erythematosus; prevention of organ rejection after transplant surgery

Adverse reactions
Blood: anemia, **bone marrow suppression, thrombocytopenia,** leukopenia
CV: pulmonary fibrosis
GI: nausea, vomiting, anorexia, **pancreatitis**
Hepatic: elevated liver enzyme levels
Other: **immunosuppression,** arthralgia, muscle weakness

Cyclophosphamide

Indications
Inflammatory diseases, such as rheumatoid arthritis, psoriatic arthritis, and systemic lupus erythematosus; cancer

Adverse reactions
Blood: anemia, **bone marrow suppression, thrombocytopenia,** leukopenia
CV: pulmonary fibrosis
GI: nausea, vomiting, **pancreatitis**
Hepatic: elevated liver enzyme levels

Cyclosporine

Indications
Prevention of organ rejection after transplant surgery; also used with corticosteroids to reduce inflammation in rheumatoid arthritis

---

Common reactions are in *italics;* life-threatening reactions are in **bold italics.**

Adverse reactions
CNS: *tremor,* headache
GI: *gum hyperplasia,* nausea, vomiting, diarrhea, abdominal distention
GU: *nephrotoxicity*
Hepatic: *hepatotoxicity*
Metabolic: hyperkalemia, hyperglycemia
Other: hypertension, *hirsutism,* sinusitis, gynecomastia, hearing loss, tinnitus, muscle pain, edema

---

Hydroxychloroquine

Indications
Severe rheumatoid arthritis and systemic lupus erythematosus; suppression and chemoprophylaxis of malaria

Adverse reactions
Blood: *aplastic anemia, thrombocytopenia,* leukopenia
CNS: irritability, headache, dizziness
GI: anorexia, nausea, vomiting, cramps
Skin: bleaching of hair, alopecia, skin eruptions, pruritus
Other: *hypersensitivity* (dermatitis, urticaria, angioedema), retinopathy

---

Lymphocyte immune globulin

Indications
Rescue therapy in transplant rejection; mild or severe aplastic anemia

Adverse reactions
Blood: leukopenia, *thrombocytopenia*
CNS: malaise, *seizures,* headache
Other: fever, chills, skin reactions

Methotrexate

Indications
Inflammatory diseases, such as rheumatoid arthritis, psoriatic arthritis, vasculitis, inflammatory bowel disease, and systemic lupus erythematosus; cancer

Adverse reactions
Blood: anemia, *bone marrow suppression, thrombocytopenia,* leukopenia

CV: pulmonary fibrosis
GI: nausea, vomiting, *pancreatitis*
Hepatic: elevated liver enzyme levels

Muromonab-CD3

Indications
Reversal of acute renal allograft rejection (not effective as a single-agent prophylaxis)

Adverse reactions
Blood: pancytopenia, *aplastic anemia,* neutropenia
CV: *cardiac arrest,* hypotension, shock
GI: *nausea, vomiting,* diarrhea
GU: renal dysfunction
Respiratory: *respiratory arrest, acute respiratory distress syndrome, pulmonary edema*
Skin: rash, urticaria, flushing, pruritus
Other: *fever, chills,* dyspnea, headache

Penicillamine

Indications
Inflammatory diseases, such as rheumatoid arthritis, psoriatic arthritis, and systemic lupus erythematosus

Adverse reactions
Blood: *bone marrow suppression, thrombocytopenia,* leukopenia
EENT: tinnitus, *reversible optic neuritis*
GI: anorexia, epigastric pain, nausea, vomiting, stomatitis, loss of taste
GU: proteinuria, *nephrotic syndrome*
Other: *allergic reactions* (pruritus, rash), lupus-like syndrome

---

Tacrolimus (Prograf)

Indications
Rescue therapy in liver transplant recipients with failing grafts who are receiving cyclosporine-based immunosuppressive therapy (investigational)

Adverse reactions
(Most prevalent with I.V. tacrolimus and during combined use with cyclosporine)

Common reactions are in *italics;* life-threatening reactions are in ***bold italics.***

CNS: neurotoxicity (headache, tremor, paresthesia, photophobia, tinnitus, sleep disturbances, mood changes)
Other: *nephrotoxicity,* hypertension, GI disturbances, impaired glucose tolerance

Biological response modifiers and colony-stimulating factors

Aldesleukin (interleukin-2, IL-2), epoetin alpha (erythropoietin), filgrastim (granulocyte colony stimulating factor, G-CSF), recombinant interferon alpha-2a, recombinant interferon alpha-2b, interferon alpha-n3, interferon gamma-1b, recombinant human interleukin-3 (IL-3, multipotential colony stimulating factor), macrophage colony-stimulating factor (M-CSF), sargramostim (granulocyte-macrophage colony-stimulating factor [GM-CSF]), tumor necrosis factor

Aldesleukin

Indications
Metastatic renal cell cancer

Adverse reactions
Blood: *anemia, thrombocytopenia, leukopenia, coagulation disorders, leukocytosis, eosinophilia*
CNS: *mental status changes* (lethargy, somnolence, confusion, agitation), *dizziness, syncope, motor dysfunction, coma*
CV: capillary leak syndrome leading to hypotension, occasional arrhythmias
Respiratory: *pulmonary edema, respiratory failure*
GI: *nausea, vomiting, diarrhea, stomatitis, anorexia, bleeding, dyspepsia, constipation*
GU: *oliguria, anuria, proteinuria, hematuria, dysuria,* urine retention, urinary frequency
Hepatic: *elevated liver enzyme levels, jaundice, hepatomegaly*
Respiratory: *pulmonary edema, respiratory failure*

Skin: *pruritus, erythema, rash,* **exfoliative dermatitis**
Other: *sepsis*

Epoetin alpha

Indications
Anemia secondary to reduced production of endogenous erythropoietin; anemia secondary to end-stage renal disease; adjunctive treatment of patients infected with human immunodeficiency virus (HIV) and anemia secondary to zidovudine (or other antiretroviral) therapy

Adverse reactions
Blood: iron deficiency, elevated platelet count
CNS: headache, *seizures*
CV: *hypertension,* clotting of the vascular access device and increased clotting in arteriovenous grafts, tachycardia
GI: nausea, vomiting, diarrhea
Metabolic: hyperkalemia
Skin: rash

Filgrastim

Indications
Reduction in duration and severity of chemotherapy-induced myelosuppression and increased circulating neutrophil counts; may allow administration of higher doses of chemotherapeutic drugs

Adverse reactions
Blood: *thrombocytopenia*
GU: hematuria, proteinuria
Skin: alopecia, exacerbation of preexisting skin conditions (such as psoriasis)
Other: bone pain and erythema at injection site; reversible elevations in levles of uric acid, lactate dehydrogenase, and alkaline phosphatase; *skeletal pain,* fever, splenomegaly, osteoporosis

---

Common reactions are in *italics;* life-threatening reactions are in ***bold italics.***

Interferon alpha-2a, recombinant; interferon alpha-2b, recombinant

Indications
- *Interferon alpha-2a:* hairy-cell leukemia, Kaposi's sarcoma related to acquired immunodeficiency syndrome (AIDS)
- *Interferon alfa-2b:* hairy-cell leukemia; Kaposi's sarcoma related to AIDS; chronic hepatitis; condylomata acuminata

Adverse reactions
Blood: *leukopenia,* mild thrombocytopenia
CNS: *dizziness,* confusion, paresthesia, lethargy, depression, nervousness, irritability, *fatigue*
CV: hypotension or hypertension, chest pain, arrhythmias, ***congestive heart failure*** (alpha-2a), edema, neutropenia
GI: anorexia, nausea, vomiting, *diarrhea*
Respiratory: ***bronchospasm*** (alpha-2a), coughing, dyspnea
Skin: *rash,* dry skin, *pruritus,* partial alopecia, urticaria
Other: pharyngitis, *flulike symptoms* (fever, headache, chills, muscle aches), elevated liver enzyme levels

Interferon alpha-n3

Indications
Condylomata acuminata

Adverse reactions
Blood: neutropenia
CNS: dizziness, light-headedness
GI: anorexia, dyspepsia, nausea, vomiting
Hepatic: elevated liver enzyme levels
Skin: rash, pruritus, partial alopecia
Other: *constitutional or flulike symptoms* (fever, myalgia, headache, chills, malaise, arthralgia)

Interferon gamma-1b

Indications
Reduction of frequency and severity of infections associated with chronic granulomatous disease

Adverse reactions
CV: occasional (dose-related) hypotension
GI: diarrhea, nausea, vomiting
Skin: rash

Interleukin-3, recombinant human

Indications
Early stem cell precursor to G-CSF or GM-CSF with possible role in treating leukemia, refractory anemia, and myelodysplastic syndromes, and combined with GM-CSF following autologous bone marrow transplant (investigational)

Adverse reactions
Mild constitutional symptoms

Macrophage colony-stimulating factor

Indications
Potent inducer of monocytosis; may enhance direct cytotoxicity against tumor targets for some cancers (investigational)

Adverse reactions
Blood: mild thrombocytopenia, decreased low-density lipoprotein levels

Sargramostim

Indications
Reduction in duration and severity of chemotherapy-induced myelosuppression and increased circulating neutrophil counts in patients with myelodysplastic syndromes, aplastic anemia, or agranulocytosis and in recipients of bone marrow transplants

Adverse reactions
Blood: *blood dyscrasia*
CNS: fatigue, malaise, CNS disorder

Common reactions are in *italics;* life-threatening reactions are in ***bold italics.***

CV: hemorrhage
GI: nausea, vomiting, diarrhea, anorexia, hemorrhage, stomatitis, liver damage
GU: urinary tract disorders, abnormal kidney function
Local: erythema at injection site
Respiratory: dyspnea, lung disorders
Skin: alopecia, rash
Other: bone pain, edema, fever, ***sepsis***

Tumor necrosis factor (TNF)

Indications
AIDS, cancers (investigational), sepsis (investigational)

Adverse reactions
Blood: anemia, neutropenia, hypertriglyceridemia
CNS: fatigue, malaise
CV: hypotension
GI: anorexia
Hepatic: elevated liver enzyme levels
Metabolic: hyperglycemia
Other: *fever, flulike symptoms*

Common reactions are in *italics;* life-threatening reactions are in ***bold italics.***

Quick reference to drugs used in infectious disorders

Anti-infective classes

Aminoglycosides, carbapenems, cephalosporins, fluoroquinolones, macrolides, monobactams, penicillins, sulfonamides, tetracyclines.

Aminoglycosides

Amikacin, gentamicin, kanamycin, neomycin, netilmicin, paromomycin, streptomycin, tobramycin

Indications

Severe gram-negative infections, such as septicemia, pneumonia, intra-abdominal infections, skin or bone infections, meningitis (requires intrathecal or intraventricular administration in addition to parenteral administration), and complicated urinary tract infections; used in combination with other antibiotics for infections caused by *Pseudomonas aeruginosa* and for endocarditis caused by *Enterococcus;* may also be used as part of a multiple drug regimen for *Mycobacterium avium* complex infection in patients with acquired immunodeficiency syndrome (AIDS).

• *Neomycin and kanamycin:* orally for hepatic encephalopathy and coma and for intestinal bacterial decontamination (preoperatively); topically for eye, ear, and skin infections (neomycin); kanamycin also used for peritoneal instillation during surgery and in other irrigation solutions

• *Paromomycin:* orally for intestinal amebiasis, hepatic coma, and parasitic infections

• *Streptomycin:* part of multidrug regimen for tuberculosis; also used for enterococcal endocarditis

• *Gentamicin and tobramycin:* administered as nebulizer therapy in respiratory tract infections (primarily associated with cystic fibrosis; efficacy has not been fully evaluated); also administered as impregnated beads imbedded into bone cement for gram-negative joint infections and orthopedic surgical procedures

Adverse reactions

Blood: *hemolytic anemia,* leukopenia, ***thrombocytopenia*** (all rare)
EENT: *ototoxicity* (vestibular and cochlear)
GI: nausea, vomiting, diarrhea (uncommon)
GU: *nephrotoxicity* (associated with serum trough levels above the normal therapeutic range; monitor serum drug levels and serum creatinine levels closely)
Other: *hypersensitivity,* enhanced neuromuscular blockade

Carbapenems

Imipenem/cilastatin sodium

Indications

Serious infections caused by a wide range of susceptible gram-positive, gram-negative, and anaerobic bacteria; useful in mixed polymicrobial infections. Spectrum of activity includes *Pseudomonas aeruginosa.*

Adverse reactions

Blood: eosinophilia, leukopenia, agranulocytosis, ***thrombocytopenia***
CNS: *seizures* (with high doses or when dose has not been adjusted for renal dysfunction), dizziness, confusion, encephalopathy
GI: nausea, vomiting, abdominal cramps, *pseudomembranous colitis*
Other: *hypersensitivity* (rash, urticaria, pruritus, ***anaphylaxis***), superinfection, cross-allergenicity between imipenem and penicillins

---

Common reactions are in *italics;* life-threatening reactions are in ***bold italics.***

Cephalosporins

- *First-generation cephalosporins:* cefadroxil, cefazolin, cephalexin, cephalothin, cephapirin, cephradine
- *Second-generation cephalosporins:* cefaclor, cefamandole, cefmetazole, cefonicid, ceforanide, cefotetan, cefoxitin, cefprozil, cefuroxime, loracarbef
- *Third-generation cephalosporins:* cefixime, cefoperazone, cefotaxime, cefpodoxime, ceftazidime, ceftizoxime, ceftriaxone

Indications

Infections of the skin, soft tissues, respiratory tract (bronchitis, pneumonia, otitis media, sinusitis), bones, joints, and urinary tract caused by a wide array of bacteria (susceptibilities depend on the generation of cephalosporin)
- *First-generation drugs:* most active against gram-positive bacteria; active against staphylococci, streptococci, *Escherichia coli*, *Klebsiella* species, and *Proteus mirabilis;* used prophylactically to reduce infections in patients undergoing surgical procedures (cardiac, orthopedic, gynecologic, gastrointestinal); commonly used to treat skin or skin-structure infections
- *Second-generation drugs:* less activity than first-generation cephalosporins against gram-positive bacteria, but expanded activity to cover more gram-negative organisms, including some ampicillin-resistant strains of *Haemophilus influenzae* and *Moraxella (Branhamella) catarrhalis* that may cause upper respiratory tract infections such as bronchitis, sinusitis, and otitis media
- *Cefuroxime:* spectrum expanded to cover *Haemophilus influenzae*
- *Cefoxitin, cefotetan, cefmetazole:* spectrum expanded to include anaerobic organisms (such as *Bacteroides fragilis*); used for suspected intra-abdominal infections (peritonitis, abscess) and gynecologic infections
- *Third-generation drugs:* spectrum of activity expanded to cover more relatively resistant gram-negative bacteria, such as *Serratia, Citrobacter, En-*terobacter, and others that are associated with nosocomial infections but varies with each third-generation cephalosporin; possess the least activity of the three generations against gram-positive bacteria; penetration into cerebrospinal fluid allows use in meningitis; also used for cervical and urethral gonorrhea caused by *Neisseria gonorrhoeae* and for serious Lyme disease
- *Ceftazidime:* serious infections caused by *Pseudomonas aeruginosa* (often in combination with aminoglycosides).

Adverse reactions

Blood: eosinophilia, reversible neutropenia or leukopenia, ***hemolytic anemia, thrombocytopenia***
CNS: ***seizures*** (at high doses)
GI: *nausea, vomiting, diarrhea,* dyspepsia, cholestasis (ceftriaxone), ***pseudomembranous colitis*** (toxigenic *Clostridium difficile* diarrhea)
GU: ***nephrotoxicity*** (rare), transient elevated blood urea nitrogen
Hepatic: elevated liver function test results
Local: *phlebitis at I.V. site, pain at I.M. site*
Other: ***hypersensitivity*** (rash, urticaria, ***Stevens-Johnson syndrome, anaphylaxis***), bacterial and fungal superinfection; disulfuram-type reactions (only with cefamandole, cefoperazone, cefotetan, and cefmetazole)

Fluoroquinolones

Ciprofloxacin, enoxacin, lomefloxacin, norfloxacin, ofloxacin

Indications

Infections of the respiratory tract (excluding *Streptococcus pneumoniae* pneumonia), skin, soft tissue, bones, or joints; urinary tract infections (including prostatitis); sexually transmitted disease (gonococcal and nongonococcal urethritis or cervicitis); and infectious diarrhea; has an extended spectrum of activity against gram-positive and gram-negative bacteria compared to other oral antibiotics; because of broad spectrum of activity, may be an appro-

---

Common reactions are in *italics;* life-threatening reactions are in ***bold italics.***

priate choice for early conversion from I.V. to oral anti-infective therapy

Adverse reactions
CNS: dizziness, headache, *seizures*
GI: *nausea, vomiting, diarrhea, abdominal pain*
Skin: rash, urticaria, pruritus, photosensitivity, *anaphylaxis*

Macrolides
Azithromycin, clarithromycin, erythromycin, troleandomycin

Indications
Respiratory, genital, GI tract, and skin or soft-tissue infections caused by susceptible gram-positive (*Streptococcus, Staphylococcus*) and "atypical" organisms (*Chlamydia, Mycoplasma, Legionella*). Azithromycin and clarithromycin extend coverage to *Haemophilus influenzae* and *Moraxella (Branhamella) catarrhalis.* Useful in community-acquired pneumonia. Also used in Lyme disease, pelvic inflammatory disease, primary syphilis (if the patient is allergic to penicillin), and as an alternative to tetracycline in nongonococcal urethritis or cervicitis.

Adverse reactions
GI: *nausea,* vomiting, *diarrhea,* abdominal pain (especially with erythromycin)
Hepatic: hepatic dysfunction, cholestatic hepatitis (erythromycin estolate)
Local: *phlebitis or pain at I.V. site* (only erythromycin is administered parenterally)
Other: fever, superinfection, *hypersensitivity* (urticaria, skin eruptions, rash, *anaphylaxis*); ototoxicity (with high I.V. doses and renal or hepatic dysfunction)

Monobactams
Aztreonam

Indications
Serious infections caused by gram-negative bacteria, including susceptible strains of *Pseudomonas aeruginosa.* Aztreonam has a narrow spectrum of activity against aerobic

gram-negative bacteria, similar to that of the aminoglycosides.

Adverse reactions
Blood: pancytopenia, anemia, neutropenia, *thrombocytopenia*
CNS: *seizures* (rare)
GI: nausea, vomiting, abdominal cramps, diarrhea, *pseudomembranous colitis*
Local: phlebitis at I.V. site, *pain at I.M. site*
Other: *hypersensitivity* (rash, urticaria, pruritus, *anaphylaxis*)

Penicillins
Natural penicillins, aminopenicillins, extended-spectrum penicillins, penicillinase-resistant penicillins

Natural penicillins
Penicillin G benzathine, penicillin G potassium, penicillin G procaine, penicillin G sodium, penicillin V potassium

Indications
Infections caused by susceptible strains of gram-positive bacteria, such as *Streptococcus pneumoniae*; groups A, B, C, D (nonenterococcal), and G streptococci; and *Streptococcus viridians;* infections caused by *Bacillus anthracis, Corynebacterium diphtheriae, Listeria monocytogenes,* and anaerobic mouth flora, such as *Peptostreptococcus* and *Fusobacterium*

Adverse reactions (for all penicillins)
Blood: *hemolytic anemia,* neutropenia, leukopenia, *thrombocytopenia,* increased bleeding time (extended-spectrum penicillins)
CNS: agitation, confusion, myoclonus, *seizures* (with high doses or when dose has not been adjusted for renal impairment)
GI: *nausea, vomiting, epigastric distress, diarrhea* (most common with ampicillin and amoxicillin/clavulanic acid), *pseudomembranous colitis*
GU: interstitial nephritis
Hepatic: elevated liver function tests
Metabolic: hyperkalemia (penicillin G potassium); hypokalemia and hyper-

---

Common reactions are in *italics;* life-threatening reactions are in ***bold italics.***

natremia (extended-spectrum penicillins and penicillin G sodium)
Local: *phlebitis at I.V. site, pain at I.M. site*
Other: *hypersensitivity* (rash, urticaria, fever, severe dermatitis, laryngospasm, angioneurotic edema, *anaphylaxis*)

Aminopenicillins
Amoxicillin, ampicillin, bacampicillin

Indications
Infections of the respiratory tract (pharyngitis, sinusitis, bronchitis, pneumonia), urinary tract, skin, soft tissue, bones, or joints; gonococcal infections (most *Neiserria gonorrhoeae* strains are resistant); endocarditis; *Listeria* infections; otitis media; Lyme disease; septicemia; and meningitis caused by susceptible organisms. Less activity against gram-positive organisms compared to natural penicillins; however, the antibacterial spectrum is broadened to include *Escherichia coli, Haemophilus influenzae* (many strains are resistant), *Proteus mirabilis, Salmonella,* and *Shigella.*

Extended-spectrum penicillins
Azlocillin, carbenicillin, carbenicillin indanyl sodium, mezlocillin, piperacillin, ticarcillin; products available in combination with a beta-lactamase inhibitor include ampicillin/sulbactam, piperacillin/tazobactam, and ticarcillin/clavulanic acid

Indications
Hospital-acquired pneumonia, septicemia, abdominal infections, fever with neutropenia, and urinary tract or gynecologic infections caused by a broad range of gram-positive, gram-negative, and anaerobic organisms; antibacterial spectrum broadened to include relatively resistant gram-negative and a few anaerobic organisms; however, provide less activity against gram-positive organisms than natural penicillins
• *Carbenicillin indanyl sodium:* urinary tract infections only; does not achieve adequate serum levels to be used for systemic infections (available as tablet only)

Penicillinase-resistant penicillins
Cloxacillin, dicloxacillin, methicillin, nafcillin, oxacillin

Indications
Systemic infections caused by penicillinase-producing staphylococci

Sulfonamides
Single agents: sulfacetamide, sulfacytine, sulfadiazine, sulfamethizole, sulfamethoxazole, sulfapyridine, sulfasalazine, sulfisoxazole
Combination products: co-trimoxazole (sulfamethoxazole-trimethoprim), erythromycin-sulfisoxazole

Indications
• *Single agents:* urinary tract infections, otitis media, nocardiosis, toxoplasmosis (with pyrimethamine), chancroid, and topically for skin and soft-tissue infections
• *Combination products:* otitis media due to gram-positive bacteria, *Haemophilus influenzae, or Moraxella (Branhamella) catarrhalis.* Co-trimoxazole is effective against a broad spectrum of bacteria and is useful in urinary tract infections, bronchitis, traveler's diarrhea, and *Pneumocystis carinii* pneumonia in patients with AIDS.

Adverse reactions
Blood: *agranulocytosis, aplastic anemia, hemolytic anemia,* megaloblastic anemia, neutropenia, leukopenia, *thrombocytopenia*
CNS: headache, dizziness, insomnia
GI: *anorexia, nausea, vomiting, abdominal pain, diarrhea*; *pseudomembranous colitis* (rare)
GU: crystalluria (can lead to renal damage, hematuria)
Other: tinnitus, *hypersensitivity* (rash, pruritus, skin eruptions, *erythema multiforme [Stevens-Johnson syndrome], fever,* serum sickness, *anaphylaxis*)

Tetracyclines
Demeclocycline, doxycycline, methacycline, minocycline, oxytetracycline, tetracycline

Indications
Lyme disease (tetracycline only), endemic typhus, chancroid, and infections caused by *Chlamydia* (nongonococcal urethritis or cervicitis, atypical pneumonia), *Mycoplasma* (atypical pneumonia), *Rickettsia* (Rocky Mountain spotted fever), and other uncommon organisms; used in acute exacerbations of chronic bronchitis and systemic treatment of acne; effective against a relatively broad spectrum of gram-positive and gram-negative activity, although resistance can occur
• *Demeclocycline:* hyponatremia due to syndrome of inappropriate antidiuretic hormone (SIADH)
• *Minocycline:* asymptomatic carriers of *Neisseria meningitidis* when rifampin is contraindicated

Adverse reactions
Blood: neutropenia, ***thrombocytopenia, hemolytic anemia*** (all rare)
CNS: light-headedness, vertigo, pseudotumor cerebri (rare in infants)
GI: anorexia, *nausea, vomiting, diarrhea,* ***pancreatitis,*** esophagitis, enterocolitis
GU: blood urea nitrogen increase
Hepatic: increased liver function test results, ***hepatotoxicity*** (rare)
Local: phlebitis at I.V. site, *pain at I.M. site*
Skin: *photosensitivity, rash, urticaria*
Other: dysphasia, glossitis, ***hypersensitivity,*** tooth discoloration

Miscellaneous anti-infectives

Chloramphenicol, lincosamides, metronidazole, vancomycin

Chloramphenicol

Indications
Serious infections caused by susceptible bacteria resistant to other agents or when other agents are contraindicated (for example, penicillin or cephalosporin allergy); drug of choice for typhoid fever *(Salmonella typhi).* Excellent CNS penetration allows use in meningitis; anaerobic activity allows use in brain abscess. Can be used in rickettsial infections (Rocky Mountain spotted fever).

Adverse reactions
Blood: *aplastic anemia* (not dose-related, irreversible, and idiopathic), hypoplastic anemia, ***granulocytopenia,*** thrombocytopenia (dose-related, reversible)
CNS: headache, mild depression, confusion, delirium, peripheral neuropathy, optic neuritis (with prolonged therapy)
CV: ***gray syndrome in neonates*** (abdominal distention, gray cyanosis, vasomotor collapse, respiratory distress, death due to accumulation of chloramphenicol)
GI: nausea, vomiting, stomatitis, diarrhea, enterocolitis
Other: jaundice, ***hypersensitivity*** (fever, rash, angioedema, ***anaphylaxis***)

Lincosamides
Clindamycin, lincomycin

Indications
Infections due to gram-positive (*Staphylococcus, Streptococcus*) or anaerobic (*Bacteroides fragilis*) organisms; particularly effective in infections caused by a mixture of these organisms, such as respiratory tract infections (aspiration pneumonia, empyema, lung abscess), intra-abdominal infections, skin and soft-tissue infections (diabetes-related foot ulcer), and pelvic inflammatory infections; lincomycin generally less active than clindamycin

Adverse reactions
Blood: *leukopenia, neutropenia,* eosinophilia, ***thrombocytopenia***
CV: ***hypotension, syncope, cardiac arrest after rapid I.V. administration*** (all with lincomycin)

Common reactions are in *italics;* life-threatening reactions are in ***bold italics.***

GI: *nausea,* vomiting, abdominal pain, *diarrhea,* **pseudomembranous colitis** (due to *Clostridium difficile*), esophagitis, metallic taste
Local: phlebitis at I.V. site, *pain and sterile abscess at I.M. site*
Other: hypersensitivity (maculopapular rash, urticaria, **erythema multiforme,** generalized morbilliform rash, **anaphylaxis**)

Metronidazole

Indications
Anaerobic bacteria and many protozoa; indicated for serious infections such as intra-abdominal infections (peritonitis, abscess), gynecologic infections (trichomoniasis and Gardnerella), bone and joint infections, lower respiratory tract infections, CNS infections, and septicemia; administered orally for pseudomembranous colitis associated with *Clostridium difficile*

Adverse reactions
Blood: transient leukopenia, neutropenia
CNS: vertigo, headache, ataxia, incoordination, depression, restlessness, insomnia, sensory neuropathy, neuromyopathy, *seizures*
GI: *nausea, vomiting, anorexia,* abdominal cramping, epigastric distress, metallic taste
GU: darkened urine, polyuria, dysuria, incontinence
Local: *thrombophlebitis after I.V. infusion*
Other: hypersensitivity (urticaria, rash, pruritus), mutagenic and carcinogenic in mice; effects on humans not fully known

Vancomycin

Indications
Gram-positive infections when bacteria are not susceptible to penicillins or when patient is allergic to penicillin; effective against *Streptococcus, Staphylococcus,* and *Corynebacterium jeikeium;* major uses: resistant staphylococcal infections, enterococcal endocardi-

tis, and orally to treat pseudomembranous colitis caused by *Clostridium difficile*

Adverse reactions
Blood: neutropenia, **thrombocytopenia**
GU: nephrotoxicity
Local: *pain or thrombophlebitis at I.V. site*
Skin: *"red-neck" syndrome with rapid I.V. infusion (hypotension associated with a maculopapular rash on face, neck, trunk, and extremities)*
Other: *chills, fever,* **anaphylaxis,** superinfection, tinnitus, ototoxicity

Antivirals

Acyclovir, amantadine, didanosine (ddI), foscarnet, ganciclovir, ribavirin, rimantadine, vidarabine, zalcitabine (ddC), zidovudine (AZT)

Acyclovir

Indications
• Parenterally for initial and recurrent mucosal or cutaneous herpes simplex virus types I and II in immunocompromised patients, severe first episodes of genital herpes infection, encephalitis caused by herpes simplex in patients over age 6 months, and varicella-zoster (chicken pox) infections in immunocompromised adults and children
• Orally for initial and recurrent genital herpes in selected patients and for acute treatment of herpes zoster (shingles) and varicella-zoster infections in patients under age 2
• Topically for mucocutaneous herpes simplex infections

Adverse reactions
CNS: *headache; encephalopathic changes,* including lethargy, obtundation, tremor, confusion, hallucinations, agitation, **seizures, coma** (with I.V. dosage)
CV: hypotension
GI: *nausea, vomiting,* diarrhea

Common reactions are in *italics;* life-threatening reactions are in **bold italics.**

GU: *increased blood urea nitrogen or serum creatinine levels,* renal dysfunction (especially with rapid I.V. infusion)
Local: *inflammation, phlebitis, and irritation at injection site*
Skin: rash, urticaria

Amantadine, rimantidine

Indications
Prophylaxis and symptomatic treatment of influenza A viral infections (not effective against influenza B infections); must be administered within 48 hours of onset of symptoms

Adverse reactions
CNS: *irritability, insomnia,* anxiety, impaired concentration (all less common with rimantadine)
CV: orthostatic hypotension, peripheral edema, ***congestive heart failure***
GI: anorexia, nausea
Skin: *livedo reticularis* (with prolonged use)

Didanosine

Indications
Human immunodeficiency virus (HIV) infections when patient is unresponsive to or cannot tolerate zidovudine

Adverse reactions
CNS: *headache, peripheral neuropathy,* asthenia, insomnia, CNS depression, seizures
GI: *diarrhea, nausea, vomiting, abdominal pain,* constipation, stomatitis, taste loss or change, ***pancreatitis*** (can be severe)
Hepatic: ***hepatotoxicity***
Skin: rash, pruritus, alopecia
Other: myalgia, arthritis, pain, cough, infection

Foscarnet

Indications
Cytomegalovirus retinitis in patients with AIDS

Adverse reactions
Blood: anemia, ***bone marrow suppression*** (rare)
CNS: *headache, fatigue, rigors, dizziness, hypoesthesia, paresthesia, **coma,*** visual field deficits, extrapyramidal reactions, ***cerebral edema***
EENT: visual abnormalities
GI: anorexia, *nausea, vomiting, diarrhea, abdominal pain,* ***pancreatitis***
GU: ***nephrotoxicity*** (in 30% of patients), ***acute renal failure***
Respiratory: *cough, dyspnea,* ***bronchospasm***
Skin: *rash, sweating*
Other: fever, mineral and electrolyte disturbances (calcium, magnesium, potassium, phosphorus)

Ganciclovir

Indications
Cytomegalovirus (CMV) retinitis in immunocompromised patients; other CMV infections (pneumonia, GI infection) in immunosuppressed patients; prevention of CMV infection in transplant patients

Adverse reactions
Blood: ***granulocytopenia, thrombocytopenia,*** anemia
CNS: ataxia, dizziness, headache, confusion, seizures
CV: arrhythmias, hypotension, hypertension
GI: nausea, vomiting, diarrhea
Hepatic: elevated liver function test results
Local: erythema, pain, and phlebitis at injection site

Ribavirin

Indications
Severe lower respiratory tract infection due to respiratory syncytial virus in infants and children

Adverse reactions
Blood: anemia, reticulocytosis
CV: hypotension, cardiac arrest
EENT: conjunctivitis, eyelid rash or erythema

Common reactions are in *italics;* life-threatening reactions are in ***bold italics.***

Respiratory: worsening respiratory status
Other: rash

Vidarabine

Indications
Herpes simplex encephalitis, neonatal herpes simplex infections, and herpes zoster in immunocompromised patients

Adverse reactions
Blood: anemia, neutropenia, ***thrombocytopenia***
CNS: tremor, dizziness, hallucinations, confusion, ataxia
GI: anorexia, nausea, vomiting, diarrhea
Skin: rash, pruritus

Zalcitabine

Indications
Advanced HIV infection in combination with zidovudine

Adverse reactions
Blood: ***bone marrow depression, granulocytopenia, thrombocytopenia***
CNS: *peripheral neuropathy,* headache, fatigue
GI: stomatitis, nausea, dysphagia, diarrhea
Hepatic: elevated liver function test results
Skin: rash, pruritus
Other: myalgia, arthralgia, night sweats, fever, ***pancreatitis***

Zidovudine

Indications
Orally for patients with symptomatic or asymptomatic HIV infections who have had two consecutive CD4+ T-cell counts of 500/mm^3 or less

Adverse reactions
Blood: ***severe bone marrow depression, granulocytopenia, thrombocytopenia, thrombocytosis,*** anemia
CNS: *headache, malaise,* fatigue, confusion, insomnia, seizures

GI: *nausea,* abdominal pain, diarrhea, vomiting
Hepatic: increases in liver function test results
Skin: *rash*
Other: myalgia, fever, necrotizing myopathy

Systemic antifungals

Amphotericin B, fluconazole, flucytosine, griseofulvin, itraconazole, ketoconazole, miconazole, nystatin

Amphotericin B

Indications
CNS (may require intrathecal intraventricular injection in addition to I.V. administration), pulmonary, hepatic, renal, and other systemic fungal infections; blastomycosis, histoplasmosis, cryptococcosis, candidiasis, sporotrichosis, aspergillosis, phycomycosis (mucormycosis), and coccidioidomycosis

Adverse reactions
Blood: anemia (normochromic, normocytic)
CNS: headache, peripheral neuropathy
CV: hypotension, arrhythmias, asystole
GI: *anorexia, weight loss, nausea,* vomiting, abdominal pain
GU: ***nephrotoxicity*** (in 80% of patients)
Local: *thrombophlebitis, pain at injection site*
Metabolic: hypokalemia, hypomagnesemia
Other: *fever, chills,* myalgia, arthralgia (*Note:* Risk of fever, chills, nausea, vomiting, and myalgia may be minimized by pretreating patient with antihistamines, antiemetics, and antipyretics.)

Common reactions are in *italics;* life-threatening reactions are in ***bold italics.***

Fluconazole, itraconazole, ketoconazole

Indications
• *Fluconazole:* oropharyngeal, esophageal, and systemic candidiasis; cryptococcal meningitis (including prophylaxis in AIDS patients)
• *Itraconazole:* orally for systemic blastomycosis and histoplasmosis (includes HIV- positive patients)
• *Ketoconazole:* some systemic fungal infections, recalcitrant cutaneous dermatophyte infections, oral and esophageal candidiasis

Adverse reactions
CNS: headache
GI: nausea, vomiting, diarrhea
Hepatic: *hepatotoxicity* (rarely fatal), elevated liver enzyme levels (both with ketoconazole)
Skin: rash; *Stevens-Johnson syndrome* (with fluconazole; rare)

Flucytosine

Indications
Serious infections caused by *Candida, Cryptococcus* (including meningitis); usually administered with amphotericin B for systemic fungal infections because of rapid development of resistance when flucytosine is used alone; can be used as monotherapy for fungal urinary tract infections

Adverse reactions
Blood: anemia, *bone marrow suppression, aplastic anemia,* pancytopenia, *thrombocytopenia*
CNS: dizziness, drowsiness, confusion, headache, vertigo
GI: *nausea, vomiting, diarrhea*
Metabolic: elevated blood urea nitrogen, serum creatinine, and serum alkaline phosphatase levels
Skin: rash, pruritus

Griseofulvin

Indications
Tinea infections of skin, nails, and hair that do not respond to topical agents.

Because griseofulvin is not effective against other fungal infections, the organism should be identified as a dermatophyte before therapy is initiated.

Adverse reactions
CNS: headache (early in treatment), transient decrease in hearing, fatigue (with large doses), mental confusion, psychoses, dizziness, insomnia, paresthesias (hands, feet)
GI: nausea, vomiting, excessive thirst, diarrhea
Skin: rash, urticaria, photosensitivity
Other: estrogen-like effects in children, oral thrush

Miconazole

Indications
Systemic fungal infections (coccidioidomycosis, candidiasis, cryptococcosis, and paracoccidioidomycosis); topically for vaginal and other cutaneous fungal infections

Adverse reactions
CNS: dizziness, drowsiness
CV: tachycardia, arrhythmias
GI: *nausea, vomiting,* diarrhea
Local: *phlebitis at injection site*
Skin: *pruritic rash*
Other: fever, chills

Nystatin

Indications
Oral, GI, and vaginal (topical) infections (such as oral thrush) caused by *Candida albicans* and other candidal organisms

Adverse reactions
GI: transient nausea, vomiting, diarrhea (usually with large oral doses)
Skin: contact dermatitis (topical)

Antituberculins

Capreomycin sulfate, cycloserine, ethambutol, ethionamide, isoniazid, pyrazinamide, rifampin, streptomycin (see aminoglycosides)

Common reactions are in *italics;* life-threatening reactions are in *bold italics.*

Capreomycin sulfate

Indications
Tuberculosis (usually as part of a multi-drug regimen)

Adverse reactions
Blood: eosinophilia, leukocytosis, leukopenia
CNS: headache, *neuromuscular blockade*
GU: *nephrotoxicity*
Other: *ototoxicity* (eighth cranial nerve)

Cycloserine

Indications
Tuberculosis (usually as part of a multi-drug regimen)

Adverse reactions
CNS: drowsiness, headache, vertigo, confusion, psychoses, *seizures, nervousness, hallucinations, depression*
Other: rash

Ethambutol

Indications
Tuberculosis (usually as part of a multi-drug regimen)

Adverse reactions
CNS: headache, dizziness, mental confusion
EENT: optic neuritis
GI: anorexia, nausea, vomiting
Metabolic: elevated uric acid levels, precipitation of gout
Other: *anaphylaxis,* fever, malaise

Ethionamide

Indications
Tuberculosis (usually as part of a multi-drug regimen)

Adverse reactions
CNS: depression, asthenia, *peripheral neuritis*
GI: *anorexia, epigastric distress,* nausea, vomiting
Hepatic: increased liver function test results, hepatitis

Skin: rash, *exfoliative dermatitis*

Isoniazid

Indications
Tuberculosis (usually as part of a multi-drug regimen); may be used alone for prophylaxis (6 months to a year) in patients with a significant reaction to the Mantoux test

Adverse reactions
Blood: *agranulocytosis, hemolytic anemia, aplastic anemia, thrombocytopenia,* leukopenia, neutropenia, eosinophilia
CNS: *peripheral neuropathy* (preventable by using pyridoxine during isoniazid therapy)
GI: nausea, vomiting, epigastric distress
Hepatic: *hepatitis* (may be severe or fatal; highest incidence in individuals over age 35)
Other: *hypersensitivity* (fever, skin eruptions)

Pyrazinamide

Indications
Tuberculosis (usually as part of a multi-drug regimen)

Adverse reactions
GI: anorexia, nausea, vomiting, diarrhea
Hepatic: *hepatotoxicity*
Metabolic: *hyperuricemia;* occasionally, precipitation of gout
Other: fever, myalgia, arthralgia

Rifampin

Indications
Tuberculosis (usually as part of a multi-drug regimen); also used to treat staphylococcal infections in combination with other antibiotics, for prophylaxis in persons exposed to *Haemophilus influenzae* type B infections, and to eradicate *Neisseria meningitidis* from the nasopharynx of asymptomatic carriers

---

Common reactions are in *italics;* life-threatening reactions are in ***bold italics.***

Adverse reactions
Blood: eosinophilia, transient leukopenia, ***thrombocytopenia, hemolytic anemia***
CNS: headache, fatigue, *drowsiness,* ataxia, dizziness
GI: anorexia, nausea, vomiting, abdominal pain, diarrhea
Hepatic: ***hepatotoxicity***, transient elevations in liver function test results
Skin: rash, urticaria
Other: flulike syndrome, discoloration of body fluids (red-orange tears, feces, urine, sputum, sweat)

Drugs associated with selected AIDS infections

Atovaquone, co-trimoxazole (sulfamethoxazole-trimethoprim), dapsone, pentamidine, primaquine, pyrimethamine, rifabutin, sulfadiazine, trimetrexate

Atovaquone

Indications
Mild to moderate *Pneumocystis carinii* pneumonia in patients who can't tolerate co-trimoxazole

Adverse reactions
CNS: *headache, insomnia,* asthenia, dizziness
GI: *nausea, vomiting, diarrhea,* constipation
Skin: *rash,* pruritus
Other: *fever,* oral monilia

Co-trimoxazole

Indications
Treatment or prophylaxis of *P. carinii* pneumonia

Adverse reactions
Blood: ***agranulocytosis, hemolytic anemia,*** megaloblastic anemia, neutropenia, leukopenia, ***thrombocytopenia***
CNS: headache, dizziness, tinnitus, insomnia

GI: *nausea, vomiting, diarrhea,* abdominal pain; pseudomembranous colitis (rare)
GU: ***toxic nephrosis with oliguria and anuria,*** crystalluria, hematuria, increased serum creatinine levels
Skin: rash, pruritus, *skin eruptions, **erythema multiforme (Stevens-Johnson syndrome), epidermal necrolysis, exfoliative dermatitis,*** photosensitivity
Other: ***hypersensitivity,*** *(fever, serum sickness, **anaphylaxis**)*

Dapsone

Indications
Treatment or prophylaxis of *P. carinii* pneumonia; used in combination with trimethoprim for treatment; for prophylaxis, may be used as monotherapy or in combination with trimethoprim or pyrimethamine

Adverse reactions
Blood: ***aplastic anemia, agranulocytosis, hemolytic anemia*** (especially in patients with glucose-6-phosphate dehydrogenase deficiency), methemoglobinemia, cyanosis
CNS: insomnia, psychosis, headache, dizziness, severe malaise, paresthesia
GI: anorexia, nausea, vomiting
Hepatic: hepatitis, cholestatic jaundice
Skin: rash
Other: tinnitus, allergic rhinitis

Pentamidine

Indications
Treatment or prophylaxis of *P. carinii* pneumonia

Adverse reactions
Blood: *leukopenia, **thrombocytopenia,*** anemia,
CV: ***hypotension,*** tachycardia, arrhythmias
Endocrine: ***hypoglycemia,*** hyperglycemia, hypocalcemia
GI: nausea, anorexia, metallic taste
GU: *elevated serum creatinine levels,* renal failure, ***nephrotoxicity*** (in 25% of patients)

Common reactions are in *italics;* life-threatening reactions are in ***bold italics.***

Skin: rash, facial flushing, pruritus
Other: *pancreatitis,* orthostatic hypotension

Primaquine

Indications
Treatment or prophylaxis of *P. carinii* pneumonia in combination with clindamycin

Adverse reactions
Blood: *hemolytic anemia* (in glucose-6-phosphate dehydrogenase deficiency), leukopenia, leukocytosis, mild anemia, *agranulocytosis* (rare), methemoglobinemia
GI: nausea, vomiting, diarrhea, abdominal cramps
Skin: urticaria
Other: headache, disturbances of visual accommodation

Pyrimethamine

Indications
Toxoplasmosis in combination with sulfadiazine or clindamycin; prophylaxis of *P. carinii* pneumonia in combination with dapsone (second line choice)

Adverse reactions
Blood: *agranulocytosis, aplastic anemia,* megaloblastic anemia, *bone marrow suppression,* leukopenia, *thrombocytopenia,* pancytopenia, depletion of folic acid stores
CNS: stimulation and *seizures* (acute toxicity)
GI: anorexia, vomiting, diarrhea, atrophic glossitis
Skin: rash, *erythema multiforme, toxic epidermal necrolysis*

Rifabutin

Indications
Prevention of disseminated *Mycobacterium avium* complex in patients with advanced HIV infection (CD4+ T-cell count less than 100/mm^3)

Adverse reactions
Blood: neutropenia, leukopenia, *thrombocytopenia,* eosinophilia
GI: dyspepsia, eructation, flatulence, nausea, vomiting, abdominal pain
GU: *discolored urine*
Skin: rash
Other: uveitis, fever, myalgia, myositis, taste distortion

Sulfadiazine

Indications
Adjunctive treatment of toxoplasmosis

Adverse reactions
Blood: *agranulocytosis, aplastic anemia,* megaloblastic anemia, *thrombocytopenia,* leukopenia, *hemolytic anemia*
CNS: headache, mental depression, seizures, hallucinations
GI: *nausea, vomiting, diarrhea,* abdominal pain, anorexia, stomatitis
GU: *toxic nephrosis* with oliguria and anuria, crystalluria, hematuria
Skin: urticaria, pruritus, photosensitivity, *erythema multiforme,* skin eruptions, *epidermal necrolysis, exfoliative dermatitis*
Other: jaundice, *hypersensitivity (serum sickness, fever, anaphylaxis)*

Trimetrexate

Indications
Moderate to severe cases of *P. carinii* pneumonia in patients intolerant of or refractory to co-trimoxazole therapy. (*Note:* Leucovorin must be used daily throughout trimetrexate therapy and for 72 hours after discontinuation of this drug.)

Adverse reactions
Blood: neutropenia, *thrombocytopenia*
Skin: rash
Other: *hepatotoxicity,* peripheral neuropathy

Common reactions are in *italics;* life-threatening reactions are in ***bold italics.***

Transmission prevention guidelines

To prevent the transmission of infectious diseases in hospitals and other clinical settings, the Centers for Disease Control and Prevention has published a *category-specific* isolation system, which describes six of its seven categories of isolation precautions according to major modes of transmission. The seventh category, *universal precautions*, has been expanded to cover *all* patients — not just those with known or suspected blood-borne diseases. Because of the special concern about the risk of transmitting human immunodeficiency virus, this category is covered separately. (See *Universal precautions,* pages 346 and 347.)

Type of isolation and diseases requiring isolation	Private room	Mask	Gown	Gloves	Special handling
Strict isolation Prevents transmission of contagious or virulent infections by air or contact. Special ventilation is required. ***Diseases:*** pharyngeal diphtheria, viral hemorrhagic fevers, pneumonic plague, smallpox, varicella-zoster virus (localized in immunocompromised patient or disseminated)	X with door closed	X	X	X	X
Contact isolation Prevents transmission of epidemiologically important infections that don't require strict isolation. Health care workers should wear masks, gowns, and gloves for direct or close contact, depending on the infection. ***Diseases in any age-group:*** Group A streptococcal endometritis; impetigo; pediculosis; *Staphylococcus aureus* or *Streptococcus pneumoniae* infection; rabies; rubella; scabies; staphylococcal scalded skin syndrome; major skin, wound, or burn infection (draining and not adequately covered by dressing); vaccinia; primary disseminated herpes simplex; cutaneous diphtheria; infection or colonization with bacteria that resist antibiotic therapy ***Diseases in infants and young children:*** acute respiratory infections, influenza, infectious pharyngitis, viral pneumonia, group A streptococcal infection ***Diseases in neonates:*** gonococcal conjunctivitis, staphylococcal furunculosis, neonatal disseminated herpes simplex	X	O	S	S	X

Type of isolation and diseases requiring isolation	Private room	Mask	Gown	Gloves	Special handling
Respiratory isolation Prevents transmission of infections spread primarily through the air by droplets ***Diseases:*** *Haemophilus influenzae* epiglottitis, erythema infectiosum, measles; *H. influenzae* or meningococcal pneumonia, meningococcemia, mumps, pertussis	X with door closed	O	—	—	X
Acid-fast bacillus isolation Prevents patient with active pulmonary or laryngeal tuberculosis from transmitting acid-fast bacillus to other patients. Patient requires special ventilation. ***Disease:*** tuberculosis	X with door closed	O	S	—	X
Enteric precautions Prevents transmission of infection through direct or indirect contact with feces ***Diseases:*** amebic dysentery; cholera; coxsackievirus disease; acute diarrhea with suspected infection; echovirus disease; encephalitis unless known not to be caused by enteroviruses; *Clostridium difficile* or enterocolitis caused by *Staphylococcus;* enteroviral infection; gastroenteritis caused by *Campylobacter* species, *Cryptosporidium* species, *Dientamoeba fragilis, Escherichia coli, Giardia lamblia, Salmonella* species, *Shigella* species, *Vibrio parahaemolyticus,* viruses, and *Yersinia enterocolitica;* hand-foot-and-mouth disease; hepatitis A; herpangina; necrotizing enterocolitis; pleurodynia; poliomyelitis; typhoid fever; viral pericarditis, viral myocarditis, and viral meningitis unless known not to be caused by enteroviruses	D	—	S	S	X
Drainage and secretion precautions Prevents transmission of infection from direct or indirect contact with purulent material or drainage ***Diseases:*** conjunctivitis; minor or limited abscess; minor or limited burn, skin, wound, or pressure ulcer infection; herpes zoster (shingles)	—	—	S	S	X

Key

X = Always necessary

S = Necessary if soiling of hands or clothing is likely

O = Necessary for close contact or if patient is coughing and doesn't reliably cover mouth

D = Desirable but optional; necessary only if patient has poor hygiene

Universal precautions

Because the medical history and physical examination cannot reliably identify all patients infected with human immunodeficiency virus (HIV) or other blood-borne pathogens, the Centers for Disease Control and Prevention recommends that universal blood and body-fluid precautions be used for *all* patients. Using universal precautions is especially important in emergency care settings, where the risk of blood exposure is increased and the infection status of the patient is usually unknown. Implementation of universal precautions doesn't eliminate the need for other category- or disease-specific isolation precautions, such as enteric precautions for infectious diarrhea or acid-fast bacillus isolation precautions for pulmonary tuberculosis.

Sources of potential exposure

Universal precautions apply to blood, semen, vaginal secretions, cerebrospinal fluid, synovial fluid, pleural fluid, peritoneal fluid, pericardial fluid, and amniotic fluid. Universal precautions also pertain to all body fluids — including feces, nasal secretions, saliva, sputum, sweat, tears, vomitus, or breast milk — if they contain *visible* blood. When these body fluids contain no visible blood, experts presume that they won't transmit HIV or hepatitis B virus (HBV) infections.

Barrier precautions

If you anticipate contact with the blood or body fluids of any patient, use appropriate barrier precautions to prevent exposure of skin and mucous membranes:
• Wear gloves when touching blood and body fluids, mucous membranes, or broken skin of all patients; when handling items or touching surfaces soiled with blood or body fluids; and when performing venipuncture and other vascular access procedures.

• Change gloves and wash hands after contact with each patient.
• Wear a mask and protective eyewear or a face shield to prevent exposure of mucous membranes of the mouth, nose, and eyes during procedures that are likely to generate droplets of blood or other body fluids.
• Wear a gown or an apron during procedures that are likely to generate splashing of blood or other body fluids.
• After removing gloves, thoroughly wash hands and other skin surfaces that may be contaminated with blood, body fluids containing visible blood, or other body fluids to which universal precautions apply.

Precautions for invasive procedures

If you participate in invasive procedures, expect to routinely use appropriate barrier precautions to prevent skin and mucous-membrane contact with blood and other body fluids of all patients.
• During all invasive procedures, wear gloves, a surgical mask, and goggles or a face shield.
• During procedures that commonly generate droplets or splashes of blood or other body fluids, or that generate bone chips, wear protective eyewear and a mask, or a face shield.
• During invasive procedures that are likely to cause splashing or splattering of blood or other body fluids, wear a gown or an impervious apron.
• If you perform or assist in vaginal or cesarean deliveries, wear gloves and a gown when handling the placenta or the infant (until blood and amniotic fluid are removed from the infant's skin) and during postdelivery care of the umbilical cord.

Work practice precautions

Take steps to prevent injuries caused by needles, scalpels, and other sharp instruments or devices used during procedures; when cleaning used instruments; when disposing of used needles; and when handling sharp instruments after procedures.

• To prevent needle-stick injuries, do not recap used needles, bend or break needles, remove them from disposable syringes, or otherwise manually manipulate them.

• Place disposable syringes and needles, scalpel blades, and other sharp items in puncture-resistant containers for disposal; make sure that puncture-resistant containers are located as close as practical to the area of use.

• Place large-bore reusable needles in a puncture-resistant container for transport to the reprocessing area.

• If a glove tears or a needle stick or other injury occurs, remove the glove and put on a new one as quickly as patient safety permits; remove the needle or instrument involved in the incident from the sterile field.

Additional precautions

• To minimize the need for emergency mouth-to-mouth resuscitation, make sure mouthpieces, one-way valve masks, resuscitation bags, or other ventilation devices are available for use in areas in which the need for resuscitation is likely. *Note:* Saliva has not been implicated in HIV transmission.

• If you develop exudative lesions or weeping dermatitis, refrain from all direct patient care and from handling patient care equipment until the condition resolves.

Guidelines for minimizing infection

The table below lists the minimum requirements for using gloves, gowns, masks, and protective eyewear to avoid contacting and spreading pathogens. Refer to your hospital's guidelines and use your own judgment when assessing the need for barrier protection in specific situations. Practice thorough hand washing in all cases.

Procedure	Gloves	Gown	Mask	Eyewear
Bathing, for patient with open lesions	✓	—	—	—
Bedding, changing visibly soiled	✓	If soiling likely	—	—
Bleeding or pressure application to control it	✓	If soiling likely	If splattering likely	If splattering likely
Blood glucose (capillary) testing	✓	—	—	—
Breathing treatment, routine	If soiling likely	—	If airborne infection	—
Cardiopulmonary resuscitation	✓	If splattering likely	If splattering likely	If splattering likely
Central venous line insertion and venesection	✓	✓	✓	✓
Central venous pressure measurement	✓	—	—	—
Cervical cauterization	✓	—	—	—
Chest drainage system change	✓	If splattering likely	If splattering likely	If splattering likely
Chest tube insertion	✓	If soiling likely	If splattering likely	If splattering likely
Chest tube removal	✓	If soiling likely	If splattering likely	If splattering likely
Cleaning, anal	✓	—	—	—
Cleaning (feces, spilled blood or body substances, or surfaces contaminated by blood or body fluids)	✓	If soiling likely	—	—
Cleaning, urine	✓	—	—	—
Colonoscopy, flexible sigmoidoscope	✓	✓	—	—

Note: ✓ indicates that barrier is necessary; — indicates that barrier typically is not necessary.

Procedure	Gloves	Gown	Mask	Eyewear
Coughing, frequent and forceful by patient; direct contact with secretions	—	—	✓	✓
Dialysis, peritoneal				
Initiating acute treatment	✓	✓	If splattering likely	If splattering likely
Performing an exchange	✓	✓	If splattering likely	If splattering likely
Terminating acute treatment	✓	✓	If splattering likely	If splattering likely
Dismantling tubing from cycler	✓	✓	If splattering likely	If splattering likely
Discarding peritoneal drainage	✓	✓	If splattering likely	If splattering likely
Irrigating peritoneal catheter	✓	✓	If splattering likely	If splattering likely
Collecting specimens	✓	—	—	—
Changing tubes	✓	✓	If splattering likely	If splattering likely
Performing skin care (catheter site)	✓	✓	✓	✓
Assisting with insertion of acute peritoneal catheter (outside sterile field)	✓	✓	If splattering likely	If splattering likely
Dressing change for burns	✓	✓	—	—
Dressing removal or change for wounds with little or no drainage	✓	—	—	—
Dressing removal or change for wounds with large amount of drainage	✓	If soiling likely	—	—
Emptying drainage receptacles, including suction containers, urine receptacles, bedpans, and emesis basins	✓	If soiling likely	If splattering likely	If splattering likely
Emptying wastebaskets	✓	—	—	—
Enema	✓	If soiling likely	—	—
Fecal impaction, removal of	✓	If soiling likely	—	—
Fecal incontinence, placement of indwelling urinary catheter for, and emptying bag	✓	If splattering likely	—	—

(continued)

Note: ✓ indicates that barrier is necessary; — indicates that barrier typically is not necessary.

Procedure	Gloves	Gown	Mask	Eyewear
Gastric lavage	✓	If soiling or splattering likely	—	—
Incision and drainage of abscess	✓	If splattering likely	—	—
Intravenous or intra-arterial line				
Insertion	✓	—	—	—
Removal	✓	—	—	—
Tubing change at catheter hub	✓	—	—	—
Intubation or extubation	✓	If splattering likely	If splattering likely	If splattering likely
Invasive procedures (lumbar puncture, bone marrow aspiration, paracentesis, liver biopsy) outside sterile field	✓	—	—	—
Irrigation				
Indwelling urinary catheter	✓	—	—	—
Vaginal	✓	If soiling likely	—	—
Wound	✓	If soiling likely	If splattering likely	If splattering likely
Joint or nerve injection	✓	—	—	—
Lesion biopsy or removal	✓	—	—	—
Medication administration				
Eye, ear, and nose drops	✓	—	—	—
I.M. or S.C.	✓	—	—	—
I.V. (direct or into hub of catheter or heparin lock)	✓	—	—	—
Oral (directly into patient's mouth)	✓	—	—	—
Rectal or vaginal suppository	✓	—	—	—
Topical medication for lesion	✓	—	—	—
Nasogastric tube, insertion or irrigation	✓	If soiling likely	If splattering likely	If splattering likely
Oral and nasal care	✓	—	—	—
Ostomy care, irrigation, and teaching	✓	If soiling likely	—	—
Oxygen tubing, drainage of condensate	✓	—	—	—
Pelvic exam and Papanicolaou test	✓	—	—	—
Perineal cleaning	✓	—	—	—

Note: ✓ indicates that barrier is necessary; — indicates that barrier typically is not necessary.

Procedure	Gloves	Gown	Mask	Eyewear
Postmortem care	✓	If soiling likely	—	—
Pressure ulcer care	✓	—	—	—
Shaving	✓	—	—	—
Specimen collection (blood, stool, sputum, wound)	✓	—	—	—
Suctioning Nasotracheal or endotracheal	✓	If soiling likely	If splattering likely	If splattering likely
Oral or nasal	✓	—	—	—
Temperature, rectal	✓	—	—	—
Tracheostomy suctioning and cannula cleaning	✓	If soiling likely	If splattering likely	If splattering likely
Tracheostomy tube change	✓	—	If splattering likely	If splattering likely
Urine and stool testing	✓	—	—	—
Wound packing	✓	If soiling likely	—	—

Note: ✓ indicates that barrier is necessary; — indicates that barrier typically is not necessary.

Checklist of reportable diseases

Because disease reporting laws vary from state to state and some diseases do not need to be reported in all states, this list isn't conclusive and may change periodically. Local agencies report certain diseases to state health departments, which in turn determine which diseases are reported to the Centers for Disease Control and Prevention.

☐ Acquired immunodeficiency syndrome
☐ Amebiasis
☐ Animal bites
☐ Anthrax (cutaneous or pulmonary)
☐ Arbovirus
☐ Aseptic meningitis
☐ Botulism (food-borne, infant)
☐ Brucellosis
☐ Campylobacteriosis
☐ Chancroid
☐ Chlamydial infections
☐ Cholera
☐ Diarrhea of the newborn, epidemic
☐ Diphtheria (cutaneous or pharyngeal)
☐ Encephalitis (postinfectious or primary)
☐ Food poisoning
☐ Gastroenteritis (hospital outbreak)
☐ Giardiasis
☐ Gonococcal infections
☐ Gonorrhea
☐ Group A beta-hemolytic streptococcal infections (including scarlet fever)
☐ Guillain-Barré syndrome
☐ Hepatitis A, infectious (include suspected source)
☐ Hepatitis B, serum (include suspected source)
☐ Hepatitis C, formerly called non-A, non-B (include suspected source)
☐ Hepatitis, unspecified (include suspected source)
☐ Histoplasmosis
☐ Influenza
☐ Kawasaki disease
☐ Lead poisoning
☐ *Legionella* infections (Legionnaires' disease)
☐ Leprosy
☐ Leptospirosis
☐ Listeriosis
☐ Lyme disease

☐ Lymphogranuloma venereum
☐ Malaria
☐ Measles (rubeola)
☐ Meningitis (specify etiology)
☐ Meningococcal disease
☐ Mumps
☐ Neonatal hypothyroidism
☐ Pertussis (whooping cough)
☐ Phenylketonuria
☐ Plague (bubonic or pneumonic)
☐ Poliomyelitis (spinal paralytic)
☐ Psittacosis (ornithosis)
☐ Rabies
☐ Reye's syndrome
☐ Rheumatic fever
☐ Rickettsial diseases (including Rocky Mountain spotted fever)
☐ Rubella (German measles) and congenital rubella syndrome
☐ Salmonellosis (excluding typhoid fever)
☐ Shigellosis
☐ Staphylococcal infections (neonatal)
☐ Syphilis (congenital < 1 year)
☐ Syphilis (primary or secondary)
☐ Tetanus
☐ Toxic shock syndrome
☐ Toxoplasmosis
☐ Trichinosis
☐ Tuberculosis
☐ Tularemia
☐ Typhoid and paratyphoid fever
☐ Typhus (flea- and tick-borne)
☐ Varicella (chicken pox)
☐ Yellow fever

Index

A

ABO blood typing, 21
   transplant rejection and,
      156
Acid-fast stain, 169
Acquired immunodeficiency
   syndrome, 52-71
   assessing, 56-57, 59,
      65-66
   causes of, 54, 56
   classifying, 55-56
   complications of, 57, 59
   course of, 54
   discharge preparation for,
      70
   evaluating patient's re-
      sponse to therapy for,
      71
   groups at risk for, 57
   interventions for, 67-71
   nursing diagnoses for, 66
   opportunistic diseases as-
      sociated with, 60-65t
   patient outcomes for,
      66-67
   patient teaching for, 69-71
   psychosocial support for
      patients with, 69
   treatment of, 68
Activity intolerance as nursing
   diagnosis, 28, 172
   rheumatoid arthritis and,
      111, 112
   systemic lupus erythemato-
      sus and, 122, 123
Acute pyelonephritis, 269-274
   assessing, 271-272
   causes of, 270-271
   complications of, 269
   discharge preparation for,
      274
   evaluating patient's re-
      sponse to therapy for,
      274
   interventions for, 272-274
   nursing diagnoses for, 272
   pathophysiology of, 270i
   patient outcomes for, 272
   patient teaching for,
      273-274
   risk factors for, 271
   treatment of, 273
Acyclovir, 205
Adenovirus, 279
AIDS. *See* Acquired immunodeficiency syndrome.
Airway clearance, ineffective,
   as nursing diagnosis,
   173
   asthma and, 95, 96
   pneumonia and, 277, 278
   tuberculosis and, 260
Alkaline phosphatase levels
   transplant rejection and,
      157
   viral hepatitis and, 192

Allergic bronchopulmonary aspergillosis, asthma and,
   93
Allergic transfusion reaction,
   treatment of, 104. *See
   also* Blood transfusion
   reaction.
Allograft, 155
Amantadine, 199, 200
Anaphylaxis, 82-88
   assessing, 84-85
   causes of, 82, 84
   discharge preparation for,
      88
   evaluating patient's re-
      sponse to therapy for,
      87-88
   interventions for, 86-87
   nursing diagnoses for, 85
   patient outcomes for,
      85-86
   patient teaching for, 87
   progression of, 83i
   treatment of, 87
Anergy panel, 23-24
Antidiarrheals, 308
Antiemetics, 308
Antigen-antibody tests,
   herpes zoster and, 208
Antimicrobial therapy, 77
Antinuclear antibodies test,
   21
Antiretroviral therapy, 68
Antithymocyte globulin
   (equine), 153t
Antitubercular therapy, 261
Antiviral therapy, herpes zoster and, 210
Anxiety
   anaphylaxis and, 85-86
   asthma and, 96
   blood transfusion reaction
      and, 104, 105
Assessment. *See also specific
   disorders.*
   of immune disorders, 2,
      5-9, 10-15i, 16, 17i,
      18, 19-21t, 21,
      22-23t, 23-24
   of infectious disorders,
      162, 164-169, 170t,
      171
Asthma, 92-102
   assessing, 93-95
   causes of, 92, 93
   discharge preparation for,
      101
   evaluating patient's re-
      sponse to therapy for,
      101-102
   interventions for, 96-97,
      98-99i, 100-101
   nursing diagnoses for,
      95-96
   pathophysiology of, 94-95i

Asthma *(continued)*
   patient outcomes for, 96
   patient teaching for,
      100-101
   preventing attacks of, 100
   treatment of, 97
Atopic dermatitis, 88-92
   assessing, 89
   causes of, 89
   complications of, 88
   discharge preparation for,
      91
   evaluating patient's re-
      sponse to therapy for,
      92
   interventions for, 90-92
   nursing diagnoses for, 89
   patient outcomes for,
      89-90
   patient teaching for, 91-92
   treatment of, 90
Autoantibodies, detecting,
   22-23t
Autograft, 155
Autoimmune disorders,
   108-146
Autoimmune hemolytic ane-
   mia, detecting autoantibodies in, 22t
Autoimmune thrombocyto-
   penic purpura, 134-140
   assessing, 135-136,
      138-139i
   causes of, 134-135
   complications of, 134
   discharge preparation for,
      140
   evaluating patient's re-
      sponse to therapy for,
      139-140
   interventions for, 136-139
   nursing diagnoses for, 136
   patient outcomes for, 136
   patient teaching for,
      137-139
   treatment of, 137
Automated reagin test, syphilis and, 239
Azathioprine, 152t

B

Bacteria
   classifying, 226
   disorders related to, 163t
Bacterial infections, 226-242,
   245-274
   mechanisms of, 227i
Bacterial pneumonias,
   280-281. *See also* Pneumonia.
Bilirubin levels, serum
   transplant rejection and,
      157
   viral hepatitis and, 192

Blood culture, pneumonia and, 277
Blood glucose levels
  transplant rejection and, 157
  transplant-related immuno-suppression and, 150
Blood tests, 18, 19-21t, 21, 23
  acute pyelonephritis and, 272
  Hashimoto's disease and, 142
  Lyme disease and, 252
  systemic sclerosis and, 129
Blood transfusion reaction, 102-106
  assessing, 103-104
  causes of, 102-103
  discharge preparation for, 106
  evaluating patient's response to therapy for, 106
  implementing interventions for, 105-106
  nursing diagnoses for, 104
  patient outcomes for, 105
  patient teaching for, 106
  signs of, 102
  treatment of, 104
Blood typing, 21, 23
Blood urea nitrogen levels
  transplant rejection and, 157
  transplant-related immuno-suppression and, 149
Body image disturbance as nursing diagnosis, 28
  atopic dermatitis and, 89, 90
  genital warts and, 212, 213
  systemic lupus erythematosus and, 122
Body temperature, altered, high risk for, transplant rejection and, 158
Bone marrow aspiration and biopsy, 24
  autoimmune thrombocytopenic purpura and, 136
Bone marrow transplantation, immunodeficiency and, 74
Breathing pattern, ineffective, as nursing diagnosis, 28, 174
  pneumonia and, 277-278
Bronchoscopy, tuberculosis and, 260
Brudzinski's sign, 296i
Bruton's hypogammaglobulinemia, 53t
Butterfly rash, systemic lupus erythematosus and, 121

C

Cancer, immunodeficiency and, 71-80. *See also* Immu-

nodeficiency caused by cancer and its treatment.
Candidiasis, AIDS and, 61t
Cardiac output, decreased, as nursing diagnosis, 173
  anaphylaxis and, 85, 86
  blood transfusion and, 104, 105
  Hashimoto's disease and, 142
Cardiovascular syphilis, 239. *See also* Syphilis.
Caregiver role strain as nursing diagnosis, 28
  high risk for, AIDS and, 66, 67
Care planning. *See* Planning.
Cell counts, 18, 19-20t. *See also* White blood cell count.
Cell-mediated immunity, 4-5i
Cerebral tissue perfusion, altered
  meningitis and, 295
  viral encephalitis and, 220, 221
Cerebrospinal fluid analysis, syphilis and, 239
Cervical neoplasm, AIDS and, 65t
Cervicitis, signs of, 248. *See also* Pelvic inflammatory disease.
Chemotherapy, immunodeficiency and, 74, 75
Chest X-rays
  meningitis and, 295
  systemic lupus erythematosus and, 122
  tuberculosis and, 257, 259
Chicken pox, 279
Chief complaints
  immune disorders and, 5, 40-50
  infectious disorders and, 164, 184-188
Chlamydiae, disorders related to, 163t
Chlamydial infection, 242-245
  assessing, 242-243
  causes of, 242
  complications of, 242
  discharge preparation for, 245
  evaluating patient's response to therapy for, 245
  interventions for, 244
  nursing diagnoses for, 243
  patient outcomes for, 243-244
  patient teaching for, 244
  prevalence of, 242
  transmission of, 242
  treatment of, 244
Chronic mucocutaneous candidiasis, 53t
Coccidioides, AIDS and, 61t
Common variable immune deficiency, 53t

Complement assay, 18, 21t
  systemic lupus erythematosus and, 121
Complete blood count
  rheumatoid arthritis and, 111
  systemic lupus erythematosus and, 121
  transplant-related immuno-suppression and, 149
Computed tomography
  meningitis and, 295
  rheumatoid arthritis and, 111
  tuberculosis and, 260
  viral encephalitis and, 220
Condylomata acuminata. *See* Genital warts.
Congenital immunodeficiencies, 53-54t
C-reactive protein test, rheumatoid arthritis and, 111
Creatinine levels, serum
  transplant rejection and, 157
  transplant-related immuno-suppression and, 149
CREST syndrome, 128. *See also* Systemic sclerosis.
Crossmatching, 23
  transplant rejection and, 156
Cryptococcosis, AIDS and, 61t
Cryptosporidiosis, AIDS and, 62t
Cultures, 169, 171
  collecting specimens for, 170t
  meningitis and, 295
Cyclosporine, 152t
Cystitis, 301t. *See also* Lower urinary tract infection.
Cytologic examination, 169
Cytomegalovirus, 279
  AIDS and, 63t
Cytotoxic hypersensitivity reactions, 82

D

Darkfield microscopy
  genital warts and, 212
  syphilis and, 239
Delayed hypersensitivity reactions, 82
Diagnostic test results. *See also specific disorders.*
  immune disorders and, 16, 18, 19-21t, 21, 22-23t, 23-24
  infectious disorders and, 168-169, 170t, 171
Diarrhea
  AIDS and, 66, 67
  gastroenteritis and, 307-308
  infectious, causes of, 305-306
  as nursing diagnosis, 173
  toxic shock syndrome and, 229, 230

Didanosine, 68
Diffuse systemic sclerosis, 128. *See also* Systemic sclerosis.
DiGeorge syndrome, 53t
Discoid lupus erythematosus, 119
Drug therapy
  for immune disorders, 326-331
  for infectious disorders, 332-343
DTH test, 23

E
Ecchymoses, 138i
Electrocardiography
  systemic lupus erythematosus and, 122
  systemic sclerosis and, 129
Endometritis, signs of, 248. *See also* Pelvic inflammatory disease.
Erythrocyte sedimentation rate, 18, 21t
  rheumatoid arthritis and, 111
Evaluation. *See also specific disorders.*
  immune disorders and, 35, 36i, 37-38
  infectious disorders and, 180-182

F
Facial exercises, systemic sclerosis and, 132i
Fatigue
  AIDS and, 66-67
  assessing, 42-43
  causes of, 42
  infectious mononucleosis and, 216
  influenza and, 198
  Lyme disease and, 253
  as nursing diagnosis, 25
  rheumatoid arthritis and, 111, 112
  tuberculosis and, 260-261
  viral hepatitis and, 192, 193
Fear
  autoimmune thrombocytopenic purpura and, 136
  immunodeficiency (secondary) and, 77
  transplant rejection and, 158, 159
  viral hepatitis and, 192, 193
Febrile nonhemolytic transfusion reaction, treatment of, 104. *See also* Blood transfusion reaction.
Fever
  assessing, 40-42
  causes of, 41
  classifying, 40
Flu. *See* Influenza.

Fluid volume deficit
  gastroenteritis and, 307
  high risk for, 174
  influenza and, 198
  sepsis and, 312, 316
  toxic shock syndrome and, 229, 230
  wound infection and, 288, 289
Fungal pneumonia, 282
Fungi, disorders related to, 163t

G
Gas exchange, impaired
  asthma and, 96
  pneumonia and, 277, 278
Gastroenteritis, 304-310
  assessing, 307
  causes of, 304, 305-306
  complications of, 304
  discharge preparation for, 310
  evaluating patient's response to therapy for, 309
  interventions for, 308-309
  nursing diagnoses for, 307
  patient outcomes for, 307-308
  patient teaching for, 309
  risk factors for, 307
  sites of, 306i
  treatment of, 308
Genital herpes simplex virus, 204. *See also* Herpes simplex.
Genital warts, 211-214
  assessing, 211-212
  classifying, 212
  complications of, 212
  evaluating patient's response to therapy for, 214
  implementing interventions for, 213-214
  nursing diagnoses for, 212
  patient outcomes for, 212-213
  patient teaching for, 214
  preventing, 212
  transmission of, 212
  treatment of, 213
GI endoscopy, *Helicobacter pylori* infection and, 266
Gonorrhea, 231-237
  assessing, 232-233
  causes of, 232
  complications of, 231-232
  discharge preparation for, 235
  evaluating patient's response to therapy for, 236-237
  interventions for, 235-236
  incidence of, 232
  nursing diagnoses for, 233
  patient outcomes for, 233-235
  patient teaching for, 235-236
  treatment of, 234

Goodpasture's syndrome, detecting autoantibodies in, 22t
Grafts, types of, 155
Graft-versus-host disease, transplant rejection and, 155
Gram stain, 169
  pelvic inflammatory disease and, 247
  pneumonia and, 277
Grieving, anticipatory, AIDS and, 66
Grippe. *See* Influenza.

H
Hashimoto's disease, 141-146
  assessing, 141-142, 142i, 143
  causes of, 141
  complications of, 141
  discharge preparation for, 145
  evaluating patient's response to therapy for, 145-146
  interventions for, 143-145
  incidence of, 141
  nursing diagnoses for, 142
  patient outcomes for, 142-143
  patient teaching for, 144-145
  prognosis for, 141
  thyroid enlargement in, 142i
  treatment of, 144
Hashimoto's thyroiditis, detecting autoantibodies in, 22t
HBV vaccine, viral hepatitis and, 195
Health history. *See also specific disorders.*
  immune disorders and, 2, 5-7
  infectious disorders and, 162, 164
Heart rejection, signs of, 158. *See also* Transplant rejection.
Helicobacter pylori infection, 266-269
  assessing, 266-267
  causes of, 266
  discharge preparations for, 269
  evaluating patient's response to therapy for, 268-269
  interventions for, 267-268
  nursing diagnoses for, 267
  patient outcomes for, 267
  patient teaching for, 268
  treatment of, 267
Helminths, disorders related to, 163t
Hematomas, 139i
Hematopoiesis, 72i
Hemolytic transfusion reaction, 102-103, 104. *See*

also Blood transfusion
reaction.
Herpes simplex, 202-207
AIDS and, 63t
assessing, 202, 204
causes of, 203
complications of, 203
discharge preparation for,
207
evaluating patient's re-
sponse to therapy for,
206
interventions for, 203,
205-206
nursing diagnoses for, 202
patient outcomes for,
202-203
patient teaching for, 205-206
transmission of, 203
treatment of, 205
Herpes zoster, 207-211
assessing, 207-208
causes of, 207
complications of, 208
discharge preparation for,
211
evaluating patient's re-
sponse to therapy for,
210-211
interventions for, 209-210
incidence of, 208
nursing diagnoses for, 209
patient outcomes for, 209
patient teaching for, 209-210
prognosis for, 208
treatment of, 210
Heterograft, 155
Heterophil antibodies, infectious mononucleosis and,
216
Histoplasmosis, AIDS and, 62t
HIV. *See* Human immunodeficiency virus infection.
Homograft, 155
Human immunodeficiency virus infection
classifying, 55-56
immunodeficiency and,
58-59i
transmission of, 56
Human leukocyte antigen test,
23
Humoral immunity, 4-5i
Hypersensitivity disorders,
82-106
classifying, 82
Hyperthermia as nursing diagnosis, 174
acute pyelonephritis and,
272
blood transfusion reaction
and, 104, 105
infectious mononucleosis
and, 216
influenza and, 198
Lyme disease and, 253
meningitis and, 295, 297
pneumonia and, 277, 278
toxic shock syndrome and,
229
viral encephalitis and, 220

Hyperthyroidism, signs of,
143
Hypothyroidism, signs of, 143

I

Iatrogenic factors, immunodeficiency and, 52
Idiopathic thrombocytopenic
purpura. *See* Autoim-
mune thrombocytopenic
purpura.
IgA deficiency, selective, 53t
Immune complex-mediated
hypersensitivity reac-
tions, 82
Immune globulin, viral hepatitis and, 195
Immune response, mechanics
of, 4-5i
Immunodeficiency
classifying, 52
HIV infection and, 58-59i
Immunodeficiency caused by
cancer and its treat-
ment, 71-80
assessing, 74-76
causes of, 71, 74, 75
discharge preparation for,
80
evaluating patient's re-
sponse to care for,
79-80
interventions for, 77-79
nursing diagnoses for, 77
patient outcomes for, 77
patient teaching for, 79
treatment of, 77
Immunodeficiency disorders,
52-80
Immunodeficiency with
ataxia-telangiectasia, 54t
Immunodiagnostic testing,
171
Immunoglobulin levels, 18, 20t
Immunosuppressants, transplant-related, 148,
152-153t
transplant rejection and,
156
Immunosuppression
cancer-related. *See* Immunodeficiency caused
by cancer and its
treatment.
transplant-related. *See*
Transplant-related im-
munosuppression.
Implementation. *See also* spe-
cific disorders.
immune disorders and,
33-35
infectious disorders and,
178-180
Inability to sustain spontaneous ventilation, ana-
phylaxis and, 85, 86
Indirect immunofluorescence,
infectious mononucleosis
and, 216
Individual coping, ineffective,
as nursing diagnosis, 25

Individual coping, ineffective
(continued)
systemic sclerosis and, 129
transplant-related immunosuppression and, 150
Infection, high risk for, as
nursing diagnosis, 24-25
AIDS and, 66
atopic dermatitis and,
89-90
autoimmune thrombocyto-
penic purpura and,
136
gonorrhea and, 233, 234
herpes simplex and, 202,
203
lower urinary tract infection
and, 301
transplant rejection and,
158
wound infection and,
288-289
Infection, minimizing, guidelines for, 348-351
Infection prophylaxis, 151
Infectious diarrhea, causes of,
305-306
Infectious disorders
microorganisms responsible
for, 163t
risk factors for, 164
signs and symptoms of,
184
Infectious mononucleosis,
214-218
assessing, 215-216
causes of, 215
complications of, 215
discharge preparation for,
218
evaluating patient's re-
sponse to therapy for,
218
implementing interventions
for, 216-218
incidence of, 215
nursing diagnoses for, 216
patient outcomes for, 216
patient teaching for,
217-218
prognosis for, 215
transmission of, 215
treatment of, 217
Inflammation, signs of, 3i
Inflammatory response, mechanics of, 3i
Influenza, 197-202, 279-280
assessing, 197-198
causes of, 197
complications of, 197
evaluating patient's re-
sponse to therapy for,
201-202
interventions for, 199, 201
nursing diagnoses for, 198
patient outcomes for, 198
patient teaching for, 199,
201
preventing, 200-201
treatment of, 199

Influenza virus vaccine, 200
Inhaler, how to use, 98-99i
Injury, high risk for
    herpes zoster and, 208
    meningitis and, 295, 297
    pelvic inflammatory disease
        and, 248, 249
Interventions, developing. *See
    also specific disorders.*
    for immune disorders, 32-33
    for infectious disorders,
        178
Intravenous pyelography, lower
    urinary tract infection
    and, 301
Isograft, 155
Isosporiasis, AIDS and, 63t
Itching, herpes zoster and, 208

J

Joint pain
    assessing, 46-48
    causes of, 47
Joint replacement, teaching
    about, 116-117i

K

Kaposi's sarcoma, AIDS and,
    64t
Kernig's sign, 296i
Kidney rejection, signs of,
    158. *See also* Transplant
    rejection.
Klebsiella pneumonia, 280
Knowledge deficit as nursing
    diagnosis, 28, 173
    anaphylaxis and, 85, 86
    asthma and, 96
    atopic dermatitis and, 89,
        90
    chlamydial infection and,
        243, 244
    genital warts and, 212,
        213
    Hashimoto's disease and,
        142-143
    Helicobacter pylori infection
        and, 267
    syphilis and, 239-240
    toxic shock syndrome and,
        229, 230
    transplant rejection and,
        158-159

L

Legionella pneumophila pneu-
    monia, 280-281
Legionnaires' disease, 280-281
Liver enzyme levels
    transplant-related immuno-
        suppression and,
        149-150
    viral hepatitis and, 192
Liver rejection, signs of, 158.
    See also Transplant re-
    jection.
Lower urinary tract infection,
    299-304
    assessing, 299-301, 301t

Lower urinary tract infection
    (continued)
    causes of, 299
    discharge preparation for,
        304
    evaluating patient's re-
        sponse to therapy for,
        303-304
    interventions for, 302-303
    nursing diagnoses for, 301
    patient outcomes for,
        301-302
    patient teaching for,
        302-303
    preventing, 303
    risk factors for, 300
    treatment of, 302
Lumbar puncture
    herpes zoster and, 208
    Lyme disease and, 253
    meningitis and, 295
    viral encephalitis and, 220
Lung rejection, signs of, 158.
    See also Transplant re-
    jection.
Lupus-like syndrome, drug-
    induced, 122
Lyme disease, 251-255
    assessing, 251-253
    causes of, 251
    complications of, 251
    discharge preparation for,
        255
    evaluating patient's re-
        sponse to therapy for,
        255
    interventions for, 253-255
    nursing diagnoses for, 253
    patient outcomes for, 253
    patient teaching for,
        254-255
    preventing, 254
    transmission of, 251
    treatment of, 253
Lymphadenopathy
    assessing, 45-46
    causes of, 45
Lymph node biopsy, 24
Lymph nodes, assessing, 9,
    10-15i, 168
Lymphocyte immune globulin,
    153t

M

Magnetic resonance imaging,
    rheumatoid arthritis and,
    111
Malignant lymphomas, AIDS
    and, 65t
Malnutrition, immunodefi-
    ciency and, 52
Mantoux test, 256-257, 259i
Measles, 280
Meningitis, 292-299
    assessing, 293, 295, 296i
    causes of, 292-293
    complications of, 292
    discharge preparation for,
        298
    evaluating patient's re-
        sponse to therapy for,
        299

Meningitis *(continued)*
    interventions for, 297-299
    nursing diagnoses for, 295
    patient outcomes for, 295,
        297
    patient teaching for,
        298-299
    risk factors for, 293
    treatment of, 297
Microscopic examination, di-
    rect, 169
Muromonab-CD3, †53t
Myasthenia gravis, detecting
    autoantibodies in, 22t
Mycobacterium avium com-
    plex, AIDS and, 60t
Mycobacterium tuberculosis,
    AIDS and, 60t
Mycoplasma, disorders related
    to, 163t
Mycoplasmal pneumonia,
    281-282

N

Nasal cannula, how to use,
    285i
Neurosyphilis, 238. *See also*
    Syphilis.
Neutropenia, 73i
Neutrophil count
    calculating, 76
    transplant rejection and,
        157
Noncompliance as nursing di-
    agnosis, 173
Nosocomial infection
    incidence of, 276
    risk factors for, 277
Nursing diagnosis. *See also
    specific disorders.*
    immune disorders and,
        24-25, 26-27i, 28-29
    infectious disorders and,
        171-174
Nursing process, application
    of
    to immune disorders, 2-38
    to infectious disorders,
        162-182
Nutrition, altered, as nursing
    diagnosis, 25
    Helicobacter pylori infection
        and, 267
    systemic sclerosis and,
        129, 130
    tuberculosis and, 260
    viral hepatitis and, 192

O

Ocular herpes simplex virus,
    204. *See also* Herpes
    simplex.
Opportunistic diseases associ-
    ated with AIDS, 60-65t
Oral mucous membrane, al-
    tered, as nursing diagno-
    sis, 28, 173
    herpes simplex and,
        202-203

Osteomyelitis, 318-322
  assessing, 318-319
  causes of, 318, 319
  complications of, 319
  discharge preparation for,
    321
  evaluating patient's re-
    sponse to therapy for,
    322
  interventions for, 320-322
  infection sites for, 319
  nursing diagnoses for, 319
  patient outcomes for,
    319-320
  patient teaching for, 321-322
  treatment of, 320

PQ

Pain as nursing diagnosis, 28,
    172-173
  acute pyelonephritis and,
    272
  assessing, 184-185, 187
  causes of, 185
  chlamydial infection and,
    243-244
  gonorrhea and, 233, 234
  Helicobacter pylori infection
    and, 267
  herpes simplex and, 202,
    203
  herpes zoster and, 208
  infectious mononucleosis
    and, 216
  influenza and, 198
  lower urinary tract infection
    and, 301, 302
  Lyme disease and, 253
  meningitis and, 295
  pelvic inflammatory disease
    and, 248, 249
  referred sites of, 186i
  rheumatoid arthritis and,
    111-112
  systemic lupus erythemato-
    sus and, 122-123
  toxic shock syndrome and,
    229-230
Pancreas rejection, signs of,
  158. *See also* Transplant
  rejection.
Patient outcomes. *See* Planning.
Patient teaching, 34, 179. *See
  also specific disorders.*
Pelvic inflammatory disease,
  245-251
  assessing, 247-248
  causes of, 246-247
  complications of, 246
  discharge preparation for,
    251
  evaluating patient's re-
    sponse to therapy for,
    250-251
  interventions for, 249-250
  nursing diagnoses for,
    248-249
  pathophysiology of, 246i
  patient outcomes for, 249

Pelvic inflammatory disease
    (continued)
  patient teaching for,
    249-250
  risk factors for, 247
  treatment of, 250
Pemphigus vulgaris, detecting
  autoantibodies in, 22t
Perioral herpes simplex virus,
  204. *See also* Herpes
  simplex.
Peripheral tissue perfusion,
  altered, systemic scle-
  rosis and, 129
Pernicious anemia, detecting
  autoantibodies in, 22t
Petechiae, 138i
Physical examination. *See
  also specific disorders.*
  immune disorders and, 7-9,
    10-15i, 16, 17i
  infectious disorders and,
    165-168
Physical mobility, impaired, as
  nursing diagnosis, 28
  rheumatoid arthritis and,
    111
  systemic lupus erythemato-
    sus and, 122
  viral encephalitis and, 220,
    221
PID. *See* Pelvic inflammatory
  disease.
Planning. *See also specific
  disorders.*
  immune disorders and,
    29-33
  infectious disorders and,
    174-178
Platelet count
  autoimmune thrombocyto-
    penic purpura and,
    135-136
  transplant rejection and,
    157
Pleural fluid analysis, pneumonia and, 277
Pneumococcal pneumonia,
  281
Pneumocystis carinii pneumonia, 282
  AIDS and, 62t
Pneumonia, 276-287
  assessing, 276-277,
    279-282
  causes of, 276
  classifying, 276
  complications of, 278
  discharge preparation for,
    286
  evaluating patient's re-
    sponse to therapy for,
    286-287
  interventions for, 278, 282,
    284, 286
  nursing diagnoses for, 277
  patient outcomes for,
    277-278
  patient teaching for, 284,
    286
  risk factors for, 278
  transmission of, 278

Pneumonia *(continued)*
  treatment of, 283
  types of, 279-282
Polymerase chain reaction,
  171
Posttransplantation infections,
  monitoring, 150
Prednisone, 152t
Primary biliary cirrhosis, detecting autoantibodies in,
  22t
Progressive multifocal leukoencephalopathy, AIDS
  and, 64t
Protection, altered
  autoimmune thrombocyto-
    penic purpura and,
    136
  autoimmunity and, 27i
  hypersensitivity and, 27i
  immunodeficiency and, 26i,
    77
  as nursing diagnosis, 28-29
  sepsis and, 312, 315
  systemic lupus erythemato-
    sus and, 122, 123
  systemic sclerosis and, 129
  transplant-related immuno-
    suppression and, 150
Prothrombin time, viral hepatitis and, 192
Protozoa, disorders related to,
  163t
Protozoan pneumonia, 282
Pseudomonas aeruginosa
  pneumonia, 281
Pulmonary function tests,
  systemic sclerosis and,
  129
Pulse oximetry, pneumonia
  and, 277
Purpuric lesions, identifying,
  138-139i
Purulent discharge
  assessing, 187-188
  causes of, 188

R

RA. *See* Rheumatoid arthritis.
Radiation therapy
  immunodeficiency and, 74
  transplant rejection and,
    156
Radioallergosorbent test, 18,
  21
Radiographic testing, 171
Rapid plasma reagin test,
  syphilis and, 239
Rash
  assessing, 48-50
  causes of, 49
  classifying, 48-49
Reassessment, 35, 37, 181
Renal biopsy, systemic lupus
  erythematosus and, 122
Reportable diseases, 352
Respiratory syncytial virus,
  280
Rheumatoid arthritis,
  108-119
  assessing, 109-111
  causes of, 108-109

Rheumatoid arthritis
(continued)
  complications of, 108
  detecting autoantibodies in,
    22t
  discharge preparation for,
    118
  evaluating patient's re-
    sponse to therapy for,
    118-119
  interventions for, 112, 114,
    116-117i, 117-118
  incidence of, 110
  joint replacement and,
    116-117i
  nursing diagnoses for, 111
  patient outcomes for,
    111-112, 113-114
  patient teaching for, 114,
    116-117i, 117-118
  treatment of, 115
Rheumatoid factor test, 111
Rh typing, 21, 23
Rickettsiae, disorders related
  to, 163t
Role performance, altered,
  rheumatoid arthritis and,
  111
Rubeola, 280

S
Salmonellosis, AIDS and, 60t
Salpingo-oophoritis, signs of,
  248. *See also* Pelvic inflammatory disease.
Scleroderma. *See* Systemic
  sclerosis.
Sensitivity testing, 171
Sepsis, 310-318
  assessing, 310, 312,
    313-314
  causes of, 310
  differentiating stages of,
    311-312i
  discharge preparation for,
    317
  interventions for, 316-317
  monitoring, 315
  nursing diagnoses for, 312
  patient outcomes for, 312,
    315-316
  patient teaching for, 317
  treatment of, 316
Septic shock, 312i. *See also*
  Sepsis.
Serologic testing, *Helicobacter
  pylori* infection and, 266
Serum tests, 18, 19-21t, 21
Severe combined immunodeficiency, 53t
Sexuality patterns, altered, as
  nursing diagnosis, 28,
  173
  genital warts and, 212-213
  gonorrhea and, 233
  pelvic inflammatory disease
    and, 248, 249
  syphilis and, 239
Sexually transmitted disease,
  preventing, 232. *See
  also specific diseases.*

Shingles. *See* Herpes zoster.
Skin biopsy
  systemic lupus erythemato-
    sus and, 122
  systemic sclerosis and, 129
Skin integrity, impaired
  AIDS and, 66, 67
  atopic dermatitis and, 89
  herpes zoster and, 208
  syphilis and, 239
  systemic sclerosis and,
    129, 130
Skin integrity, impaired, high
  risk for, as nursing diagnosis, 28, 173
  pelvic inflammatory disease
    and, 248, 249
  viral hepatitis and, 192,
    193
  wound infection and, 288,
    289
SLE. *See* Systemic lupus erythematosus.
Social isolation as nursing diagnosis, 173
  atopic dermatitis and, 89,
    90
  tuberculosis and, 260, 261
Spleen, assessing, 17i
Sputum smear, tuberculosis
  and, 259-260
Staining techniques, 169
Staphylococcus pneumonia,
  281
Status asthmaticus, treatment of, 97
Streptococcus pneumonia,
  281
Stress, immunodeficiency and,
  52
Surgery, immunodeficiency
  and, 74
Swallowing, impaired, Hashimoto's disease and, 142
Syngeneic graft, 155
Synovial fluid analysis, rheumatoid arthritis and, 111
Syphilis, 237-242
  assessing, 237-239
  causes of, 237
  complications of, 237
  discharge preparation for,
    241
  evaluating patient's re-
    sponse to therapy for,
    241-242
  interventions for, 240-241
  nursing diagnoses for, 239
  patient outcomes for,
    239-240
  patient teaching for,
    240-241
  stages of, 237-238
  transmission of, 237
  treatment of, 240
Syphilitic chancre, 238i
Systemic inflammatory re-
  sponse syndrome,
  311-312i
Systemic lupus erythematosus, 119-127
  assessing, 120-122

Systemic lupus erythematosus
(continued)
  causes of, 119
  complications of, 119
  detecting autoantibodies in,
    22t
  discharge preparation for,
    126
  evaluating patient's re-
    sponse to therapy for,
    125-127
  interventions for, 123, 125
  nursing diagnoses for, 122
  patient outcomes for,
    122-123
  patient teaching for, 125
  treatment of, 124
Systemic scleroderma. *See*
  Systemic sclerosis.
Systemic sclerosis, 127-134
  assessing, 128-129, 129i
  causes of, 127
  complications of, 127
  discharge preparation for,
    133
  evaluating patient's re-
    sponse to therapy for,
    134
  facial exercises for, 132i
  forms of, 128
  interventions for, 130-134
  nursing diagnoses for, 129
  patient outcomes for,
    129-130
  patient teaching for,
    130-134, 132i
  treatment of, 131

T
Tacrolimus, 153t
TB. *See* Tuberculosis.
Temperature, altered, sepsis
  and, 312, 315
Therapeutic regimen, ineffective management of
  transplant rejection and,
    158, 159
  tuberculosis and, 260
Thought processes, altered
  AIDS and, 66, 67
  Lyme disease and, 253
  viral encephalitis and,
    220-221
Thyroid enlargement, Hashimoto's disease and, 141,
    142i
Thyroid hormone levels,
  serum, Hashimoto's dis-
  ease and, 142
Tissue biopsies, transplant rejection and, 157
Tissue integrity, impaired, as
  nursing diagnosis, 173
  herpes simplex and, 202,
    203
Tissue typing, 21, 23
  transplant rejection and,
    156
Toxic shock syndrome,
  226-231
  assessing, 229
  causes of, 228

i refers to an illustration; t, to a table

Toxic shock syndrome *(continued)*
complications of, 226, 228
discharge preparation for, 231
evaluating patient's response to therapy for, 231
interventions for, 230-231
nursing diagnoses for, 229
patient outcomes for, 229-230
patient teaching for, 230-231
preventing, 228
treatment of, 230
Toxoplasmosis, AIDS and, 63t
Transaminase levels, serum transplant rejection and, 157
Transfusion, safe administration of, 105
Transfusion reaction. *See* Blood transfusion reaction.
Transient hypogammaglobulinemia of infancy, 53t
Transmission prevention guidelines, 344-345
Transplant complications, 148-160
Transplant rejection, 154-160
assessing, 155-158
causes of, 155
discharge preparation for, 160
evaluating patient's response to therapy for, 159-160
graft-versus-host disease and, 155
interventions for, 159
nursing diagnoses for, 158
patient outcomes for, 158-159
patient teaching for, 159
preventing, 156
types of, 157
Transplant-related immunosuppression, 148-154
assessing, 148-150
discharge preparation for, 154
evaluating patient's response to therapy for, 153-154
interventions for, 151-152
nursing diagnoses for, 150
patient outcomes for, 150
patient teaching for, 151-152
Treponemal serologic tests, syphilis and, 239
Tubercle bacilli, types of, 257i
Tuberculin skin testing, tuberculosis and, 256-257, 259i
Tuberculosis, 255-266
assessing, 256-260, 259i
causes of, 256
complications of, 256
discharge preparation for, 264

Tuberculosis *(continued)*
evaluating patient's response to therapy for, 265-266
interventions for, 261-265
nursing diagnoses for, 260
patient outcomes for, 260-261
patient teaching for, 263-265
treatment of, 261
Tzanck smear
herpes simplex and, 202
herpes zoster and, 208

U

Universal precautions, 346-347
Urea breath test, *Helicobacter pylori* infection and, 267
Urethritis, 301t. *See also* Lower urinary tract infection.
Uric acid levels, serum, transplant-related immunosuppression and, 150
Urinalysis
acute pyelonephritis and, 271
lower urinary tract infection and, 300-301
systemic lupus erythematosus and, 122
systemic sclerosis and, 129
Urinary elimination pattern, altered, as nursing diagnosis, 173
acute pyelonephritis and, 272
chlamydial infection and, 243
gonorrhea and, 233-234
lower urinary tract infection and, 301
Urine amylase levels, transplant rejection and, 157
Urine pH, transplant rejection and, 157
UTI. *See* Lower urinary tract infection.

V

Varicella, 279
Varicella zoster, AIDS and, 64t
VDRL slide test, syphilis and, 239
Venereal warts. *See* Genital warts.
Venturi mask, how to use, 285i
Viral encephalitis, 218-224
assessing, 219-220, 223
causes of, 219
complications of, 219
discharge preparation for, 224
evaluating patient's response to therapy for, 223-224
interventions for, 221-223
nursing diagnoses for, 220
patient outcomes for, 220-221
patient teaching for, 223

Viral encephalitis *(continued)*
treatment of, 222
Viral hepatitis, 190-197
assessing, 190, 192
causes of, 190
complications of, 190
discharge preparation for, 196
evaluating patient's response to therapy for, 196-197
interventions for, 193-196
nursing diagnoses for, 192
patient outcomes for, 192-193
patient teaching for, 194-196
treatment of, 194
types of, 191t
Viral infections, 190-224
Viral meningitis, risk factors for, 293. *See also* Meningitis.
Viral pneumonias, 279-280. *See also* Pneumonia.
Virus, disorders related to, 163t
Voiding cystoureterography, lower urinary tract infection and, 301

W

Weight loss
assessing, 43-45
causes of, 44
White blood cell count
with differential, 168-169
infectious mononucleosis and, 216
meningitis and, 295
pneumonia and, 277
Wiskott-Aldrich syndrome, 54t
Wound infection, 287-292
assessing, 287-288
causes of, 287
complications of, 287
discharge preparation for, 291
evaluating patient's response to therapy for, 291-292
interventions for, 289-290
nursing diagnoses for, 288
patient outcomes for, 288-289
patient teaching for, 289-290
risk factors for, 287
treatment of, 290

XYZ

Xenograft, 155
X-rays
acute pyelonephritis and, 272
rheumatoid arthritis and, 111
systemic sclerosis and, 129
Zalcitabine, 68
Zidovudine, 68

i refers to an illustration; t, to a table